T0263131

Obesity: A Multidisciplinary Approach

Editorial Advisor

JOEL J. HEIDELBAUGH

ELSEVIER

1600 John F. Kennedy Boulevard • Suite 1800 • Philadelphia, Pennsylvania, 19103-2899

http://www.theclinics.com

CLINICS COLLECTIONS
ISSN 2352-7986, ISBN-13: 978-0-323-35962-7

Editor: Patrick Manley (p.manley@elsevier.com)
Developmental Editor: John Vassallo (j.vassallo@elsevier.com)

© 2014 Elsevier Inc. All rights reserved.

This periodical and the individual contributions contained in it are protected under copyright by Elsevier, and the following terms and conditions apply to their use:

Photocopying
Single photocopies of single articles may be made for personal use as allowed by national copyright laws. Permission of the Publisher and payment of a fee is required for all other photocopying, including multiple or systematic copying, copying for advertising or promotional purposes, resale, and all forms of document delivery. Special rates are available for educational institutions that wish to make photocopies for non-profit educational classroom use. For information on how to seek permission visit www.elsevier.com/permissions or call: (+44) 1865 843830 (UK)/(+1) 215 239 3804 (USA).

Derivative Works
Subscribers may reproduce tables of contents or prepare lists of articles including abstracts for internal circulation within their institutions. Permission of the Publisher is required for resale or distribution outside the institution. Permission of the Publisher is required for all other derivative works, including compilations and translations (please consult www.elsevier.com/permissions).

Electronic Storage or Usage
Permission of the Publisher is required to store or use electronically any material contained in this periodical, including any article or part of an article (please consult www.elsevier.com/permissions). Except as outlined above, no part of this publication may be reproduced, stored in a retrieval system or transmitted in any form or by any means, electronic, mechanical, photocopying, recording or otherwise, without prior written permission of the Publisher.

Notice
No responsibility is assumed by the Publisher for any injury and/or damage to persons or property as a matter of products liability, negligence or otherwise, or from any use or operation of any methods, products, instructions or ideas contained in the material herein. Because of rapid advances in the medical sciences, in particular, independent verification of diagnoses and drug dosages should be made.

Although all advertising material is expected to conform to ethical (medical) standards, inclusion in this publication does not constitute a guarantee or endorsement of the quality or value of such product or of the claims made of it by its manufacturer.

Clinics Collections (ISSN 2352-7986) is published by Elsevier Inc., 360 Park Avenue South, New York, NY 10010-1710. Business and editorial offices: 1600 John F. Kennedy Boulevard, Suite 1800, Philadelphia, PA 19103-2899. **POSTMASTER:** Send address changes to *Clinics Collections*, Elsevier Health Sciences Division, Subscription Customer Service, 3251 Riverport Lane, Maryland Heights, MO 63043. **Customer Service: Telephone: 1-800-654-2452** (U.S. and Canada); **1-314-447-8871** (outside U.S. and Canada). **Fax: 314-447-8029. E-mail: journalscustomerserviceusa@elsevier.com** (for print support); **journalsonlinesupport-usa@elsevier.com** (for online support).

Reprints. For copies of 100 or more of articles in this publication, please contact the Commercial Reprints Department, Elsevier Inc., 360 Park Avenue South, New York, NY 10010-1710. Tel.: 212-633-3874; Fax: 212-633-3820; E-mail: reprints@elsevier.com.

Contributors

EDITORIAL ADVISOR

JOEL J. HEIDELBAUGH, MD, FAAFP, FACG
Clinical Associate Professor, Departments of Family Medicine and Urology; Clerkship Director, Department of Family Medicine, University of Michigan Medical School, Ann Arbor, Michigan; Ypsilanti Health Center, Ypsilanti, Michigan

AUTHORS

JO APPLEBAUM, MPH
Children's Health Fund and Community Pediatric Programs, Montefiore Medical Center, Bronx, New York

SANDRA AREVALO, MPH, RD, CDE
Center for Child Health and Resiliency, Montefiore Medical Center, Bronx, New York

SEAN J. BARNETT, MD, MS, FACS, FAAP
Assistant Professor of Surgery and Pediatrics, Division of Pediatric General & Thoracic Surgery, Cincinnati Children's Hospital Medical Center, Cincinnati, Ohio

ALLEN F. BROWNE, MD
Division of Pediatric Surgery, Children's Hospital of Illinois, Order of St. Francis Medical Center, University of Illinois College of Medicine-Peoria, Peoria, Illinois

KENNETH R. CARSON, MD
Division of Hematology and Oncology, Department of Internal Medicine; Division of Public Health Sciences, Department of Surgery, Washington University in St. Louis, St Louis, Missouri

MAURIZIO CASSADER, PhD
Department of Medical Sciences, University of Turin, Turin, Italy

PAUL CHANG, MD
Professor of Medicine, Section of Gastroenterology, Temple University School of Medicine, Philadelphia, Pennsylvania

EDMOND H.L. CHAU, MD
Resident, Department of Anesthesiology, Toronto Western Hospital, University Health Network, University of Toronto, Toronto, Ontario, Canada

FRANCES CHUNG, MBBS, FRCPC
Professor, Department of Anesthesia, Toronto Western Hospital, University Health Network, University of Toronto, Toronto, Ontario, Canada

NANCY L. CLOAK, MD
Staff Psychiatrist, Oregon Center for Clinical Investigations; Private Practice, Portland, Oregon

CAROLYN DAVIS, PhD
Founder/Director of the Tennessee Institute for Performance and Sport Psychology, Core Faculty in the College of Social and Behavioral Sciences, Department of Counseling Psychology, Walden University, Minneapolis, Minnesota

RITA DOUMIT, PhD, MPH, RN
Assistant Professor, Alice Ramez Chagoury School of Nursing, Lebanese American University, Byblos, Lebanon

FRANK FRIEDENBERG, MD, MS (Epi)
Senior Fellow, Section of Gastroenterology, Temple University School of Medicine, Philadelphia, Pennsylvania

ROBERTO GAMBINO, PhD
Department of Medical Sciences, University of Turin, Turin, Italy

ANTJE GARTEN, PhD
Department of Women and Child Health, Hospital for Children and Adolescents, Center for Pediatric Research Leipzig (CPL), University Hospitals, Leipzig, Germany

NICOLAS GOOSSENS, MD, MSc
Clinical Fellow, Division of Gastroenterology and Hepatology, Geneva University Hospital, Geneva, Switzerland

PATRICK R. HARRISON, BS, MA
Department of Psychology, Loyola University Chicago, Chicago, Illinois

MELANIE HINGLE, PhD, MPH, RD
Assistant Research Professor, Department of Nutritional Sciences, University of Arizona, Tucson, Arizona

MARK J. HOLTERMAN, MD, PhD
Professor, Division of Pediatric Surgery, Children's Hospital of Illinois, Order of St. Francis Medical Center, University of Illinois College of Medicine-Peoria, Peoria, Illinois

MATTHEW M. HUTTER, MD, MPH
Director, The Codman Center for Clinical Effectiveness in Surgery; Division of General and Gastrointestinal Surgery, Department of Surgery, Massachusetts General Hospital, Boston, Massachusetts

TIMOTHY D. JACKSON, MD, MPH
The Codman Center for Clinical Effectiveness in Surgery, Massachusetts General Hospital, Boston, Massachusetts; Assistant Professor of Surgery, Department of Surgery, University of Toronto, Toronto, Ontario, Canada

JONATHAN JUN, MD
Assistant Professor, Division of Pulmonary and Critical Care Medicine, Johns Hopkins University School of Medicine, Baltimore, Maryland

EMILY S. JUNGHEIM, MD, MSCI
Division of Reproductive Endocrinology and Infertility, Department of Obstetrics and Gynecology, Washington University in St. Louis, St Louis, Missouri

WIELAND KIESS, MD
Department of Women and Child Health, Hospital for Children and Adolescents, Center for Pediatric Research Leipzig (CPL), University Hospitals, Leipzig, Germany

JOANNE KOUBA
Assistant Professor, Niehoff School of Nursing, Loyola University Chicago, Chicago, Illinois

DALE KUNKEL, PhD
Professor, Department of Communication, University of Arizona, Tucson, Arizona

AI-XUAN LE HOLTERMAN, MD
Professor, Division of Pediatric Surgery, Children's Hospital of Illinois, Order of St. Francis Medical Center, University of Illinois College of Medicine-Peoria, Peoria, Illinois

HILDRED MACHUCA, DO
Center for Child Health and Resiliency, Montefiore Medical Center, Bronx, New York

AMY MANION, PhD, RN, PNP
Instructor, College of Nursing, Rush University, Chicago, Illinois

CHRISTINE MARIC-BILKAN, PhD, FASN, FAHA
Associate Professor, Department of Physiology and Biophysics, University of Mississippi Medical Center, Jackson, Mississippi

OMAR MESARWI, MD
Postdoctoral Fellow, Division of Pulmonary and Critical Care Medicine, Johns Hopkins University School of Medicine, Baltimore, Maryland

LISA K. MILITELLO, MSN, MPH, CPNP
College of Nursing, Arizona State University, Phoenix, Arizona

BABAK MOKHLESI, MD, MSc
Associate Professor, Section of Pulmonary and Critical Care Medicine, Department of Medicine, Sleep Disorders Center, University of Chicago Pritzker School of Medicine, Chicago, Illinois

KELLE H. MOLEY, MD
Division of Reproductive Endocrinology and Infertility, Department of Obstetrics and Gynecology, Washington University in St. Louis, St Louis, Missouri

FEDERICA MOLINARO, MD
Department of Medical Sciences, University of Turin, Turin, Italy

VINCENT MORELLI, MD
Associate Professor, Department of Family and Community Medicine, School of Medicine, Sports Medicine Fellowship Director, Meharry Medical College, Nashville, Tennessee

GIOVANNI MUSSO, MD
Department of Emergency Medicine, Gradenigo Hospital, Turin, Italy

FRANCESCO NEGRO, MD
Professor, Divisions of Gastroenterology and Hepatology, and Clinical Pathology, Geneva University Hospital, Geneva, Switzerland

ELENA PASCHETTA, MD
Department of Medical Sciences, University of Turin, Turin, Italy

JAN POLAK, MD, PhD
Postdoctoral Fellow, Division of Pulmonary and Critical Care Medicine, Johns Hopkins University School of Medicine, Baltimore, Maryland

VSEVOLOD Y. POLOTSKY, MD, PhD
Associate Professor, Division of Pulmonary and Critical Care Medicine, Johns Hopkins University School of Medicine, Baltimore, Maryland

PAULINE S. POWERS, MD
Professor of Psychiatry and Behavioral Medicine, Department of Pediatrics; Director, Center for Eating and Weight Disorders, College of Medicine, University of South Florida, Tampa, Florida

SUSANNE SCHUSTER
Department of Women and Child Health, Hospital for Children and Adolescents, Center for Pediatric Research Leipzig (CPL), University Hospitals, Leipzig, Germany

ALAN SHAPIRO, MD
Children's Health Fund and Community Pediatric Programs, Montefiore Medical Center, Bronx, New York

LORALEI L. THORNBURG, MD
Assistant Professor of OB/GYN, Division of Maternal Fetal Medicine, Department of OB/GYN, University of Rochester Medical Center, University of Rochester, Rochester, New York

ALTAGRACIA TOLENTINO, MD
Center for Child Health and Resiliency, Montefiore Medical Center, Bronx, New York

JENNIFER L. TRAVIESO, BS
Division of Reproductive Endocrinology and Infertility, Department of Obstetrics and Gynecology, Washington University in St. Louis, St Louis, Missouri

BARBARA VELSOR-FRIEDRICH, PhD, RN
Professor and Faculty Scholar, Niehoff School of Nursing, Loyola University Chicago, Chicago, Illinois

YUSUF YILMAZ, MD
Department of Gastroenterology, School of Medicine, Marmara University, Pendik; Institute of Gastroenterology, Marmara University, Maltepe, Istanbul, Turkey

ZOBAIR M. YOUNOSSI, MD, MPH, FACG, FACP, AGAF
Chairman, Department of Medicine, Inova Fairfax Hospital; Vice President for Research, Inova Health System; Professor of Medicine, VCU-Inova Campus; Betty and Guy Beatty Center for Integrated Research, Falls Church, Virginia

Contents

Pediatric Obesity

> Although childhood obesity rates have stabilized in the last decade, 17%
> of US children are obese, and poor minority children remain disproportion-
> ately affected. Community health centers, with their family-centered
> approach, are ideally situated to play a leading role in prevention and
> intervention of childhood obesity in the poor communities they serve.
> Public–private partnerships enhance resources for community health
> centers, enabling more intensive focus on interventions that address the
> most prevalent health conditions in these communities. Starting Right,
> an example of such a partnership, is a guideline-based, multidisciplinary,
> multicomponent initiative for screening, prevention, and treatment of pedi-
> atric obesity at an inner city community health center. The initiative aims to
> build capacity at the individual, family, health center, and community level.
> Universal screening, messaging throughout the life cycle, and innovative
> interventions appear to be making an impact.

> Widely researched as separate entities, our understanding of the comorbid
> effects of childhood obesity and asthma on quality of life is limited. This
> article discusses the effects of childhood obesity and asthma on self-
> reported quality of life in low-income African American teens with asthma.
> When controlling for the influence of symptom frequency, asthma classifi-
> cation, asthma self-efficacy, and asthma self-care levels, body mass index
> remains a most important factor in determining self-reported quality of life
> among teens with asthma. Although overweight and obesity did not
> change the effectiveness of the asthma intervention program, obesity did
> affect participants quality of life scores.

> This review discusses the evidence base for medications that are currently
> used for obesity and eating disorders, including their Food and Drug
> Administration approval status by disorder and age group, contraindica-
> tions, and major adverse effects. Investigational agents currently being

considered, issues related to psychiatric and medical comorbidity, limitations of pharmacologic strategies, and recommendations for treatment are also addressed.

Childhood obesity is a tremendous burden for children, their families, and society. Obesity prevention remains the ultimate goal but rapid development and deployment of effective nonsurgical treatment options is not currently achievable given the complexity of this disease. Surgical options for adolescent obesity have been proven to be safe and effective and should be offered. The development of stratified protocols of increasing intensity should be individualized for patients based on their disease severity and risk factors. These protocols should be offered in multidisciplinary, cooperative clinical trials to critically evaluate and develop optimal treatment strategies for morbid obesity.

This article assesses the role played by media in contributing to the current epidemic of childhood obesity. Electronic media use, often referred to as screen time, is significantly correlated with child adiposity. Although the causal mechanism that accounts for this relationship is unclear, it is well established that reducing screen time improves weight status. Media advertising for unhealthy foods contributes to obesity by influencing children's food preferences, requests, and diet. Industry efforts have failed to improve the nutritional quality of foods marketed on television to children, leading public health advocates to recommend government restrictions on child-targeted advertisements for unhealthy foods.

Obesity and Secondary Disorders

Obesity is strongly associated with the prevalence of nonalcoholic fatty liver disease (NAFLD) in adult and pediatric populations. Nutrition, physical activity, and behavioral modifications are critical components of the treatment regimen for all obese patients with NAFLD. Bariatric surgeries that affect or restrict the flow of food through the gastrointestinal tract may improve liver histology in morbidly obese patients with nonalcoholic steato-hepatitis (NASH), although randomized clinical trials and quasi-randomized clinical studies are lacking. Early detection of NASH and hepatic fibrosis using noninvasive biochemical and imaging markers that may replace liver biopsy is the current challenge.

Epidemiologic data have demonstrated that obesity is an important risk factor for the development of gastroesophageal reflux disease (GERD).

There is also accumulating data that obesity is associated with complications related to longstanding reflux such as erosive esophagitis, Barrett esophagus, and esophageal adenocarcinoma. Central obesity, rather than body mass index, appears to be more closely associated with these complications. Surgical data are confounded by the concomitant repair of prevalent hiatal hernias in many patients.

Normal sleep is characterized both by reduced glucose turnover by the brain and other metabolically active tissues, and by changes in glucose tolerance. Sleep duration has decreased over the last several decades; data suggest a link between short sleep duration and type 2 diabetes. Obstructive sleep apnea (OSA) results in intermittent hypoxia and sleep fragmentation, and also is associated with impaired glucose tolerance. Obesity is a major risk factor for OSA, but whether OSA leads to obesity is unclear. The quality and quantity of sleep may profoundly affect obesity and glucose tolerance, and should be routinely assessed by clinicians.

Asthma is one of the most common chronic illnesses in the world, affecting an estimated 300 million people. Globally, the prevalence of asthma has continued to spread as economic improvements in developing countries create a population trend toward urbanization and adoption of a western lifestyle. Research supports an association between obesity and asthma. Only by making weight management a priority in the treatment of asthma can the rising prevalence of both diseases be hindered and global health improved.

Patients with obesity hypoventilation syndrome (OHS) have a higher burden of co-morbidities and increased risk for perioperative morbidity and mortality. Therefore, a thorough plan of evaluation and management is essential for patients with OHS who undergo surgery. Currently, information on the perioperative management of OHS is extremely limited in the literature. As the prevalence of OHS is likely to increase as a result of the current global obesity epidemic, it is crucial for physicians to recognize and manage patients with this syndrome. This review examines the current data on OHS and discusses its optimal perioperative management.

Obesity and diabetes are major health concerns worldwide. Along with other elements of the metabolic syndrome, including hypertension, they contribute to the development and progression of renal disease, which, if not treated, may lead to end-stage renal disease (ESRD). Although early intervention and management of body weight, hyperglycemia, and hypertension are imperative, novel therapeutic approaches are also necessary to reduce the high morbidity and mortality associated with renal disease. This review provides perspectives regarding the mechanisms by which obesity may lead to ESRD and discusses prevention strategies and treatment of obesity-related renal disease.

Obesity is associated with multiple adverse reproductive outcomes, but the mechanisms involved are largely unknown. Obesity has been referred to as a "complex system," defined as a system of heterogeneous parts interacting in nonlinear ways to influence the behavior of the parts as a whole. Human reproduction is also a complex system; hence the difficulty in identifying the mechanisms linking obesity and adverse reproductive function. This review discusses the adverse reproductive outcomes associated with obesity and the mechanisms involved and concludes with a discussion of public health policy with respect to the treatment of infertility in obese women.

Metabolic Disorders

The metabolic syndrome and the hepatitis C virus (HCV) infection are 2 global health care challenges with a complex interaction. Insulin resistance, a central component of the metabolic syndrome, is epidemiologically and pathophysiologically intrinsically linked to HCV infection. Insulin resistance and diabetes affect clinical outcomes in patients with liver disease related to HCV, namely, incidence of hepatocellular carcinoma, liver-related mortality, fibrosis progression rate, response to antiviral therapy, and possibly the incidence of cardiovascular events. Viral and metabolic steatosis and its interactions with HCV and the metabolic syndrome are discussed. Management and the need for further research conclude the article.

Adipose tissue has been recognized as a major target of growth hormone (GH) action. GH was shown to inhibit adipocyte differentiation but stimulated preadipocyte proliferation in vitro. GH acts directly via its receptor or via upregulating insulin-like growth factor (IGF)-I, which is a critical mediator of preadipocyte proliferation, differentiation, and survival. Results from clinical studies on GH treatment in patients with GH deficiency or GH insensitivity syndrome can be used to dissect GH and IGF as well as IGF-binding protein (IGFBP) actions in vivo. In this article, changes of the GH/IGF system during adipocyte differentiation in vitro as well as related signaling pathways and their impact on adipose tissue growth and function are discussed. Clinical considerations include the effects of GH and IGF-I on adipose tissue during treatment of GH deficiency, differences in the IGF system between visceral and subcutaneous adipose tissue depots as well as the recently emerging role for adipose tissue in the regulation of glucose homeostasis.

Dietary Approaches

Obesity-related disorders derive from a combination of genetic susceptibility and environmental factors. Recent evidence supports the role of gut microbiota in the pathogenesis of obesity, type 2 diabetes mellitus, and insulin resistance by increasing energy harvest from diet and by inducing chronic, low-grade inflammation. Several studies describe characteristic differences between composition and activity of gut microbiota of lean individuals and those with obesity. Despite this evidence, some pathophysiological mechanisms remain to be clarified. This article discusses mechanisms connecting gut microbiota to obesity and fat storage and the potential therapeutic role of probiotics and prebiotics.

Surgical Options

Morbid obesity continues to see a rapid increase in pediatric and adolescent populations. Morbidly obese adolescents develop significant comorbidities that continue on into adulthood. Although medical management in the overweight population of children can be helpful, morbidly obese adolescents do not show significant long-term weight reduction with lifestyle modification. Bariatric surgery is a safe and long-term solution in selected morbidly obese adolescents who are physically and psychosocially mature. Adolescent bariatric surgical patients require lifelong dietary modification and follow-up to ensure adequate nutritional supplementation. Roux-en-Y gastric bypass (RYGB) remains the gold standard operation but sleeve gastrectomy (SG) continues to gain rapid prominence, given its simplicity and reduced post-operative complication rates. The adjustable gastric band (AGB) in the adolescent population can be efficacious compared with medical therapy but has demonstrated significantly higher complication and reoperation rates compared with its use in adults. More long-term, longitudinal studies are necessary to firmly establish guidelines for patient selection and optimal procedure choice.

Laparoscopic sleeve gastrectomy (LSG), laparoscopic adjustable gastric band (LAGB) and laparoscopic Roux-en-Y gastric bypass (LRYGB) are all considered acceptable contemporary surgical options for the treatment of morbid obesity. Recent quality improvement efforts have significantly reduced the morbidity and mortality associated with modern bariatric surgical procedures. LRYGB appears to be most effective although is associated with more risk when compared to both LAGB and LSG. LSG is positioned between the LRYGB and LABG in associated morbidity and effectiveness although long-term outcome data is lacking.

Special Considerations

Sports psychologists play an important role in enhancing performance among athletes. In conjunction with team physicians, they can also shed light on psychological disorders common in athletes, such as mood and eating disorders, and overtraining syndrome. Sports psychologists can also lend their expertise to assist with injury prevention and recovery and compliance issues. Sports psychology has a role in helping to reverse the growing obesity epidemic among school-aged children. These professionals, working with coaches, can increase children's levels of physical activity. Cognitive-behavioral techniques could lead to enhanced enjoyment, increased participation, improved school performance, and a reduction in obesity.

This article updates the obstetric community on the limitation of ultrasound scan in the obese patient, and the data regarding optimizing ultrasound care for this population. Special attention is given to the limitations of ultrasound scan for performing first-trimester genetic screening, genetic ultrasound scan, and anatomic evaluation and the limitations of ultrasound scan to predict birth weight in the obese patient.

Preface

Clinics Review Articles have been a part of the library of physicians, nurses, and residents for nearly 100 years. This trusted resource covers over 50 medical disciplines every year, producing thousands of articles focused on the most current concepts and techniques in medicine. This collection of articles, devoted to obesity, draws from the database of the *Clinics* to provide multidisciplinary teams with practical clinical advice on comorbidities and complications of this highly prevalent disease.

A multidisciplinary perspective is key to effective team-based management. Featured articles from the *Endocrinology and Metabolism Clinics, Pediatric Clinics, Medical Clinics, Gastroenterology Clinics, Clinics in Liver Disease*, and *Nursing Clinics* reflect the wide range of clinicians who manage patients with obesity-related disorders.

I encourage you to share this volume with your colleagues in hopes that it may promote more collaboration, new perspectives, and informed, effective care for your patients.

Joel J. Heidelbaugh, MD, FAAFP, FACG
Ypsilanti, Michigan
October 2014

Clinics Collections 3 (2014) xiii
http://dx.doi.org/10.1016/j.ccol.2014.09.027
2352-7986/14/$ – see front matter © 2014 Published by Elsevier Inc.

Prevention and Management of Pediatric Obesity

A Multipronged, Community-Based Agenda

Alan Shapiro, MD[a], Sandra Arevalo, MPH, RD, CDE[b],
Altagracia Tolentino, MD[b], Hildred Machuca, DO[b],
Jo Applebaum, MPH[a],*

KEYWORDS

- Pediatric obesity • Prevention • Intervention • Primary care • Nutrition education

KEY POINTS

- Although childhood obesity rates have stabilized in the last decade, 17% of US children are obese, and poor minority children remain disproportionately affected.
- Community health centers, with their family-centered approach, are ideally situated to play a leading role in prevention and intervention of childhood obesity in the poor communities they serve. Public–private partnerships enhance resources for community health centers, enabling more intensive focus on interventions that address the most prevalent health conditions in these communities.
- Starting Right, an example of such a partnership, is a guideline-based, multidisciplinary, multicomponent initiative for screening, prevention, and treatment of pediatric obesity at an inner city community health center. The initiative aims to build capacity at the individual, family, health center, and community level. Universal screening, messaging throughout the life cycle, and innovative interventions appear to be making an impact.

INTRODUCTION

National surveillance data show that obesity prevalence among US children has stabilized over the past decade at nearly 17% [1]. Although encouraging, these rates place millions of children at risk for associated chronic health conditions, and poor minority children are disproportionately affected. According to 2009 to 2010 national data, 24% of non-Hispanic black and 21% of Hispanic children were obese compared

This article originally appeared in Advances in Pediatrics, Volume 61, 2014.
[a] Children's Health Fund and Community Pediatric Programs, Montefiore Medical Center, 853 Longwood Avenue, Bronx, NY 10459, USA; [b] Center for Child Health and Resiliency, Montefiore Medical Center, 890 Prospect Avenue, Bronx, NY 10459, USA
* Corresponding author. Community Pediatric Programs, Montefiore Medical Center, 853 Longwood Avenue, 2nd Floor, Bronx, NY 10459.
E-mail address: jappleba@montefiore.org

2352-7986/14/$ – see front matter © 2014 Elsevier Inc. All rights reserved.

with 14% of non-Hispanic white children. These disparities persist across all age groups, and present as early as 2 to 5 years of age. Recent reports suggest childhood obesity rates are decreasing in New York City, but predominantly among white children [2]. From 2010 to 2011, the highest obesity rates were seen in Hispanic (27%) and black (21%) children living in high-poverty neighborhoods (ie, ≥30% of residents living below federal poverty level).

Developed by the Children's Health Fund (CHF) in partnership with the Children's Hospital at Montefiore, the Center for Child Health and Resiliency (CCHR) and the South Bronx Health Center (SBHC) are federally qualified health centers serving the nation's poorest congressional district. In this community, a staggering 47% of families with children live below the federal poverty level; 71% of residents are Hispanic, and 26% are black. Thirty-one percent are children under age 18 years (vs 22% in NYC overall) [3]. The South Bronx has among the lowest concentration of grocery stores, and smallest proportion of land used for parks and recreation, of any New York City neighborhood [4,5]. Furthermore, children in this community engage in less physical activity than recommended [6], spending more time at home while parents work long hours and/or multiple jobs—a 21st century version of the latchkey kids. Not surprisingly given this context, the South Bronx has a disproportionately high prevalence of obesity and type 2 diabetes, and low rates of health-promoting behaviors [7]. Of 42 New York City neighborhoods, the communities served by CCHR rank last in most key health indicators [8,9].

To advance the community health center's mission of closing the gap in health disparities, CCHR develops and evaluates interventions that address these conditions in the community it serves [10]. In response to the surge in childhood obesity, Starting Right was launched in 2001 as a guideline-based, multidisciplinary, multicomponent initiative designed as front-line screening, prevention, and treatment of pediatric obesity in a busy primary care setting [11–13]. The initiative consists of interventions that build capacity at the individual, family, health center, and community level. This report describes the elements of Starting Right adopted by an inner city community health center and the population served, consisting of children and families living primarily in public housing in the South Bronx. It also discusses preliminary outcome findings.

SETTING

The South Bronx Health Center (SBHC) was established in 1993 by CHF/Montefiore to serve children and their families in one of New York City's most densely concentrated public housing neighborhoods and a federally designated Health Provider Shortage Area. In 2011, CHF and Montefiore opened the Center for Child Health and Resiliency, providing family-focused, comprehensive primary care to approximately 3500 pediatric patients (0–19 years) annually. In 2010, 42% of children aged 10 to 19 years seen at this clinic were overweight (18%) or obese (24%), and 70% of them had multiple risk factors for type 2 diabetes. In addition to primary care, CCHR provides colocated nutrition, mental health, health education, and case management services.

STARTING RIGHT

Starting Right's goals are to intervene as early as possible to prevent childhood obesity. Primary care providers are well-positioned for front-line identification of children at risk, yet clinician adoption of screening guidelines remains suboptimal in primary care practice [14,15]. Studies show that providers believe obesity prevention and treatment are important and that they have a role to play in intervention [16,17]. However, pediatric primary care providers are reluctant to address obesity due to lack of time and resources, unfamiliarity with guidelines, and the perception that interventions are either unavailable or ineffective [17].

The Starting Right initiative addresses these barriers with its 4 key components: tools and training for improved screening and treatment, culturally appropriate nutrition education materials and counseling, targeted group interventions, and community partnerships. The multidisciplinary team includes primary care providers, nurses, registered dietitians, a health educator, and public health professionals to support intervention design and evaluation. CCHR has a dedicated evaluation team to conduct continuous quality improvement and assess intervention effectiveness, with an emphasis on using health information technology.

INITIATIVE COMPONENTS
Pediatric primary care screening and treatment

At the core of Starting Right is putting into practice complex, nationally accepted guidelines in a primary care setting in which patients have multiple medical and psychosocial issues. Starting Right's clinical leadership, a pediatrician and a registered dietitian, conduct trainings on the latest guidelines and develop tools to facilitate screening, assessment, and referral in the primary care visit. Protocols have been implemented to: (1) universally screen for overweight/obesity by determining body mass index (BMI) percentile; (2) counsel families about nutrition and physical activity regardless of children's weight status; (3) assess risk factors for obesity-related comorbid conditions, such as cardiovascular disease, type 2 diabetes, and nonalcoholic fatty liver disease; and (4) refer to subspecialty care as appropriate [12,13,18].

In 2003, based on then-current American Diabetes Association and Expert Committee recommendations for screening and treatment of pediatric obesity [11,19], the Starting Right team developed a template that was incorporated into the paper medical record to guide providers through the screening process. The template was then revised according to 2007 Expert Committee recommendations [12]. In response to guidelines issued by the National Heart, Lung, and Blood Institute in 2011 for screening and management of cardiovascular risk in children, the authors developed a new algorithm to translate the latest evidence into routine primary care (**Fig. 1**) [13,20,21]. To the authors' knowledge, an algorithm reflecting these guidelines has not been published previously. These guidelines have been incorporated into templates for the electronic medical record adopted by CCHR and its hospital affiliate.

As part of performance improvement, chart reviews were conducted before and after provider training and implementation of each version of the screening protocol. Providers received feedback and retraining as needed to improve screening and documentation, which are essential components of performance improvement. Results show a marked increase in documentation of BMI percentile after implementation of the Starting Right template from 2004 to 2005 (**Fig. 2**); by 2008, 99% of children aged 2 to 19 years had BMI percentile documented at their well child care visit. As of 2012, HRSA requires federally qualified health centers to report annually on the percentage of children aged 3 to 17 years seen for any type of primary care visit, with BMI percentile documented [14]. Using standardized measures enables comparison with national averages. For children seen at CCHR in 2012, 93% had their BMI percentile documented, compared with 46% of Medicaid and 45% of commercially insured patients (2011 data) [14].

Nutrition education and counseling

CCHR primary care providers counsel families about nutrition and physical activity across the lifecycle, from pregnancy through adolescence and adulthood,

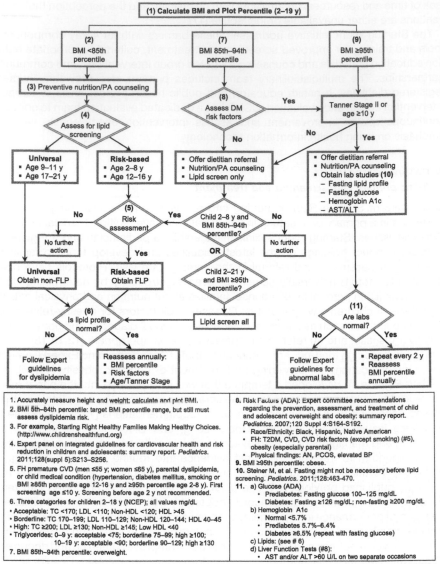

Fig. 1. Screening algorithm for childhood overweight, obesity, and comorbidities based on 2011 Guidelines for Cardiovascular Health and Risk Reduction in Children and Adolescents National Heart, Lung, and Blood Institute. *Abbreviations:* ALT, alanine aminotransferase; AN, acanthosis nigricans; AST, aspartate aminotransferase; BMI, body mass index; BP, blood pressure; CVD, cardiovascular disease; DM, diabetes mellitus; FH, family history; FLP, fasting lipid profile; HDL, high-density lipoprotein; LDL, low-density lipoprotein; PA, physical activity; PCOS, polycystic ovary syndrome; TC, total cholesterol. (*Courtesy of* The National Heart, Lung, and Blood Institute, Bethesda, MD.)

using Starting Right's low-literacy, culturally appropriate health education materials published in English and Spanish (available at childrenshealthfund.org) [22]. These materials target pregnant women, families with young children, and adolescents.

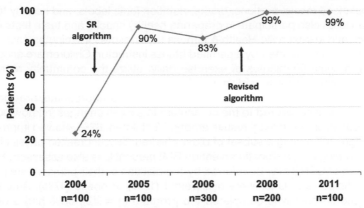

Fig. 2. Percentage of children with BMI percentile documentation before and after implementing the Starting Right (SR) screening protocol and template. Analyses of random samples of children, aged 2 to 19 years, seen for a well child care visit in the measurement year.

Children and their families also are referred internally to a registered dietitian for nutrition and lifestyle counseling. Using motivational interviewing techniques [12,23], the dietitian assesses family members' readiness to make changes and helps them set relevant, attainable, and measurable goals. Counseling is informed by years of experience providing care for a diverse community and results of qualitative research conducted among overweight youth and their parents at CCHR. Focus groups emphasized numerous barriers to healthy eating and physical activity: conflicting family needs/preferences; lack of knowledge/skills; financial constraints; limited access to healthy foods and safe outdoor spaces; long work hours; and emotional distress as both a contributor and consequence of overeating and overweight [24]. Moreover, in the local community, cultural norms favor larger body types and discourage weight loss, which could signify poverty, weakness, illness, or drug use.

To enhance acceptance of nutrition referral, the dietitian is called into the examination room by the primary care provider to meet the child and his or her family (meet and greet model) and, when feasible, the dietician conducts a nutrition counseling session immediately following the primary care visit. Tandem visits jump start individual nutrition education and enhance adherence to nutrition-related recommendations. Results of preliminary analysis among 96 overweight/obese children with at least 2 nutrition counseling sessions suggest that over an average of 9.7 months, BMI percentile decreased in 60.4% of patients (mean change of −1.7 percentile).

Group interventions

Health & Fitness Group

Concomitant with universal BMI screening, Starting Right launched a community-based intervention in 2005 to address nutrition education and physical activity among overweight or obese children aged 10 to 14 years. To destigmatize the program, and broaden its reach as obesity prevention and treatment, Health & Fitness was expanded in 2010 to include children aged 6 to 14 years regardless of weight status and integrated into an after-school program at a local public housing community center. The program is open to health center patients and nonpatient public housing residents. This community partnership connects CCHR patients with a free recreational facility and provides essential nutrition education to children and families living in public housing.

Over the 12 weekly sessions, the program's health educator delivers 45-minute age-appropriate, interactive, culturally sensitive nutrition lessons that address food groups, balanced meals, portions, drinks, nutrition facts labels, and healthy fast food options. Children also participate in preparing healthy snacks and taste tests of fruits, vegetables, and low-fat milk. Health & Fitness then devotes 45 minutes each session to physical activity facilitated by a certified fitness instructor. Children are encouraged to perform at least 60 minutes of exercise daily, utilize the community recreational center throughout the week, and limit sedentary activity [12].

To evaluate effectiveness, all children complete an age-appropriate, pre-/postintervention questionnaire tailored to the curriculum to assess changes in knowledge and behavior. Based on preliminary results among 92 children, 82% showed improvement in knowledge, and among a subset of older children, 59% increased physical activity behaviors. Change in pre-/postintervention BMI percentile is also assessed. Because children seen at CCHR may be referred by the dietitian or their primary care provider, 59% of participants thus far were overweight (12%) or obese (47%). Among overweight/obese children who completed the program (n = 42), 60% had a decrease in BMI percentile (mean change of −2.6 percentile). Among healthy weight children, 92% maintained BMI below the 85th percentile. This evaluation is ongoing; the authors also plan to assess the effect on BMI status of individual nutrition counseling and group intervention compared with primary care visits alone.

Group prenatal and well baby care
A paradigm shift from traditional one-on-one care to a group primary care model for pregnant women and in early childhood affords a key prevention strategy to address healthy lifestyle for both mother and baby. Group care provides pregnant women and new mothers with intensive health education, social support, and more time with health professionals than traditional visits. CCHR offers group prenatal care and group well baby care as an alternative to one-on-one prenatal and pediatric visits for the first 18 months. The group care model is based on Centering Pregnancy [25], adapted for the needs and priorities of the CCHR population. During 90- to 120-minute sessions, groups of 8 to 10 women receive prenatal care from women's health providers, and 8 to 10 mother/baby dyads receive well child care from pediatricians, following the routine schedule for prenatal and well child care visits. Fathers or coparents, other family members, and friends are encouraged to attend. Multidisciplinary specialists, including mental health professionals, cofacilitate the group at predetermined sessions to foster stress management, coping, and conflict resolution skills. The registered dietitian has a critical role in providing nutrition messaging, including breastfeeding, introduction of solid foods, and healthy eating for the entire family, and conducting interactive cooking demonstrations at every session.

To date, approximately 400 pregnant women and 90 mother/baby dyads have participated in group care. Outcomes being tracked include breastfeeding initiation and duration, appropriate introduction of solid foods, prenatal weight gain, postpartum weight retention, and children's BMI percentile. Preliminary analyses suggest more favorable results for group compared with traditional care at SBHC/CCHR and with national averages. Of note, among children who participated in group well baby care (n = 36), 2.8% were overweight or obese (≥85th percentile) at age 2 years compared with 15.7%% of 2-year-olds seen at CCHR (n = 356) over the same time period. Ongoing evaluation will further elucidate the effect of group compared with traditional care on primary obesity prevention and other key outcomes.

Partnerships

Partnerships with community-based organizations, private foundations, and local and federal government agencies are essential to developing and sustaining childhood obesity programs. Starting Right's Health & Fitness Group has been conducted at a police athletic league, a local middle school, and since 2010 in a public housing recreation center. Each partnership permitted children from the host site (nonpatients) to participate, increasing community access to nutrition education and physical activity. Such partnerships build community capacity, promoting healthier communities at the population level [26]. Partnerships with private foundations and government agencies also help to generate resources for the program. Recently, CCHR was chosen to participate in a collaboration of hospital-affiliated community health centers, the New York City Department of Health and Mental Hygiene, and other key stakeholders to improve the health of local communities by increasing access to healthy foods and safe environments for physical activity.

IMPLICATIONS

In addressing health disparities, community health centers, the original medical home, have the unique vantage point as agents of change at the individual, family, and community level. Functioning as beacons in underserved neighborhoods, community health centers garner trust that can be leveraged to tackle etiologically complex conditions such as obesity. Creating culturally sensitive, interactive educational materials helps to narrow the information gap between primary care providers and the population served and encourages behavior change. Moreover, public-private partnerships enhance resources for often financially strapped health centers, enabling more intensive focus on prevalent health conditions that disproportionately affect poor communities.

Starting Right is an example of such a partnership. This multicomponent initiative that provides universal screening, messaging throughout the life cycle, and innovative interventions appears to be making an impact. Governmental, medical, public health, and other nongovernmental bodies have put into action policies and recommendations to reverse the obesity epidemic and mitigate the rise of comorbid conditions. Community health centers, with their family-centered approach, should play a leading role in the prevention and intervention of childhood obesity in the poor communities they serve. Failure to do so will widen the gap in health disparities and result in adverse health outcomes for generations to come.

REFERENCES

[1]. Ogden CL, Carroll MD, Kit BK, et al. Prevalence of obesity and trends in body mass index among US children and adolescents, 1999-2010. JAMA 2012; 307(5):483–90.
[2]. Centers for Disease Control and Prevention (CDC). Obesity in K-8 students - New York City, 2006-07 to 2010-11 school years. MMWR Morb Mortal Wkly Rep 2011;60(49):1673–8.
[3]. U.S. Census Bureau, 2008-2010 American Community Survey. Available at: http://www.nyc.gov/html/dcp/html/neigh_info/bx02_info.shtml. Accessed January 8, 2013.
[4]. New York City, Department of City Planning. Going to market: New York City's neighborhood grocery store and supermarket shortage. Available at: http://www.nyc.gov/html/dcp/html/supermarket/index.shtml. Accessed January 8, 2013.
[5]. New York City, Department of City Planning. Community district needs for fiscal year 2010: the Bronx. DCP #08–05, December 2008. Available at: http://home2.nyc.gov/html/dcp/pdf/pub/bxneeds_2010.pdf. Accessed January 8, 2013.

[6]. Matte T, Ellis JA, Bedell J, et al. Obesity in the South Bronx: a look across generations. New York: New York City Department of Health and Mental Hygiene; 2007.

[7]. Goranson C, Jasek J, Olson C, et al. New York city community health survey atlas, 2009. New York: New York City Department of Health and Mental Hygiene; 2010.

[8]. Olson EC, Van Wye G, Kerker B, et al. Take care Hunts Point and Mott Haven. NYC community health profiles. 2nd edition. 2006;7(42):1–16. Available at: http://www.nyc.gov/html/doh/downloads/pdf/data/2006chp-107.pdf. Accessed April 16, 2014.

[9]. Olson EC, Van Wye G, Kerker B, et al. Take care Highbridge and Morrisania. NYC community health profiles. 2nd edition. 2006;6(42):1–16. Available at: http://www.nyc.gov/html/doh/downloads/pdf/data/2006chp-107.pdf. Accessed April 16, 2014.

[10]. Shapiro A, Gracy D, Quinones W, et al. Putting guidelines into practice: improving documentation of pediatric asthma management using a decision-making tool. Arch Pediatr Adolesc Med 2011;165(5):1–7.

[11]. Barlow SE, Dietz WH. Obesity evaluation and treatment: expert committee recommendations. The Maternal and Child Health Bureau, Health Resources and Services Administration and the Department of Health and Human Services. Pediatrics 1998;102(3):E29.

[12]. Barlow SE, Expert Committee. Expert committee recommendations regarding the prevention, assessment, and treatment of child and adolescent overweight and obesity: summary report. Pediatrics 2007;120(Suppl 4):S164–92.

[13]. Expert Panel on Integrated Guidelines for Cardiovascular Health and Risk Reduction in Children and Adolescents, National Heart, Lung, and Blood Institute. Expert panel on integrated guidelines for cardiovascular health and risk reduction in children and adolescents: summary report. Pediatrics 2011; 128(Suppl 5):S213–56.

[14]. National Committee for Quality Assurance. The state of healthcare quality. 2012. Available at: http://www.ncqa.org/Portals/0/State%20of%20Health%20Care/2012/SOHC_Report_Web.pdf. Accessed April 16, 2014.

[15]. Liang L, Meyerhoefer C, Wang J. Obesity counseling by pediatric health professionals: an assessment using nationally representative data. Pediatrics 2012; 130(1):67–77.

[16]. Leverence RR, Williams RL, Sussman A, et al. Obesity counseling and guidelines in primary care: a qualitative study. Am J Prev Med 2007;32(4):334–9.

[17]. Klein JD, Sesselberg TS, Johnson MS, et al. Adoption of body mass index guidelines for screening and counseling in pediatric practice. Pediatrics 2010;125(2):265–72.

[18]. American Diabetes Association. Standards of medical care in diabetes—2012. Diabetes Care 2012;35(Suppl 1):S11–63.

[19]. American Diabetes Association. Type 2 diabetes in children and adolescents. Pediatrics 2000;105(3):671–80.

[20]. Daniels SR, Greer FR, Committee on Nutrition. Lipid screening and cardiovascular health in childhood. Pediatrics 2008;122(1):198–208.

[21]. Steiner MJ, Skinner AC, Perrin EM. Fasting might not be necessary before lipid screening: a nationally representative cross-sectional study. Pediatrics 2011; 128(3):463–70.

[22]. Children's Health Fund. Starting Right health education materials. Available at: http://www.childrenshealthfund.org/healthcare-for-kids/health-education-materials/starting-right. Accessed March 18, 2014.

[23]. Schwartz RP, Hamre R, Dietz WH, et al. Office-based motivational interviewing to prevent childhood obesity: a feasibility study. Arch Pediatr Adolesc Med 2007;161(5):495–501.

[24]. Larkin M, Applebaum J, Goldsmith S, et al. Double drama: emotional aspects of obesity and behavior change among parents and teens in the South Bronx. Presented at the American Academy of Pediatrics, Future of Pediatrics Conference. Chicago, July 29–31, 2011.

[25]. Rising SS, Kennedy HP, Klima CS. Redesigning prenatal care through Centering Pregnancy. J Midwifery Womens Health 2004;49(5):398–404.

[26]. Mistry KB, Minkovitz CS, Riley AW, et al. A new framework for childhood health promotion: the role of policies and programs in building capacity and foundations of early childhood health. Am J Public Health 2012;102(9):1688–96.

Pediatric Obesity and Asthma Quality of Life

Barbara Velsor-Friedrich, PhD, RN[a],*,
Lisa K. Militello, MSN, MPH, CPNP[b], Joanne Kouba[c],
Patrick R. Harrison, BS, MA[d], Amy Manion, PhD, RN, PNP[e],
Rita Doumit, PhD, MPH, RN[f]

KEYWORDS

- Asthma • Obesity • Youth • Quality of life

KEY POINTS

- The literature to date highlights existing gaps and provides several outlets for future research.
- The comorbid prevalence of obesity and asthma in youth is clearly an area requiring additional research.
- It is evident that health disparities exist for both asthma and obesity, especially in both Hispanic and African American youth.
- It is suggested that for these at-risk populations, weight-management and weight-reduction education should be included in every health-related visit.
- In addition, because of the negative effect of asthma and obesity on quality of life, tools such as the Pediatric Asthma Quality of Life Questionnaire should be used at every asthma evaluation visit and quality-of-life issues discussed, and incorporated into the asthma treatment plan.

BACKGROUND AND SIGNIFICANCE
Adult Obesity

The phenomenon of unhealthy weight status in the United States has captured the attention of health professionals and the public alike. Dramatic increases in body mass index (BMI; weight in kilograms divided by height in meters squared, ie, kg/m^2)

This article originally appeared in Nursing Clinics of North America, Volume 48, Issue 2, June 2013.
[a] Niehoff School of Nursing, Loyola University Chicago, Granada Center Room 355B, 1032 West Loyola Avenue, Chicago, IL 60626, USA; [b] College of Nursing, Arizona State University, 500 North 3rd Street, Phoenix, AZ 85004-0698, USA; [c] Niehoff School of Nursing, Loyola University Chicago, 2160 South First Avenue, Maywood, IL 60153, USA; [d] Department of Psychology, Loyola University Chicago, 1032 West Loyola Avenue, Coffee Hall, Chicago, IL 60626, USA; [e] College of Nursing, 600 South Paulina Avenue Suite 440, Amour Academic Center, Chicago, IL 60612, USA; [f] Alice Ramez Chagoury School of Nursing, Lebanese American University, Byblos, Lebanon
* Corresponding author.
E-mail address: bvelsor@luc.edu

Clinics Collections 3 (2014) 11–22
http://dx.doi.org/10.1016/j.ccol.2014.09.029
2352-7986/14/$ – see front matter © 2014 Elsevier Inc. All rights reserved.

have been reported through public health surveillance programs such as the National Health and Nutrition Examination Survey (NHANES) starting in the 1970s to the 1990s for both adults and youth, making obesity and overweight common conditions in the United States. According to the most recent NHANES reports, using data from 2009 to 2010, age-adjusted obesity prevalence for adults is 35.7% and overweight prevalence for this group is 33.1%. In other words, 68.8% of adults in the United States have a BMI greater than is considered healthy.[1]

The burden of high BMI is not equally distributed among all segments of the adult population. Analysis of NHANES trends from 1999 to 2010 suggests that significant increases in obesity prevalence have occurred for white, non-Hispanic black, and Mexican American men, and non-Hispanic black and Mexican American women.[1]

Obesity in Youth

The obesity phenomenon in youth parallels that of adults in the United States. Childhood obesity has tripled in the last 4 decades. Current estimates are that 16.9% of youth between 2 and 19 years of age are obese (BMI $\geq$95th percentile for age) and 14.9% are overweight (BMI between the 85th and 94th percentile for age), which results in a total of 31.8% of youth in the United States meeting criteria for unhealthy weight.[2] As a child's age increases, so does their likelihood of being overweight or obese, as shown in **Table 1**. Preschool children aged 2 to 5 years have lower odds (0.58 for males; 0.62 for females) of obesity compared with adolescents aged 12 to 19 years.[2] Similar to disparities in adults, the burden of excess weight is more prevalent in black and Hispanic youth, and in both genders, as shown in **Table 1**. For youth combined between 2 and 19 years old, males have a significantly higher prevalence of obesity (18.6%) than females (15%)[2]; this holds true for white but not Hispanic or non-Hispanic black youth.

Youth Obesity and Asthma

The prevalence of both asthma and obesity has increased dramatically over the last several decades, which has led to an increase in the number of studies examining the relationship between these 2 variables.[3,4] However, despite the increased interest in these comorbidities, much of the research in this area has focused on adults.[3,5–7]

A study examining the prevalence of obesity among adults, using data from the NHANES I, II, and III, showed that adults with asthma are far more likely to be obese than adults without asthma.[3] In a retrospective study of 143 adult individuals aged 18 to 88 years, the prevalence of obesity increased along with increasing asthma severity in adults.[5] Furthermore, the results showed that females with asthma were significantly more overweight than males, with a mean BMI of 35.9 versus 32.14

Table 1
Prevalence of high body mass index (BMI; $\geq$85th percentile) in United States youth: both genders combined for selected groups

BMI $\geq$85th Percentile	2–19 Years Old	2–5 Years Old	6–11 Years Old	12–19 Years Old
All racial/ethnic groups	31.8	26.7	32.6	33.6
Non-Hispanic white	27.9	23.8	27.6	30.0
Mexican American	39.4	33.3	39	43.4
Non-Hispanic black	39.1	41.8	42.7	41.2

Data from Ogden CL, Carroll MD, Kit BK, et al. Prevalence of obesity and trends in body mass index among US children and adolescents, 1999–2010. JAMA 2012;307(5):483–90.

(P = .01). These findings suggest that obesity may be a potentially modifiable risk factor for asthma.[5]

The relationship between asthma and high BMI has also been examined in youth. Much of this research has focused on low-income urban and minority populations, owing to the higher prevalence of asthma and obesity in these groups. In a sample (N = 171) of predominantly Hispanic (78%) youth, 45.9% of those with asthma were overweight or obese compared with 30.2% of those without asthma who were overweight or obese (P = .04).[8] It was unclear whether exercise-induced asthma symptoms resulted in exercise avoidance and obesity, or if obesity exacerbated asthma symptoms with exercise. Belamarich and colleagues[9] examined inner-city children with asthma and determined that there was a higher incidence of obesity in Latino study subjects. In addition, obese children with asthma used more asthma medications, wheezed more, and had a greater proportion of unscheduled visits to the emergency department (ED).

A cross-sectional study using data from the 1988 to 1994 NHANES documented that 2 of the highest-risk groups for developing asthma were children older than 10 years with a BMI greater than or equal to the 85th percentile, and children with a parental history of asthma who were 10 years or younger and of African American ethnicity.[10] A subsequent study of NHANES data between 1999 and 2006 included 16,074 youth between the ages of 2 and 19 years.[11] The odds of asthma for those categorized as overweight and obese were 1.32 and 1.68, respectively, after adjustment for age, survey period, race/ethnicity, gender, and other social factors. Overweight and obesity were also associated with a higher likelihood for an asthma attack, visits to the ED, wheezing episodes, missed school, or ambulatory care visit in the last year. Limitations of studies based on NHANES data are the cross-sectional study design and the self-reporting of asthma.

A large cross-sectional study examined relationships between current asthma diagnosis, weight status, and race/ethnicity using information from 681,122 electronic medical records of youth in the Kaiser Permanente health system between 2007 and 2009.[12] The prevalence of current physician-diagnosed asthma with current medication use was 10.9%. Black youth were more likely to have asthma than non-Hispanic white youth (odds ratio = 1.93). When asthma diagnosis was examined for various weight categories, a dose-response relationship was noted, with increasing odds of asthma for those who were classified as overweight, obese, or extremely obese reported as 1.22, 1.37, and 1.68, respectively (P<.001 for trend).

When the data were further stratified by race/ethnicity and weight status, differences were noted. The dose-response relationship between weight status and risk of asthma was most pronounced in the Native American/Alaskan population, with odds of asthma for the extremely obese being 3.65 times that of asthma for normal-weight Native Americans/Alaskan youth. However, because of the small sample size (n = 610), statistical significance was not established. This dose-response relationship was statistically significant for the white sample, with odds of 1.3, 1.47, and 1.93 for those who were overweight, obese, and extremely obese in comparison with normal weight. This relationship was also identified in black youth, although with smaller and narrower odds. Also interesting was that the odds for asthma with increasing weight status was less in Hispanic youth with high BMI than in white youth with high BMI, though still higher than in normal-weight Hispanic youth. Researchers also found that those with extreme obesity were 18% more likely to use oral corticosteroids (P<.001), and 9% more likely to use inhaled corticosteroids (P<.001) than normal-weight youth. Extremely obese youth with asthma made 274 more ambulatory care visits per 1000 youth (P<.001) and 23 more ED visits (P<.001) than normal-weight youth with asthma. Strengths of this study included physician-diagnosed asthma and the large sample.

International studies report similar findings. A study conducted in Taiwan examined the relationship between asthma, lung function, and BMI in more than 15,000 school-aged children. The prevalence of asthma increased as BMI increased in both males and females.[13] A similar result was found in a study conducted in Nova Scotia, Canada, which examined 3804 students 10 to 11 years of age. Controlling for socioeconomic factors, there was a linear association between BMI and asthma, with a 6% increase in prevalence per unit increase of BMI.[14]

The consistency of the studies noted offer promising support of the correlation between high BMI and asthma. However, many used a cross-sectional design aiding in hypothesis generation but not adding to insights about causation.

The systematic review of Noal and colleagues[15] provides insights into the temporal relationship between BMI and asthma and the causal path. Ten longitudinal studies examined the relationship between weight status in early childhood and the development of asthma in adolescence. With one exception, all studies reported sample sizes greater than 1000. The majority (8 of 10) of the studies reported a positive association between overweight or obesity in early childhood and the development of asthma in adolescence. For example, Mannino and colleagues[16] followed 4393 asthma-free children for up to 14 years. Analysis of the data showed that boys with a BMI at or greater than the 85th percentile at age 2 to 3 years and boys with a BMI consistently at or above the 85th percentile were at higher risk for subsequent asthma development. Three of the studies reported in the systematic review by Noal and colleagues[15] reported higher risk for females, 3 studies reported higher risk for males, and 2 reported that the relationship was independent of gender. Although this review provides support for the causative role of high BMI in asthma incidence because of its longitudinal study design, the mechanisms for this relationship are still unclear. Proposed hypotheses have included a mechanical effect of obesity on respiratory function, the role of obesity in fueling inflammatory responses leading to asthma and/or obesity-induced immune changes that trigger genetic or hormonal pathways for asthma. Environmental factors that promote obesity, such as sedentary lifestyle, diet, and low birth weight, may also promote asthma development.[15] Clearly the rising incidence of asthma and obesity, and their combined impact on youth's quality of life (QOL), requires additional investigation.

REVIEW OF THE LITERATURE
Pediatric Asthma Quality of Life

The need to address QOL issues in chronically ill youth has become a priority in the United States.[17] There are several reasons for examining QOL in adolescents with asthma as a unique group distinct from young children and adults. Adolescence is a period of emergence of independent thinking and behavior which, along with various stressors, such as peer pressure, may affect the interpretation of asthma symptoms and adherence to prescribed asthma therapy.[18–20] This concept was supported in a study by Bruzzese and colleagues,[20] which found that early adolescents' asthma self-management was suboptimal. Although they perceive themselves to have greater responsibility for managing their asthma, early adolescents did less to care for their asthma, suggesting they may be given responsibility for asthma care prematurely.

Clinicians and researchers routinely use QOL as an indicator of successful management of asthma in youth. Measures of QOL are thought to indicate how much an adolescent's illness interferes with daily life and how well the teenager is adapting to his or her illness across several areas of functioning such as social, emotional, and physical.

A systematic review by Everhart and Fiese[21] found that asthma severity was a correlate of QOL in youth with asthma. Youth whose asthma symptoms were not well managed were more likely to experience an impaired level of QOL. Everhart and Fiese[21] concluded that researchers and health care providers basing clinical outcomes on QOL assessments should consider asthma severity in their evaluations.

These findings were supported by another study conducted with 533 Dutch adolescents. Symptom severity affected overall and positive QOL, both directly and indirectly, via coping. The lifestyle restricted by coping strategies and worrying about asthma were associated with poorer overall QOL. The use of the coping strategies-restricted lifestyle, positive reappraisal, and information seeking was related to increased scores on the positive QOL domain, whereas hiding asthma was related to lower scores on the positive QOL domain.[22]

Burkhart and colleagues[18] explored the predictors of QOL among adolescents from the United States and Iceland. Statistically significant predictors of higher asthma QOL were a better rating of overall health ($P<.01$), not having had a severe asthma attack in the last 6 months ($P<.01$), and lower depressive symptoms ($P<.01$). The researchers concluded that interventions designed to decrease depression and prevent asthma exacerbations might improve QOL for adolescents with asthma. In line with this study, Mohangoo and colleagues[23] evaluated health-related QOL (HRQOL) in adolescents with wheezing attacks using self-reported data, and determined independent associations between wheezing attacks and QOL. The presence of at least 4 wheezing attacks during the past year was associated with relevant deficits in QOL.

Another study conducted by Schmier and colleagues[24] evaluated asthma-related activity limitations and productivity losses among children and adolescents (age 4–18 years). Both HRQOL and productivity were significantly lower in patients with inadequately controlled asthma when compared with those with controlled asthma. Inadequately controlled asthma had a significant impact on asthma-specific HRQOL, school productivity and attendance, and work productivity of children and their caregivers.

Bruzzese and colleagues[25] tested the efficacy of an 8-week school-based intervention (Asthma Self-Management for Adolescents, ASMA) on 345 primarily Latino (46%) and African American (31%) high school students (mean age 15.1 years, 70% female) reporting an asthma diagnosis, symptoms of moderate to severe persistent asthma, and use of asthma medication in the last 12 months. Primary outcomes were asthma self-management, symptom frequency, and QOL; secondary outcomes were asthma medical management, school absences, days with activity limitations, and urgent health care use. Participants reported significant increases in confidently managing their asthma; use of controller medication and written treatment plans; fewer night awakenings, days with activity limitation, and school absences due to asthma; improved QOL; and fewer acute care visits, ED visits, and hospitalizations.

The feasibility of a motivational interviewing–based asthma self-management program (5 home visits) was developed and assessed in 37 African American adolescents with asthma (age 10–15 years). The teens had recently been seen in an inner-city ED for asthma symptoms and were prescribed an asthma controller medication.[26,27] Although there were no pre-post differences in adolescent-reported medication adherence, participants did report increased motivation and readiness to adhere to treatment. Teens and their caregivers reported statistically significant increases in their asthma QOL. The findings from this pilot study suggest that motivational interviewing is a feasible and promising approach for increasing medication adherence among inner-city adolescents with asthma, and is worthy of further evaluation in a randomized trial.

Pediatric Asthma, Obesity, and QOL

Although asthma severity has been shown to negatively affect QOL, there has been limited research conducted on the effects of both obesity and asthma on QOL despite the increasing prevalence of both diseases. The few studies that have explored QOL, asthma, and obesity in adults have demonstrated mixed results. A study of 382 adults with asthma discovered that the patients with higher BMIs reported lower QOL scores regardless of asthma severity.[25] Grammer and colleagues[28] studied 352 adults with asthma, 191 of whom were obese. Using the Asthma Quality of Life Questionnaire (AQLQ), results showed that obesity directly correlated with decreased QOL and increased health care utilization as demonstrated by ED/urgent care encounters. A second study using the AQLQ examined more than 900 patients, both adults and children, and found similar results in the adult group; obesity significantly correlated with decreased QOL. However, the researchers found no correlation between AQLQ scores and obesity in the children studied. There was no increase in health care use for either the obese adults or children.[29]

Researchers in Germany compared QOL in children with obesity, asthma/atopic dermatitis, or both, using the German KINDL QOL questionnaire. Among the 3 groups, the results showed lower QOL scores in children with obesity, which improved following obesity treatment.[30]

In another international study, Blandon and colleagues[31] examined 100 obese, overweight, and normal-weight children in Mexico with intermittent or mild persistent asthma. There were significant differences in QOL in the obese asthmatic group ($P<.000$). A third study conducted in the Netherlands by van Gent and colleagues,[32] using the Pediatric Asthma Quality of Life Questionnaire, found children with both asthma and obesity had lower (25%) QOL scores than children with either asthma alone (14%) or obesity alone (1%).

From the review of the literature, there appears to be a relationship between asthma and obesity. However, the exact nature of this relationship has yet to be fully determined.[33] Given the rising prevalence of obesity and asthma, additional studies regarding asthma, obesity, and QOL are warranted in order to better understand the interaction between the two comorbidities. In addition, the mechanism behind the link between asthma and obesity needs to be further investigated. The knowledge gained from further studies will aid in the development of more effective treatments and prevention programs for both asthma and obesity.

School-Based Asthma Education Programs

Coffman and colleagues[34] conducted a systematic review of the literature on school-based asthma education programs for youth aged 4 to 17 years with a clinical diagnosis of asthma or symptoms consistent with asthma. Synthesizing across studies was difficult because the characteristics of interventions and target populations varied widely, as did the outcomes assessed. Most studies that compared asthma education with usual care found that school-based asthma education programs improved knowledge of asthma, self-efficacy, and self-management behaviors. Fewer studies reported favorable effects on QOL, symptom days, symptom nights, and school absences.

More recently other supportive interventions, such as cognitive behavior modification strategies, have been found to be successful in treating children and adolescents with chronic illnesses. Interventions that use behavioral strategies are more effective in supporting change than are solely knowledge-based interventions.[35–37] Coping skills training (CST) is based on social cognitive theory, and stresses the use of adaptive coping methods and problem-solving skills. The goal of CST is to teach children and adolescents personal and social coping skills that can assist them in dealing with potential stressors they encounter in their daily lives and the stress reactions that may result from these situations.[38] The use of such skills can increase a teen's sense of competence and self-efficacy in dealing with a wide range of daily demands and health issues. In the youth population, CST has resulted in decreasing substance abuse,[39] increased social skills and reduction of aggressive behaviors,[40] and a decrease in negative responses to stressors.[41] It has also been used successfully in children with chronic illnesses such as cancer and diabetes[42–44] and in minority youth with diabetes.[45,46]

STUDY BY THE AUTHOR
Purpose

The purpose of this study is to report on the specific effects of childhood obesity and asthma on self-reported asthma QOL, coping, and control of asthma health outcomes in low-income African American teens with asthma. A randomized controlled trial (n = 137) was conducted to evaluate the efficacy of a school-based asthma education/management program on asthma-related QOL and other psychosocial and health outcomes in urban African American teens with asthma. The intervention components and results of the study have been reported in detail elsewhere.[47] In brief, the TEAM program (Teen Education and Asthma Management) is composed of 3 elements: (1) asthma education; (2) CST; and (3) nurse practitioner re-enforcement visits.

Methods

Students were recruited from 5 African American dominant urban high schools. Approximately 94% of students and their families received public assistance. Student assent and parent/guardian assent was obtained. Randomization occurred by school because individual randomization within schools could lead to contamination. Students in both the treatment and control groups attended 2 asthma education sessions (group format), 3 educational re-enforcement sessions (group sessions), and an individual clinic visit with the TEAM nurse practitioner at baseline and at the end of program.

Students in the intervention group participated in CST. Five CST sessions were offered once a week during the extended homeroom period for 45 minutes. A makeup session was offered at the end of the fifth session. The following skills were taught: (1) social problem solving; (2) effective communication; (3) managing stress; (4) conflict resolution; and (5) cognitive restructuring (guided self-dialogue). At each session a skill was taught and then students were asked to role-play the skill within an asthma-based scenario. Each week the previous skill was reviewed and the new skills were taught in the same manner. Data were collected at baseline and at 2, 6, and 12 months.

Measures

The Parent Questionnaire was completed by the student's parent/guardian and supplies information regarding demographics and the adolescent's current and prior asthma health status.

The Pediatric Asthma Quality of Life Questionnaire[48] is a 23-item, 7-point Likert-scale instrument that assesses both physiologic and emotional functional impairments experienced by children and adolescents. There are 3 subscales: symptoms experienced (10 items), activity limitation (5 items), and emotional functional (8 items). Total scale α values ranged from 0.93 to 0.94 across all time periods.

Coping was measured using the Kid Cope,[49,50] a 17-item inventory designed to assess 10 cognitive and behavioral strategies used by adolescents. These strategies include distraction, social withdrawal, cognitive restructuring, self-criticism, blaming others, problem-solving, emotional regulation, wishful thinking, social support, and resignation. Total scale α values ranged from 0.73 to 0.86 across time periods.

Control of Asthma Health Outcomes was operationally defined as according to the National Asthma Education and Prevention Program guidelines.[51] For this study, well-controlled was defined as meeting all of the following criteria: mean peak flow reading in the green zone, asthma symptom frequency less than 2 days a week, asthma symptom frequency less than 2 nights per month, and the use of asthma rescue medicine less than 2 days per week.

Overweight and obesity were operationally defined per the Centers for Disease Control criterion and plotted on age-appropriate and gender-appropriate growth charts. If a student had a BMI greater than or equal to 85% to 94% the diagnosis of overweight was made, and if their BMI was equal to or greater than 95% the diagnosis of obesity was made.[52]

Data analysis

Using correlation and regression analyses, relations among study variables were examined. Correlational analyses were used to examine the bivariate relations among intent to treat approach, a series of mixed-model analyses of variance examined the interaction between BMI and obesity and asthma QOL. Regression analyses were used to determine which variables predicted significant variability in asthma QOL. Finally, a series of *t*-tests were conducted to determine whether those who were overweight or obese had significantly worse outcomes than those who were of normal weight. Two-sided test were used and a *P* value of less than .05 was considered significant.

Results

At baseline, self-reported asthma QOL scores indicated a moderate level of impairment for all students, with only 53% of students determined to be in control of their asthma. Correlational results indicated that BMI was negatively associated with asthma QOL at baseline ($r = -0.16$), 2 months ($r = -0.10$), 6 months ($r = -0.09$), and 12 months ($r = -0.24$), although this relationship was only significant at 12 months ($P<.01$). These findings suggest that increased BMI is negatively associated with self-reported asthma QOL.

To further explore the nature of the relation between BMI and asthma QOL, *t*-tests were conducted to determine whether those who were overweight or obese had significantly worse asthma QOL relative to those who were of normal weight. Results indicated that those who were overweight or obese at baseline had marginally significantly lower asthma QOL (mean = 4.65, standard deviation [SD] = 1.11) compared with those who were normal weight (mean = 4.97, SD = 0.83), $t(121) = 1.78$, $P = .07$. Furthermore, at 12 months, those who were overweight or obese reported higher levels of negative coping (mean = 1.42, SD = 0.63) compared with those who were of normal weight (mean = 1.20, SD = 0.52), $t(121) = 2.06$, $P = .04$. In addition, those who were not in control of their asthma reported lower asthma QOL (mean = 4.67, SD = 1.10), $t(132) = 2.51$, $P = .01$. There were no significant differences between those who were overweight or obese and those who were normal at any other time point.

To examine the role of BMI in determining asthma QOL relative to other important predictors, a series of regression equations tested the relative importance of BMI in asthma QOL. Results indicated that when including symptom frequency, asthma classification (intermittent, mild, moderate, severe), asthma knowledge, asthma self-efficacy, and asthma self-care levels, BMI remained the strongest predictor of asthma QOL ($\beta = -0.28$, $P = .002$) along with asthma knowledge ($\beta = 0.28$, $P = .003$). These findings suggest that even when controlling for the influence of symptom frequency and asthma classification, BMI remains a most important factor in determining self-reported QOL among teens with asthma.

To determine whether BMI and obesity inhibits the effectiveness of an asthma treatment program (TEAM), an additional series or regression models were used to test the moderating role of BMI and obesity. Contrary to hypotheses, results indicated that when controlling for baseline levels of asthma QOL, neither BMI nor obesity had a significant moderating effect on the effectiveness of an asthma treatment program at 6 months ($\beta = -0.07$, $P = .82$; $\beta = 0.03$, $P = .86$, respectively). Similarly, when controlling for baseline levels of asthma QOL, neither BMI nor obesity had a significant moderating effect on the effectiveness of an asthma treatment program on asthma QOL at 12 months ($\beta = -0.05$, $P = .73$; $\beta = 0.03$, $P = .91$, respectively). These findings suggest that although BMI and obesity are important predictors of asthma-related QOL in their own right, they did not influence the effectiveness of the asthma treatment program in this study.

Discussion and Clinical Implications

Although the results showed that overweight and obesity did not change the effectiveness of the asthma treatment program, the impact obesity plays on QOL should not be ignored.

These findings support previous literature suggesting that overweight/obese adolescents experience poorer physical health than their nonoverweight peers. In a sample of 923 adolescents, Wake and colleagues[53] found that obesity was associated with a lower QOL. However, special needs related to asthma only slightly rose with increased BMI, and not to the point of significance. It was found that many adverse health and psychological effects of childhood obesity could be reversed if the obesity were treated before adolescence. However, specific health problems that would prompt a reduction in the BMI of adolescence were not reported. Although the strength of the random sampling method, parallel adolescent self-reports and parent proxy reporting, and large sample size add weight to the study findings, the study was limited by potential bias owing to attrition and a higher rate of obese participants lost.

In another study, Burkhart and colleagues[18] found that gender was statistically significantly associated with QOL in a sample of 30 adolescents with asthma. Males had a higher QOL compared with females ($P = .003$), and QOL scores were poorer with the experience of an asthma attack in the past 6 months. Asthma severity did not correlate with asthma QOL. However, the majority of the participants reported their asthma as mild (57%) and more than half said their activity was occasionally limited by asthma (56%). This study lends interesting insights into the predictors of QOL in adolescents with asthma; however, the weight of the contribution is limited by the small sample size, exploratory nature, and cross-sectional design.

The literature to date does highlight existing gaps and provides several outlets for future research. The comorbid prevalence of obesity and asthma in youth is clearly an area requiring to be understood. It is evident that health disparities exist for both asthma and obesity, especially in both Hispanic and African American youth. It is suggested that for these at-risk populations, weight-management and weight-reduction education should be included in every health-related visit. In addition, because of the negative effect of asthma and obesity on QOL, tools such as the Pediatric AQLQ should be used at every asthma evaluation visit, and QOL issues discussed as well as being incorporated into the asthma treatment plan.

REFERENCES

1. Flegal KM, Carroll MD, Kit BK, et al. Prevalence of obesity and trends in the distribution of body mass index among US adults, 1999-2010. JAMA 2012;307(5): 491–7.
2. Ogden CL, Carroll MD, Kit BK, et al. Prevalence of obesity and trends in body mass index among US children and adolescents, 1999-2010. JAMA 2012; 307(5):483–90.
3. Ford ES, Mannino DM. Time trends in obesity among adults with asthma in the United States: findings from three national surveys. J Asthma 2005;42(2): 91–5.
4. Chen AY, Kim SE, Houtrow AJ, et al. Prevalence of obesity among children with chronic conditions. Obesity 2009;17(6):1–4.
5. Akerman MJ, Calacanis CM, Madsen MK. Relationship between asthma severity and obesity. J Asthma 2004;41(5):521–6.
6. Luder E, Ehrlich RI, Lou WY, et al. Body mass index and the risk of asthma in adults. Respir Med 2004;98(1):29–37.
7. Spivak H, Hewitt MF, Onn A, et al. Weight loss and improvement of obesity-related illness in 500 U.S. patients following laparoscopic adjustable gastric banding. Am J Surg 2005;189(1):27–32.
8. Gennuso J, Epstein LH, Paluch RA, et al. The relationship between asthma and obesity in urban minority children and adolescents. Arch Pediatr Adolesc Med 1998;152:1197–2000.
9. Belamarich PF, Luder E, Kattan M, et al. Do obese inner-city children with asthma have more symptoms than nonobese children with asthma? Pediatrics 2000; 106(6):1436–41.
10. Rodriguez MA, Winkleby MA, Ahn D, et al. Identification of population subgroups of children and adolescents with high asthma prevalence: findings from the Third National Health and Nutrition Examination Survey. Arch Pediatr Adolesc Med 2005;156(3):269–75.
11. Visness CM, London SJ, Daniels JL, et al. Association of childhood obesity with atopic and non-atopic asthma: results from the National Health and Nutrition Examination Survey 1999-2006. J Asthma 2010;47:822–9.
12. Black MH, Smith N, Porter AH, et al. Higher prevalence of obesity among children with asthma. Obesity 2012;20:1041–7.
13. Chu YT, Chen WY, Wang TN, et al. Extreme BMI predicts higher asthma prevalence and is associated with lung function impairment in school-aged children. Pediatr Pulmonol 2009;44(5):472–9.
14. Sithole F, Douwes J, Burstyn I, et al. Body mass index and childhood asthma: a linear association? J Asthma 2008;45(6):473–7.
15. Noal RB, Menezes AMB, Macedo EC, et al. Childhood body mass index and risk of asthma in adolescence: a systematic review. Obes Rev 2011;12:93–104.
16. Mannino DM, Mott J, Ferdinands J, et al. Boys with high body masses have an increased risk of developing asthma: findings from the National Longitudinal Survey of Youth (NLSY). Int J Obes 2006;30:6–13.
17. Centers for Disease Control and DC. Healthy People. 2020. Available at: www.cdc.gov/nchs/healthy-people.htm. Accessed July 20, 2012.

18. Burkhart P, Svavardottir EK, Rayens MK, et al. Adolescents with asthma: predictors of quality of life. J Adv Nurs 2009;64(4):860–6.
19. Velsor-Friedrich B, Vlasses F, Moberley J, et al. Talking with teens about asthma management. J Sch Nurs 2004;20(3):140–8.
20. Bruzzese JM, Stepney C, Fiorino EK, et al. Asthma self-management is suboptimal in urban Hispanic and African American/black early adolescents with uncontrolled persistent asthma. J Asthma 2011;183:998–1006.
21. Everhart RS, Fiese BH. Asthma severity and child quality of life in pediatric asthma: a systematic review. Patient Educ Couns 2008;75:162–8.
22. Van De Ven MO, Engels RC, Sawyer SM, et al. The role of coping strategies in quality of life adolescents with asthma. Qual Life Res 2007;16:625–34.
23. Mohangoo AD, deKoning HJ, Mangunkusumg RT, et al. Health-related quality of life in adolescents with wheezing attacks. J Adolesc Health 2007;41(5):464–71.
24. Schmier JK, Manjunath R, Halpern MT, et al. The impact of inadequately controlled asthma in urban children on quality of life and productivity. Ann Allergy Asthma Immunol 2007;98(3):245–51.
25. Bruzzese JM, Sheares BJ, Vincent JE, et al. Effects of a school-based intervention for urban adolescents with asthma. Am J Respir Crit Care Med 2011;49(1):90–7.
26. Riekert KA, Borrelli B, Bilderback A, et al. The development of a motivational interviewing intervention to promote medication adherence among inner-city, African American adolescents with asthma. Patient Educ Couns 2011;82(1):117–22.
27. Lavoie KL, Bacon SL, Labrecque M, et al. Higher BMI is associated with worse asthma control and quality of life but not asthma severity. Respir Med 2006;100:648–57.
28. Grammer LC, Weiss KB, Pedicano JB, et al. Obesity and asthma morbidity in a community-based adult cohort in a large urban area: The Chicago Initiative to Raise Asthma Health Equity (CHIRAH). J Asthma 2010;47:491–5.
29. Peters JI, McKinney JM, Smith B, et al. Impact of obesity in asthma: evidence from a large prospective disease management study. Ann Allergy Asthma Immunol 2011;106:30–5.
30. Ravens-Sieberer U, Redegeld M, Bullinger M. Quality of life after in-patient rehabilitation in children with obesity. Int J Obes Relat Metab Disord 2001;25(S1):S63–5.
31. Blandon VV, del Rio Navarro B, Berber Eslava A, et al. Quality of life in pediatric patients with asthma with or without obesity: a pilot study. Allergol Immunopathol (Madr) 2004;32(5):259–64.
32. van Gent R, van der Ent CK, Rovers MM, et al. Excessive body weight is associated with additional loss of quality of life in children with asthma. J Allergy Clin Immunol 2007;119:591–6.
33. Michelson PH, Williams LW, Benjamin DK, et al. Obesity, inflammation, and asthma severity in childhood: data from the National Health and Nutrition Examination Survey 2001-2004. Ann Allergy Asthma Immunol 2009;103(5):381–5.
34. Coffman JM, Cabana MD, Yelin EH. Do school-based asthma education programs improve self-management and health outcomes? Pediatrics 2009;124:729–42, 729.
35. Cristensin H, Griffins K, Korten A. Web-based cognitive behavior therapy: analysis of site usage and changes in depression and anxiety scores. J Med Internet Res 2002;4(1):e3.

36. Wright J. Cognitive behavior therapy. Basic principles and recent advances. Focus: The Journal of Lifelong Learning in Psychiatry American Psychology Association 2006;4(2):173–8.
37. Glick B. Cognitive behavioral interventions for at-risk youth. Kingston (NJ): Civic Research Institute; 2006.
38. Forman S. Coping skills for children and adolescents. San Francisco (CA): Josey-Bass; 1993.
39. Forman S, Linney J, Brondion M. Effects of coping-skills training on adolescents at risk for substance abuse. Psychol Addict Behav 1990;4:67–76.
40. Prinz R, Blechman E, Dumas J. An evaluation of peer coping-skills training for childhood aggression. Clin Child Fam Psychol Rev 1994;23:193–203.
41. Elias MJ, Gara M, Ubriaco M, et al. Impact of a preventive social problem solving intervention children's coping with middle-school stressors. Am J Community Psychol 1986;14:259–75.
42. Grey M, Boland E, Davidson M, et al. Coping skills training for youths with diabetes on intensive therapy. Appl Nurs Res 1999;12:3–12.
43. Grey M, Whittemore R, Jaser S, et al. Efforts of coping skills training in school-age children with type 1 diabetes. Res Nurs Health 2009;32:405–18.
44. Varni JW, Katz ER, Colegrove R, et al. The impact of social skills training on the adjustment of children with newly diagnosed cancer. J Pediatr Psychol 1993;18:751–67.
45. Jefferson V, Jaser S, Lindemann E, et al. Coping skills training in a telephone health coaching program for youth at risk for type 2 diabetes. J Pediatr Health Care 2011;25:153–61.
46. Grey M, Berry D, Davidson M, et al. Preliminary testing of a program to prevent type 2 diabetes among high-risk youth. J Sch Health 2004;74:10–5.
47. Velsor-Friedrich B, Militello L, Richards M, et al. Effects of coping skills training in low-income urban African-American adolescents with asthma. J Asthma 2011;49(4):372–9.
48. Junniper E, Guyatt G, Feeny D, et al. Measuring quality of life in children with asthma. Qual Life Res 1996;5:35–46.
49. Spirito A, Star L, Willimas C. Development of a brief coping checklist for use with pediatric populations. J Pediatr Psychol 1988;13:555–74.
50. Spirito A, Stark L, Kanpp L. Stress and coping in child health. In: Wallander JL, Walker CE, editors. The assessment of coping in chronically ill children: implications for clinical practice. New York: Guilford Press; 1992. p. 327–44.
51. National Asthma Education and Prevention Program. Expert Panel report. Guidelines for the diagnosis and management of asthma update on selected topics. 2007. Available at: http://www.nhlbi.nih.gov/guidelines/asthma/asthgdln.pdf. Accessed July 20, 2012.
52. Centers for Disease Control and Prevention (CDC). About BMI for children and teens. Available at: http://www.cdc.gov/healthyweight/assessing/bmi/childrens_bmi/about_childrens_bmi.html. Accessed May 27, 2012.
53. Wake M, Canterford L, Patton GC, et al. Comorbidities of overweight/obesity experienced in adolescence: longitudinal study. Arch Dis Child 2010;95:162–8.

Psychopharmacologic Treatment of Obesity and Eating Disorders in Children and Adolescents

Pauline S. Powers, MD[a],*, Nancy L. Cloak, MD[b,c]

KEYWORDS

- Obesity • Eating disorders • Psychopharmacologic treatment • Adolescents

KEY POINTS

- Most evidence-based treatments for eating disorders are psychosocial.
- No medications are approved by the Food and Drug Administration (FDA) for the treatment of eating disorders in children and adolescents and only one is approved for the treatment of adults.
- Selective serotonin reuptake inhibitors are not effective for anorexia but may be helpful for comorbid conditions.
- Fluoxetine (Prozac) is FDA-approved for treatment of bulimia in adults, and there is a single positive open-label trial in adolescents.
- Orlistat (Xenical, Alli) is FDA approved for the treatment of obesity in children aged 12 years and older.
- Issues associated with psychiatric comorbidity in eating disorders and obesity relate to (1) accurate diagnosis and effective treatment, (2) medical complications, (3) potential for medications to exacerbate eating disorders and obesity, (4) risks of medication nonadherence or misuse, and (5) the impact of eating disorders and gastric bypass surgery on pharmacokinetics.

OVERVIEW

Obesity and eating disorders are common conditions that usually begin in childhood or adolescence and are difficult to treat. More than 110 million children are overweight or obese worldwide[1] and they have at least a 70% chance of becoming obese adults.[2]

This article originally appeared in Child and Adolescent Psychiatric Clinics of North America, Volume 21, Issue 4, October 2012.
Funding sources: None.
Conflict of interest: None.
[a] Department of Pediatrics, Center for Eating and Weight Disorders, College of Medicine, University of South Florida, 3515 East Fletcher Avenue, Tampa, FL 33613, USA; [b] Oregon Center for Clinical Investigations, 2232 NW Pettygrove Street, Portland, OR 97210, USA; [c] Private Practice, 2455 Northwest Marshall Street, Suite 7, Portland, OR 97210, USA
* Corresponding author.
E-mail address: ppowers@health.usf.edu

2352-7986/14/$ – see front matter © 2014 Elsevier Inc. All rights reserved.

The lifetime prevalence of eating disorders is about 11% in the United States.[3] One recent surveillance study in Britain[4] found that the overall incidence of eating disorders in children younger than 13 years was 3.01 per 100 000 and that 50% of these children required hospital admission.

The rates of premature mortality are significant for adolescents and children with obesity and eating disorders. The long-term consequences of obesity (diabetes, hypertension, and cardiac disease) may shorten lifespans by an average of up to 7 years,[5] although younger people may be more at risk for premature mortality.[6] Even those who lose weight are still at risk for a host of physiologic and psychological complications.[7] Standardized mortality ratios (SMRs) for obesity vary by age and sex. (The SMR is the ratio between the observed number of deaths in a study population and the number of deaths expected based on the age- and sex-specific rates in a standard population. If the ratio is more than 1, there is said to be excess deaths in the study population.) Overall, the SMR for obesity for men is 1.67 and 1.45 for women, indicating a significant excess risk of death; the SMR for young men aged 18 to 29 years is the highest at 2.46.[8] A recent meta-analysis also found elevated SMRs for anorexia nervosa (AN), bulimia nervosa (BN), and eating disorders not otherwise specified (ED NOS).[9] Thus, in addition to their high prevalence, eating disorders and obesity carry significant risks for mortality (for example, the SMR for AN is 5.86), which are comparable to mortality risks for other serious diseases of youth, such as asthma[10] and type 1 diabetes (**Fig. 1**).[11]

Most of the evidence-based treatments for eating disorders are psychotherapies (**Table 1**); only one medication is approved by the US Food and Drug Administration (FDA) for the treatment of an eating disorder (fluoxetine [Prozac] at 60 mg/d for adults with bulimia); and only one medication is approved for the treatment of obesity in youth (orlistat [Xenical, Alli]). However, other medications are frequently used off-label. In this review, the authors summarize the evidence base for medications that are currently used for obesity and eating disorders. The existing evidence in children and adolescents are reviewed, but most of the data derives from studies in adults. The authors also discuss the FDA approval status for the most commonly used medications and review their contraindications and major adverse effects (**Table 2**). Investigational agents currently being considered, issues related to psychiatric and medical comorbidity, and limitations of pharmacologic strategies are addressed, and recommendations for treatment are provided.

PHARMACOTHERAPY FOR AN

AN is associated with an intense fear of gaining weight or becoming fat that leads to energy restriction and significantly low body weight (**Table 3**). Affecting 0.3% of US

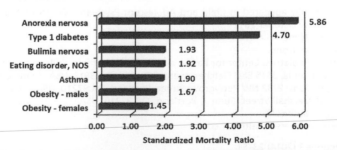

Fig. 1. Standardized mortality ratios for selected diseases in children and adolescents (references in text).

Table 1
Major evidence-based treatments for eating disorders

Disorder	Intervention	Outcome Measure	Control	Percentage Achieving		NNT[a]
				Treatment (%)	Control (%)	
AN	Family based treatment[130] (adolescents only)	Full weight restoration, normal EDE scores	Individual therapy	41.8	22.6	5
BN	CBT[131]	Abstinence from bingeing and purging	Nonspecific therapy	56.0	24.0	3
	Interpersonal psychotherapy[132]	Abstinence from bingeing and purging	Behavior therapy	44.0	20.0	4
	Self-help (CBT based)[133]	≥50% decrease in bingeing and purging	Wait list	56.3	31.0	4
	Fluoxetine[44]	≥50% decrease in bingeing and purging	Pill placebo	63.0	43.0	5
Binge-eating disorder	CBT[134]	Abstinence from binge eating	Behavioral weight loss	51.0	36.0	7
	Topiramate[84]	Abstinence from binge eating	Pill placebo	58.0	29.0	3
	Self-help (CBT based)[135]	Abstinence from binge eating	Wait list	43.0	8.0	3

Abbreviations: CBT, cognitive-behavioral psychotherapy; EDE, Eating Disorder Examination; NNT, number needed to treat.
[a] Number needed to treat is the average number of patients who need to be treated for one additional patient to benefit compared with a control or no treatment. It is calculated as the reciprocal of the absolute percentage difference between the treatment group and the control group.

Table 2
Selected medications used to treat eating disorders and obesity[a]

Medication	Drug Class	Diagnosis	FDA Approved for ED, Obesity	Dose[b]	FDA Approved for Other Dx in Children or Adolescents	Side Effects	Black-Box Warnings
Aripiprazole	Atypical antipsychotic	AN	No	2–10 mg	Schizophrenia (13 y and older); bipolar I (10 y and older); irritable autism (6 y and older)	Sedation, possible metabolic syndrome, akathisia	Suicidality in patients younger than 24 y, increased mortality in elderly with dementia
Atomoxetine	SNRI	BED	No	80–110 mg	ADHD (6 y and older)	Dry mouth, nausea, hepatotoxicity (rare)	Suicidality
Bupropion SR	Antidepressant (aminoketone class)	Obesity	No	50–400 mg	No	Seizure risk (1%), increased in patients with ED	Suicidality
Citalopram	SSRI	BED	No	60 mg[c]	No	Gastrointestinal, sexual dysfunction, risk for serotonin syndrome	Suicidality
Cyproheptadine	Antihistamine	AN	No	2–16 mg	Rhinitis (2 y and older)	Sedation	None
Diethylpropion	Appetite suppressant	Obesity	Yes	25 mg bid	Obesity (16 y and older)	Arrhythmias, gastrointestinal, addictive	Pulmonary hypertension, valvulopathy

Duloxetine	SSNRI	BED	No	60–90 mg	No	Gastrointestinal, sexual dysfunction, risk for hepatotoxicity (rare), risk for serotonin syndrome	Suicidality
Escitalopram	SSRI	BED	No	30 mg	Depression (12 y and older)	Gastrointestinal, sexual dysfunction, risk for serotonin syndrome	Suicidality
Exenatide	Glucagonlike peptide agonist	Obesity	No	5–10 mcg SQ bid	No	Nausea	Pancreatitis
Fluoxetine	SSRI	BN BED	Yes, BN in adults	60 mg	Depression (8 y and older); OCD (6 y and older)	Gastrointestinal, sexual dysfunction, risk for serotonin syndrome	Suicidality
Fluvoxamine	SSRI	BN BED	No No	100 mg bid	OCD (8 y and older)	Gastrointestinal, sexual dysfunction, risk for serotonin syndrome	Suicidality
Liraglutide	Glucagon-like peptide agonist	Obesity	No	0.6–1.8 mcg SQ	No	Nausea	C-cell tumors in animals
Lorcaserin	5-HT-2C receptor agonist	Obesity	Yes	10 mg bid	No	Headache, dizziness, fatigue, nausea	None
Metformin	Biguanide insulin sensitizer	Obesity	No	500–1000 mg bid	Type 2 diabetes mellitus (10 y and older)	Gastrointestinal symptoms	Lactic acidosis (rare but can be lethal)

(continued on next page)

Table 2
(continued)

Medication	Drug Class	Diagnosis	FDA Approved for ED, Obesity	Dose[b]	FDA Approved for Other Dx in Children or Adolescents	Side Effects	Black-Box Warnings
Naltrexone	Opioid antagonist	BN	No	200 mg	No	Avoid with opioids	Hepatotoxicity
Olanzapine	Atypical antipsychotic	AN	No	1.25–10.0 mg	Schizophrenia (13 y and older)	Sedation, possible metabolic syndrome	Increased mortality in dementia
Ondansetron	Selective 5-HT-3 antagonist	BN	No	8 mg tid	Nausea, vomiting associated with chemotherapy (4 y and older)	Visual, possible QT prolongation	None
Orlistat	Reversible lipase inhibitor	Obesity	Yes, 12 y and older	120 mg tid		Gastrointestinal, vitamin D supplement needed	Contraindicated in cholelithiasis
Phendimetrazine	Appetite suppressant	Obesity	Yes	35 mg tid	No	Tachycardia, glaucoma, addictive	Pulmonary hypertension, valvulopathy
Phentermine	Appetite suppressant	Obesity	Yes	37.5 mg	No	Cardiovascular, tachycardia, hypertension, addictive	Pulmonary hypertension, valvulopathy
Phentermine-topiramate ER	Appetite suppressant/anticonvulsant	Obesity	Yes	7.5/46 mg–15/92 mg	No	Paraesthesias, dizziness, dysgeusia	None

Pramlintide	Amylin analogue	Obesity	No	60–240 mcg SQ tid before meal		No	Hypoglycemia, gastrointestinal	Hypoglycemia (with insulin)
Quetiapine	Atypical antipsychotic	AN	No	25–300 mg		No	Sedation, possible metabolic syndrome	Suicidality, increased mortality in dementia
Sertraline	SSRI	BN BED	No	100 mg (BN), 200 mg (BED)		No	Gastrointestinal, sexual dysfunction, risk for serotonin syndrome	Suicidality
Topiramate	Anticonvulsant	BN BED	No No	100–250 mg 200–300 mg	Seizure disorder (2 y and older)	No No	Nausea, odd taste, cognitive problems; rare: metabolic acidosis, kidney stones	None
Venlafaxine XR	SSNRI	Atypical AN	No	75 mg		No	Gastrointestinal, sexual dysfunction, risk for serotonin syndrome	Suicidality

Abbreviations: ADHD, attention-deficit/hyperactivity disorder; BED, binge-eating disorder; Dx, diagnosis; ED, eating disorder; OCD, obsessive-compulsive disorder; SNRI, selective norepinephrine reuptake inhibitor; SSNRI, selective serotonin/norepinephrine reuptake inhibitor; SSRI, selective serotonin reuptake inhibitor; SQ, subcutaneously.

[a] Fluoxetine is FDA approved for BN in adults in a dosage of 60 mg/d. No other medication is approved for any eating disorder. Orlistat is the only medication that is FDA approved for obesity in children and adolescents (aged 12 years and older).

[b] Dosages are once per day unless otherwise indicated. Dosages shown are those found to be effective in clinical trials, most of which were done with adults. Clinicians should review prescribing information and use judgment when prescribing for pediatric patients.

[c] Use of citalopram at doses greater than 40 mg/day is not recommended, due to the potential for QT prolongation. Source: http://www.fda.gov/Safety/MedWatch/SafetyInformation/SafetyAlertsforHumanMedicalProducts/ucm297624.htm. Accessed August 4, 2012.

Data from www.drugs.com; www.dailymed.nlm.nih.gov; www.FDA.gov; www.dailymed.nlm.nih.gov/. Accessed March 27, 2012.

Table 3
DSM-IV TR diagnostic criteria for eating disorders and proposed DSM-V revisions[a]

	Current Criteria (DSM-IV-TR)	Proposed Changes in Criteria (DSM-V)
General	Two sections: (1) eating disorders and (2) feeding and eating disorders of infancy and early childhood	Combined into one section entitled "Eating Disorders Diagnoses"
AN	Refusal to maintain a minimally normal weight (at least 85% of ideal body weight)	Restricted intake leading to significantly low body weight for age, sex, developmental trajectory, and physical health
	Intense fear of gaining weight	Intense fear of gaining weight or persistent behavior to avoid weight gain, despite underweight
	Disturbance in way body is experienced, undue influence of body shape/weight on self-evaluation, or denial of the seriousness of current low body weight.	Disturbance in way body is experienced, undue influence of body shape/weight on self-evaluation, or persistent lack of recognition of the seriousness of low body weight
	In females, primary amenorrhea or 3 mo or more of secondary amenorrhea	Removal of amenorrhea criterion
BN	Recurrent binge eating (large amounts of food in discrete time period coupled with feeling of loss of control)	Recurrent binge eating (large amounts of food in discrete time period coupled with feeling of loss of control)
	Recurrent compensatory behavior	Recurrent compensatory behavior
	Self-evaluation unduly influenced by shape or weight	Self-evaluation unduly influenced by shape or weight
	Does not occur during episodes of AN	Does not occur during episodes of AN
	Occurs 3 times per week for last 3 mo	Occurs 1 time per week for last 3 mo
	Two types (purging and nonpurging)	Removal of 2 types
Binge-Eating Disorder	Falls under ED-NOS with research criteria for further study	Established as independent diagnosis in DSM-V
	Recurrent episodes of binge eating	Recurrent episodes of binge eating
	Binge eating is associated with 3 or more of following:	Binge-eating is associated with 3 or more of following:
	1. Eating more rapidly than normal	1. Eating more rapidly than normal
	2. Eating until uncomfortably full	2. Eating until uncomfortably full
	3. Eating large amounts when not physically hungry	3. Eating large amounts when not physically hungry
	4. Eating alone because of embarrassment	4. Eating alone because of embarrassment
	5. Feeling guilty or disgusted with self after eating	5. Feeling guilty or disgusted with self after eating
	Marked distress about binge eating	Marked distress about binge eating
	Occurs at least 2 d a wk for 6 mo	Occurs at least weekly for 3 mo

[a] Proposed revisions are indicated by italics.

adolescents,[12] AN is associated with multiple medical complications and has the highest mortality rate of any psychiatric disorder.[13] At present, no medication is approved by the FDA for the treatment of AN, although a wide variety of medications have been studied,[14] primarily antidepressants and atypical antipsychotics. However, despite initial promise in open-label studies, double-blind placebo-controlled trials have been disappointing for both classes of drugs.

Antidepressants

Initial reports indicating that the selective serotonin reuptake inhibitors (SSRIs) were effective for the core symptoms of AN were promising,[15] particularly those suggesting that fluoxetine might prevent relapse.[16] However, subsequent well-controlled studies have shown no benefit of fluoxetine for the treatment of AN, or for prevention of relapse.[17,18] SSRIs are also ineffective for the treatment of depression in acutely ill patients with AN,[19] probably because the antidepressant effect depends on adequate intake of tryptophan.[20] They may have a role in treating patients who have made progress with nutritional rehabilitation.

Antipsychotics

With the advent of atypical antipsychotics, most in the first group to be approved have been studied for the treatment of AN, at least with case reports or open-label studies. Two that have not been assessed are clozapine (Clozaril) and ziprasidone (Geodon) because of their associations with leukopenia and QT prolongation, respectively. Similar to the experience with antidepressants, early case reports and open-label studies suggested improvement with olanzapine[21] (Zyprexa) and quetiapine (Seroquel),[22] but double-blind placebo-controlled trials were less positive. One study found that among adult patients with AN already in structured treatment, there was a slightly more rapid weight gain and a lessening of obsessive compulsive symptoms with olanzapine compared with placebo.[23] Later studies with adolescents did not find a benefit for olanzapine.[24,25] Similarly, a follow-up double-blind placebo-controlled trial of quetiapine in adults found that there was no difference between quetiapine and placebo.[26] A double-blind placebo-controlled study of risperidone (Risperdal) in adolescents and young adults was also negative.[27] Case reports of aripiprazole (Abilify) are promising,[28] but a randomized trial has not yet been completed. Thus far, the antipsychotics most recently approved (asenapine [Saphris], lurasidone [Latuda], iloperidone [Fanapt], and paliperidone [Invega]) have not been studied.

There are reasons to think that antipsychotics might be helpful. For example, the common body image disturbance (the fixed false belief that one is fat when actually semistarved) meets the criteria for a psychotic symptom. For some patients, scores on the Positive and Negative Syndrome Scale are elevated and similar to those of patients with schizophrenia.[29] Also, there are studies suggesting that there are dopamine D2/D3 receptor binding abnormalities among patients with AN.[30,31] Despite these interesting observations, thus far, no antipsychotic medication has been demonstrated to be systematically effective for adult patients with AN in randomized double-blind placebo-controlled trials.[32] Results with adolescents have usually been clearly negative.

However, individual patients may benefit from atypical antipsychotics and, thus far, the evidence is slightly better for olanzapine than for the other atypical antipsychotics. A suitable patient might be an adolescent with severe AN who is hospitalized and has slightly odd thinking or a blunted or inappropriate affect or who describes what might be command hallucinations telling her (or him) not to eat. Even in this situation, very careful monitoring and discontinuation of the medication as soon as possible is wise.

Other Agents

Although there are no clearly efficacious medications for AN, anecdotally, it has been found that patients may benefit from low doses of minor tranquilizers before meals during the initial refeeding phase. Treatments for some of the physiologic complications of AN have been studied. Bone loss begins soon after the onset of the illness and is distinct from and more severe than postmenopausal osteoporosis.[33] Estrogen has not been as effective as expected,[34] although a recent study of the transdermal preparation suggested that it may be marginally helpful.[35] One problem with administering estrogen is that menses may return and obscure the positive prognostic value of a spontaneous return of menses. Hormonally induced menses may reinforce the denial that is so commonly part of AN. Neither calcium nor vitamin D has been demonstrated to be effective in treating osteoporosis associated with AN, but daily intakes of 1000 to 1300 mg of calcium and 600 IU of vitamin D are recommended for children and adolescents.[36] Bisphosphonates may be useful in some patients, particularly if they have already had a fracture, but recent reports of jaw necrosis[37] and atypical hip fractures[38] make this a questionable treatment if patients have not had a fracture. The long-term consequences of bisphosphonates in young women are unknown. New methods of diagnosing osteoporosis and new guidelines (FRAX, the WHO's fracture risk assessment tool)[39] for deciding if treatment should begin may be helpful in the future. Although it is well established that many patients have delayed gastric emptying[40] and treatment with metoclopramide may alleviate this problem, the risk for extrapyramidal symptoms or tardive dyskinesia is high, particularly in semistarved patients and, therefore, other strategies (eg, use of fluids for nutrition rather than solids at the beginning of the refeeding phase) may be more prudent.

Investigational Agents

Table 4 lists studies that are registered on the Clinical Trials Web site (http://clinicaltrials.gov/) for which results are not yet available or that are still underway. Most are studies of atypical antipsychotics or various treatments of bone loss. One exception on the list is hydroxyzine, long FDA approved for anxiety, which might help some of the common anxiety disorders that occur in AN.

PHARMACOTHERAPY FOR BN

BN is characterized by recurrent episodes of binge eating followed by compensatory behavior to avoid weight gain in an individual who is not underweight (see Table 3). Unlike AN, BN is very rare in prepubertal children. However, it affects 0.9% of adolescents in the United States and is associated with significant psychiatric comorbidity; social impairment; suicidal ideation[12]; and serious medical complications, including fluid and electrolyte disturbances and esophageal rupture.[41] Unlike AN, BN responds to pharmacotherapy, which can be an effective component of a treatment program for patients with BN, particularly for patients with comorbid symptoms of anxiety or depression, or as an initial treatment of patients who lack access to cognitive-behavioral psychotherapy (CBT) or who have failed to respond to it.[42]

Antidepressants

Because they are generally safe and well tolerated, the SSRI antidepressants are currently recommended as the pharmacotherapy of choice for BN; among these, fluoxetine is the only agent that has FDA approval for the treatment of BN (in adults), at a dosage of 60 mg/d. The exact mechanism of action is unknown but probably relates to disturbances of monoamines, particularly serotonin, that are seen in both ill and

Table 4
Selected agents in clinical trials for treatment of eating disorders and obesity

AN	BN	Binge-Eating Disorder	Obesity
Olanzapine[a]	Topiramate[a]	Topiramate[a]	Topiramate[a]
Risperidone[a]	CCK-1 Agonist	Bupropion	Orlistat[a]
Aripiprazole[a]	Baclofen	Lisdexamfetamine	Metformin[a]
Hydroxyzine[a]	Memantine	Orlistat	Exenatide[a]
Alprazolam[a]	N-acetylcysteine	Duloxetine	Liraglutide
Dronabinol	Erythromycin	Pramipexole	Tesofensine (monoamine reuptake inhibitor)
		Baclofen	Bupropion-naltrexone[b]
		Armodafinil	Bupropion-zonisamide[b]
			Beloranib (angiogenesis inhibitor)
			GSK 1521498 (opioid inverse agonist)
			MK 0557 (neuropeptide Y antagonist)
			SCH 497079 (histamine antagonist)
			SR 14778 (cannabinoid antagonist)
			V 24343 (cannabinoid antagonist)
			CP 866 087 (opioid antagonist)

Italicized agents are currently FDA approved for other indications.
[a] Under study for children and/or adolescents.
[b] Individual components are currently FDA approved for obesity (phentermine) or other indications.
Data from www.clinicaltrials.gov. Accessed March 28, 2012.

recovered individuals.[43] In the study leading to the FDA approval of fluoxetine for the treatment of BN, the proportion of patients responding, as defined by a 50% or greater decrease in binge-eating or self-induced vomiting episodes, in the 60-mg/d fluoxetine and placebo treatment groups was 63% and 43%, respectively, for binge-eating episodes per week and 57% and 26%, respectively, for vomiting episodes per week. This finding represents a number needed to treat (NNT) of 5 to achieve at least a 50% reduction in both binge-eating and vomiting behaviors.[44] A 20-mg/d dosage of fluoxetine was not effective. In this and other trials of fluoxetine for BN, there were concomitant improvements in measures of depression, eating disorder psychopathology, and global severity of symptoms. Compared with its use in the treatment of depression, the treatment of BN with fluoxetine requires higher doses, but the time to response is generally quicker; most eventual responders attain a response by 3 weeks.[45] A response seems to be independent of the presence or absence of comorbid depression.[46] Continuation of the medication after treatment response reduces but does not eliminate the probability of relapse; at the end of a 12-month placebo-controlled extension trial, previous responders to fluoxetine who continued the medication had a 33% relapse rate compared with 51% of those who were switched to placebo.[47] In this study, relapse was defined as a return to the baseline binge/purge frequency. For this reason, it is recommended that treatment be continued for at least 6 months after a response.[48]

Because fluoxetine is FDA approved for BN in adults and is FDA approved for the treatment of depression and obsessive-compulsive disorder in children and adolescents, it should be the first choice if pharmacologic treatment is considered. Support for its use in children and adolescents with BN consists of a single 8-week open trial with 10 adolescents aged 12 to 18 years in which fluoxetine (60 mg daily) was combined with supportive psychotherapy. The average weekly binges decreased from 4.1 to 0, the average weekly purges decreased from 6.4 to 0.4, and a significant improvement was noted on standard measures of eating disorder psychopathology. There were no discontinuations caused by adverse effects.[49] Although SSRIs other than fluoxetine should theoretically be of benefit, there are no trials in adolescents, and supporting evidence in adults is limited to one small placebo-controlled trial each of fluvoxamine (Luvox; 200 mg/d)[50] and sertraline (Zoloft; 100 mg/d),[51] both showing statistically and clinically significant reductions in bingeing and vomiting in comparison with placebo. However, a larger controlled trial of flexibly dosed fluvoxamine was negative,[52] as was a trial of citalopram (Celexa) up to 40 mg/d.[53] Paroxetine (Paxil) has not been studied.

The most common adverse effects of fluoxetine and other SSRIs are gastrointestinal disturbances (nausea, loose stools, or constipation), insomnia, jitteriness or agitation, and sexual dysfunction. To enhance compliance, patients should be informed that these medications are generally weight neutral. Although a recent reanalysis of the data has questioned the connection between antidepressants and suicidality,[54] at this time, informed consent should include a discussion of the black-box warning regarding the increased risk of suicidal ideation and behaviors (although not actual suicides) associated with the use of newer antidepressants in children, adolescents, and young adults,[55,56] and clinicians should follow FDA guidelines for monitoring.[57]

Other Agents

Topiramate (Topamax) is FDA approved for the treatment of partial-onset or secondarily generalized seizure disorders in children (aged 2 years and older), adolescents, and adults. Its association with appetite suppression and weight loss, probably mediated by the blockade of AMPA (α-amino-3-hydroxy-5-methyl-4-isoxazolepropionic acid)/kainate glutamate receptors in the hypothalamus,[58] has led to several trials in adult patients with BN. Two 10-week trials have shown a benefit of topiramate at dosages of 100 to 250 mg/d for reducing binge/purge episodes, weight, and overall clinical severity. Compared with placebo, 27.4%[59] and 33.4%[60] more patients experienced a response, which was defined as a 50% or greater reduction in binge/purge episodes; there were also improvements in measures of eating disorder psychopathology and quality of life. Because of its potential to induce weight loss, topiramate should be avoided in low-weight individuals with BN and patients with binge/purge-type AN. There have been reports of misuse by patients with eating disorders who are seeking weight loss.[61]

Based on observations in animals that opioid antagonists decrease stress-induced eating and a positive study of intravenous naloxone (Narcan) in patients with BN, several small trials have been conducted with naltrexone (Revia), which is approved for the treatment of opioid and alcohol dependence in adults. Dosages of 200 mg/d or more were beneficial in reducing bingeing and purging,[62,63] but it was not effective at the usual prescribed dosage of 50 mg/d,[64] and there have been concerns about hepatotoxicity at the higher doses. Ondansetron (Zofran) is a serotonin 3 receptor (5-HT-3) antagonist approved for the prevention of nausea and vomiting associated with chemotherapy or anesthesia in children and widely used for nausea and vomiting associated with other medical conditions. A single small (N = 26) randomized trial showed efficacy in patients with BN who had not responded to antidepressants or psychotherapy[65]; the medication was well tolerated, but the expense and frequency of administration have limited its use.

Investigational Agents and Light Therapy

Based on emerging evidence for the involvement of the gamma-aminobutyric acid (GABA) and glutamate systems in the reward process and the regulation of food intake,[66] the GABA-B receptor agonist baclofen (Lioresal), the NMDA receptor antagonist memantine (Namenda),[67] and the glutamate release inhibitor N-acetylcysteine[68] are being investigated (see **Table 4**). Bright-light therapy has been studied in 3 small controlled trials (total N = 69), all of which found efficacy for 30-minute exposure to 2500 to 10 000 lux per day.[69–71] Effects were seen as early as 1 week and seemed greatest in individuals who reported a seasonal pattern for their symptoms.

PHARMACOTHERAPY FOR BINGE-EATING DISORDER

Like BN, binge-eating disorder is characterized by recurrent episodes of binge eating accompanied by distress and lack of control over eating, but unlike bulimia, individuals do not compensate for their behavior (see **Table 3**). Currently, binge-eating disorder is classified in the appendix of the *Diagnostic and Statistical Manual of Mental Disorders* (Fourth Edition, Text Revision) (DSM-IV-TR) as a research diagnosis but it will be formally included as a disorder in DSM-V, with some modifications in criteria.[72] It is the most prevalent eating disorder in US adolescents, affecting 1.6% of the population between the ages of 13 and 18; like BN, it is associated with high levels of psychiatric comorbidity, social impairment, and suicidal ideation.[12] Because untreated binge-eating disorder is associated with the development of obesity over time,[73] identifying and treating children and adolescents with binge-eating disorder are important components of obesity-prevention efforts in this population. In general, treatment recommendations for binge-eating disorder are similar to those for bulimia, encompassing primarily CBT and antidepressant medications,[42] although no medications are currently FDA approved for the treatment of binge-eating disorder.

SSRIs

SSRI antidepressant medications have been studied for binge-eating disorder based on their efficacy in BN and likely work via similar actions on monoamine systems. There have been 7 randomized placebo-controlled trials of SSRIs in the treatment of adults with binge-eating disorder: 2 each of fluoxetine[74,75] and fluvoxamine[76,77] and one each of escitalopram (Lexapro),[78] citalopram,[79] and sertraline.[80] Target doses were at the higher end of the usual range (eg, 60–80 mg/d of fluoxetine, 30 mg/d of escitalopram, 300 mg/d of fluvoxamine, 200 mg/d of sertraline, and 60 mg/d of citalopram). All medications were effective in reducing binge-eating behavior and also improved other outcome measures, such as eating disorder psychopathology and depression. Although placebo-corrected binge-eating abstinence rates ranged from 12% to 39%, weight loss was modest, averaging 1.7 kg greater than placebo across the trials.

Other Monoaminergic Agents

Sibutramine (Meridia), a serotonin-norepinephrine reuptake inhibitor that was formerly approved for the treatment of obesity, was effective in reducing binge eating and weight but was removed from the market in 2010 because of concerns about cardiovascular toxicity. Another serotonin-norepinephrine inhibitor, duloxetine, was recently found to be effective in a 12-week randomized placebo-controlled trial. With an average dosage of 79 mg/d, 56% of patients on medication achieved remission of binge eating versus 30% of those taking placebo; average weight loss was 3.2 kg versus 0.3 kg.[81] A 10-week randomized placebo-controlled trial of the selective norepinephrine reuptake inhibitor atomoxetine (average dose 106 mg/d) yielded remission rates of 70% for medication versus 32% for placebo, an average weight loss of 2.7 kg versus 0 kg, and significantly greater improvements on measures of eating disorder psychopathology.[82]

Anticonvulsants

There have been 3 short-term (14–21 week) randomized placebo-controlled trials of topiramate in adults with binge-eating disorder, with each showing efficacy.[83–85] Rates of placebo-corrected binge abstinence ranged between 22.7% and 34.0%, with placebo-corrected weight losses ranging between 4.3 and 5.9 kg. A benefit for decreasing binge eating was seen by the second week of treatment. Dropout rates ranged from 30% to 42%, and there were frequent adverse effects, mainly paresthesias, taste alterations, and problems with cognitive functioning. Placebo-controlled studies of other anticonvulsants that affect the glutamatergic system, zonisamide (Zonegran)[86] and lamotrigine (Lamictal),[87] have not shown benefit.

Investigational Agents and Bariatric Surgery

As for BN, several initial investigations have focused on existing modulators of the glutamate and GABA systems, including the glutamate receptor antagonists memantine[67] and acamprosate (Campral).[88] Other existing agents that are currently being investigated include the stimulant lisdexamfetamine (Vyvanse); the stimulantlike agent armodafinil (Nuvigil); the dopamine agonist pramipexole (Mirapex); and the GABA-B agonist baclofen, which is also being evaluated for the treatment of bulimia (see **Table 3**).

Binge-eating disorder is not a contraindication to bariatric surgery,[89] although clinicians are advised to assess its severity and the need for treatment both preoperatively and postoperatively. In appropriately selected patients, bariatric surgery seems to result in the improvement of binge eating[90–92]; in a 1-year prospective follow-up study of patients undergoing bariatric surgery who were diagnosed by clinical interview based on DSM-V criteria, the presence of binge-eating disorder did not adversely impact weight loss.[93] Gastric bypass was the procedure used in each of these studies, and results may not apply with other bariatric procedures.

PHARMACOTHERAPY FOR OBESITY

Because of its increasing prevalence and growing recognition of its health consequences, obesity in children and adolescents has become a major focus in both clinical and public-policy settings.[94] Treatment guidelines focus on lifestyle changes, including diet, physical activity, and reduced screen time.[95] These interventions are of limited efficacy; one meta-analysis found effect sizes for a significant reduction in body mass index (BMI) of .02 for physical activity alone and 0.22 for diet alone. Behavioral interventions that involve the family were more effective (effect size 0.64).[96] Therefore, treatment guidelines encourage consideration of pharmacotherapy for obese children and adolescents who do not respond to lifestyle interventions.[95]

However, finding safe and effective pharmacologic interventions for obesity has been challenging. This work is probably challenging because the neurobiological systems that control food intake and energy balance are highly redundant and highly interrelated with the systems involved in the regulation of mood and the response to reward. Despite an explosion in basic research, the anatomy, chemistry, and functions of these elaborate neural systems and their interactions with the gastrointestinal system and adipose tissue remain poorly characterized.[97] The development of medications for obesity has also been hampered by the frequent occurrence of adverse effects. For example, one analysis of the proposed naltrexone-bupropion combination antiobesity agent found that to achieve a weight loss of at least 10% from baseline, 6 additional patients would need to be treated for one to benefit (NNT of 6); but 1 patient among 5 to 8 patients would withdraw because of adverse events (number needed to harm of 5–8).[98] Several agents have been removed from the market because of serious adverse effects, including phentermine-fenfluramine (cardiac valvulopathy), sibutramine (cardiovascular events), and rimonabant (withdrawn from the market in Europe and never approved in the United States because of mood changes and suicidality). For these reasons, the number of medications presently approved for the treatment of obesity is small, although there are several drugs in development.

Medications Approved for Treatment of Obesity in Children and Adolescents

Currently, orlistat is the only medication that is FDA approved for the treatment of obesity in adolescents aged 12 and older, in combination with lifestyle interventions. It is a reversible lipase inhibitor that blocks the absorption of approximately 30% of dietary fat at the prescription dosage of 120 mg 3 times a day and about 25% of fat absorption at the over-the-counter dosage of 60 mg 3 times a day. In the multicenter randomized placebo-controlled trial leading to its approval for use in adolescents, 67% of patients aged 12 to 16 years who took orlistat for 1 year in combination with diet and exercise lost 5% or more of their initial body weight compared with 21% of patients treated with diet and exercise alone (NNT of 2), although the actual difference in weight was small (2.6 kg) and the orlistat-treated patients began to regain weight at the same rate as the placebo-treated patients, beginning at about week 24 of the study. Other than decreases in waist circumference and diastolic blood pressure, and a trend toward lower fasting blood sugar, there were no significant differences in cardio-metabolic parameters. The most common adverse effects are bloating, abdominal discomfort, flatulence, and oily stools. Limiting dietary fat to 15 g per meal can minimize these adverse effects. Orlistat has been associated with reduced absorption of fat-soluble vitamins and significant decreases in serum vitamin D levels, so vitamin supplementation and monitoring of serum vitamin D is advised.[99] Clinicians should screen patients for the presence of eating disorder psychopathology because there have been several case reports of orlistat misuse as a purging agent by individuals with eating disorders.[100–102]

Medications Approved in Children and Adolescents for Other Indications and Studied for Treatment of Obesity

Among the medications approved in pediatric populations for other uses, metformin (Glucophage) has been studied for the treatment of obesity in children and adolescents, and topiramate has been evaluated in obese adults. Neither is currently FDA approved for the treatment of obesity. Metformin is a biguanide that increases sensitivity of various tissues (muscle, liver, adipose) to the uptake and action of insulin. It is FDA approved for the treatment of type 2 diabetes in adults and children aged 10 years and older. In 2008, a meta-analysis was conducted of 5 placebo-controlled trials with a total of 365 obese patients aged 6 to 19 years. All trials lasted 6 months and 3 used lifestyle interventions in both arms. Metformin at dosages of 1000 to 2000 mg/d reduced BMI by an average of 1.42 kg/m^2. Overall, because its benefits for both weight loss and diabetes prevention are modest in comparison with lifestyle interventions,[103] it should probably be reserved for obese adolescents who also have diabetes or insulin resistance.

Although it has not been studied in obese children and adolescents, several investigators have studied topiramate for obesity in adults. A meta-analysis of 10 trials involving 3320 adults showed significant efficacy, with an average placebo-corrected weight loss of 5.3 kg.[104] Topiramate dosages ranged from 64 mg/d to 400 mg/d, and both weight loss and adverse effects were dose dependent. Topiramate may be an effective alternative to orlistat for obese children and adolescents who have comorbid seizure disorders or who fail to respond to orlistat or do not tolerate it.

Medications Approved for Treatment of Obesity in Adults

In addition to orlistat, the appetite suppressants phentermine (Adipex-P, Ionamin), diethylpropion (Durad, Tenuate), and phendimetrazine (Bontril) are FDA approved for short-term (12 weeks) use in adults. All are controlled substances with addiction potential, and all carry FDA warnings regarding the potential for development of pulmonary hypertension and valvular heart disease if used for more than 12 weeks. A meta-analysis found average placebo-adjusted weight losses of 3.6 kg for phentermine and 3.0 kg for diethylpropion; phendimetrazine was not included because of limited data.[105] With one exception,[106] these agents have not been studied in children and adolescents and because of their potentials for addiction and serious cardiovascular side effects, they should probably not be used. Two newly FDA-approved medications (lorcaserin [Belviq] and phentermine-topiramate ER [Qsymia]; see **Table 5**) have not been studied in children or adolescents.

Medications Approved in Adults for Other Indications and Studied for Treatment of Obesity

Among these medications are one antidepressant and several agents used to treat diabetes. Bupropion is approved for depression and smoking cessation in adults and has some structural similarity to older agents used for weight loss. However, a meta-analysis showed a modest average placebo-corrected weight loss of 2.77 kg.[107] Pramlintide (Symlin), a synthetic analogue of amylin, a peptide that is cosecreted by islet cells with insulin, reduces postprandial glucose and increases satiety. A meta-analysis of 8 adult studies that reported effects on weight showed modest placebo-adjusted weight losses of 2.57 kg in obese patients with type 2 diabetes and 2.27 kg in obese patients without diabetes.[108] Two glucagonlike peptide 1 agonists, exenatide (Byetta) and liraglutide (Victoza), have been approved for the treatment of type 2 diabetes in adults and are being evaluated for the treatment of obesity (**Table 5**).

Medications in Development

In addition to the existing antidiabetic agents liraglutide and exenatide, antiobesity medications in advanced stages of development include one novel monoaminergic agent, tesofensine, and two combinations of existing medications: Contrave, a combination of sustained-release bupropion and naltrexone; and Empatic, a combination of sustained-release bupropion and zonisamide. Details are provided in **Table 5**.

As reviewed elsewhere,[109,110] many of the medications in earlier stages of development target known components of the complex systems that regulate appetite and weight (see **Table 4**). Bariatric surgery is increasingly used in adolescents and results in much greater weight losses than behavioral interventions or medications but can be associated with significant medical complications and, in some patients, adverse psychological outcomes.[111] A detailed discussion of this topic is beyond the scope of this article, but reviews of guidelines,[112] outcomes,[113] and adverse effects[114] are available.

COMORBIDITY

Issues associated with psychiatric comorbidity in eating disorders and obesity relate to (1) the negative impacts of the eating disorder on accurate diagnosis and effective treatment, (2) implications of medical complications of eating disorders for choices of pharmacotherapeutic agents, (3) the potential for some psychotropic medications to exacerbate eating disorders and obesity, (4) the risk of medication nonadherence or misuse in patients with eating disorders, and (5) the impact of eating disorders and gastric bypass surgery on pharmacokinetics.

Diagnosis and Treatment

Many psychiatric conditions are commonly comorbid with eating disorders; for example, among adolescents with BN, 50%, 66%, and 19% met criteria for a mood disorder, anxiety disorder, and/or substance use disorder, respectively.[12] However, accurate diagnosis is a key issue: starvation alone can produce anxiety, depression, cognitive impairment, and obsessive-compulsive symptoms.[115] Despite being at normal weight, patients with bulimia also show metabolic signs of starvation,[116] which can produce depression and mood lability in combination with chaotic eating patterns. All patients can have adjustment reactions related to the significant impact of their symptoms on school, work, and relationships. Therefore, most patients should have a period of 4 to 6 weeks of normal eating before treatment is initiated.[117]

There is very limited evidence regarding the effectiveness of pharmacotherapy for comorbid conditions in individuals with eating disorders because improvement in comorbid conditions has been assessed only as a secondary outcome. As discussed, SSRIs are not effective for depression or anxiety in acute AN, but most studies of SSRIs in BN and binge-eating disorder have shown improvement in depression scores. Venlafaxine has been shown to be superior to fluoxetine in reducing anxiety in a small trial of patients with atypical AN,[118] but there has not been a double-blind placebo-controlled trial in patients with typical AN. Obsessive compulsive disorder that is not just related to food and eating and that does not resolve when patients are weight restored[119] may respond to SSRIs and clomipramine, although the latter should be avoided until patients are weight restored because of the potential for worsening of hypotension, constipation, and cardiac conduction abnormalities in underweight patients.

Medical Complications of Eating Disorders and Choice of Pharmacotherapy

Although eating disorders are associated with many medical complications, cardiovascular problems are the most immediately life threatening. These problems include bradycardia, hypotension, and arrhythmias, especially those related to the prolongation of the QT interval.[120] Clinicians should use caution when administering medications that also affect the cardiovascular system. For example, agents that have alpha-receptor blocking actions, such as trazodone (Desyrel), risperidone, clozapine, low potency typical antipsychotics, and tricyclics, can exacerbate hypotension; and lithium, carbamazepine (Tegretol), tricyclics, and many antipsychotics can worsen cardiac conduction abnormalities. Baseline electrocardiograms (EKGs) should be considered for all patients with eating disorders and obesity, and practice guidelines specifically recommend EKG monitoring for more severely ill patients who are significantly underweight and/or purging frequently.[42] Because electrolyte abnormalities are also associated with arrhythmias, electrolytes should be monitored in patients with known or suspected purging. Dehydration and constipation are other conditions frequently seen in patients with eating disorders. Therefore, lithium should be avoided in patients who purge because of the potential for toxicity with fluid shifts, and patients who are likely to have malnutrition-related gastrointestinal slowing should probably not receive medications with anticholinergic properties.

Medication-related Weight Changes and Eating Disorders

Clinicians have long observed that weight changes caused by external factors (eg, oral surgery,[121] pancreatitis[122]) can be associated with new onset or worsening of eating

Table 5
Medications for obesity that are newly approved or in advanced stages of development

Agent	Mechanism	Study: Placebo-Adjusted Weight Loss (Duration)	Adverse Effects	Status
Exenatide (Byetta)	Glucagonlike peptide 1 agonist	Rosenstock et al,[136] 2010: 3.3 kg (24 wk) Dushay et al,[137] 2012: 2.9 kg (35 wk) Kely et al,[138] 2012: 3.9 kg (26 wk)[a]	Nausea, warning regarding pancreatitis	Phase III trial completed
Liraglutide (Victoza)	Glucagon-like peptide 1 agonist	Astrup et al,[139] 2009: 4.4 kg (20 wk)	Nausea, warnings about pancreatitis, increased C-cell tumors in animals	Phase III trial in process
Lorcaserin (Belviq)	Serotonin 2C receptor agonist	Smith et al,[140] 2010: 3.6 kg (52 wk) Fidler et al,[141] 2011: 3.1 kg (52 wk) O'Neil et a,[142] 2012: 4.5–5.0 kg (52 wk)	Fatigue, dizziness, headache, nausea	FDA approved for adults on June 27, 2012; release for marketing is pending DEA review
Tesofensine	Dopamine, serotonin, and norepinephrine reuptake inhibitor	NeuroSearch: 4.5, 9.1, and 10.6 kg with doses of 0.25, 0.5, and 1.0 mg, respectively[143] (24 wk)	Dry mouth, nausea, dizziness, dose-dependent increases in heart rate and blood pressure	Phase III studies planned

Phentermine-topiramate ER (Qsymia)	Monoamine releaser, NMDA receptor antagonist	Vivus, Inc: 7.5 kg[144] (28 wk); Allison et al,[145] 2012: 10.9 kg (52 wk); Gadde et al,[146] 2011: 8.9 kg (52 wk)	Paresthesias, dry mouth, disturbed taste, constipation, poor concentration	FDA approved for adults on July 17, 2012
Bupropion-naltrexone (Contrave)	ϒ-melanocyte-stimulating hormone releaser; opioid antagonist	Greenway et al,[147] 2009: 5.4–5.9 kg (24 wk); Greenway et al,[148] 2010: 6.1 kg (56 wk); Wadden et al,[149] 2011: 4.2 kg (approximate[b]; 56 wk)	Nausea, headache, constipation, dizziness, dry mouth, transient increase in blood pressure	NDA not approved because of concerns about long-term cardiovascular safety in February 2012. Manufacturer will be conducting a large randomized cardiovascular outcomes trial with anticipated resubmission in about 2 y
Bupropion-zonisamide (Empatic)	ϒ-melanocyte-stimulating hormone releaser; NMDA receptor antagonist	Orexigen[150]: 360 mg bupropion/120 mg zonisamide: 5.3 kg (24 wk); 360 mg bupropion/360 mg zonisamide: 7.8 kg (24 wk)	Insomnia, headache, nausea	Phase IIb trial completed

Abbreviation: NDA, New Drug Application.

[a] Trial conducted in pediatric patients (aged 9–16 years).
[b] Weight losses in this study were reported only as percentages of baseline weight.

disorders. As reviewed elsewhere,[123] this has also been reported in the context of weight changes associated with various medications, including many psychotropics. The association is often indirect; weight gain associated with medication will lead to intensified restricting and/or purging, but 2 atypical antipsychotics have also been directly associated with new onset of binge eating.[124] Although not studied specifically in individuals with eating disorders, medication-related weight gain is an important contributor to nonadherence in psychiatric patients in general.[125] Patients with strong drives for thinness are also at risk for misusing medications to produce weight loss. Insulin omission is the most well-known and dangerous example,[126] but there are also reports of topiramate[61] and fluoxetine[127] overuse for the purpose of weight loss. Clinicians should be mindful of the potential impact of psychotropic medications on eating behavior and weight when choosing pharmacologic interventions, discuss this openly with patients, and closely monitor weight, adherence, and the appropriate use of weight-altering medications after they are initiated.

Eating Disorders, Obesity Surgery, and Pharmacokinetics

There have been no studies of pharmacokinetics in patients with eating disorders. However, patients with AN frequently have delayed gastric emptying,[128] which could

---

Summary of psychopharmacologic treatment of obesity and eating disorders in children and adolescents

Most evidence-based treatments for eating disorders are psychosocial. No medications are FDA approved for the treatment of eating disorders in children and adolescents and only one is approved for the treatment of adults (fluoxetine 60 mg/d for BN).

For AN, although clinical trials in adolescents have been negative, olanzapine anecdotally may be helpful for severely ill patients whose symptoms have delusional and hallucinatory qualities and interfere with the benefits from usual treatment. SSRIs are not effective for anorexia either acutely or for relapse prevention and are not beneficial for depression in acutely ill patients, but they may be helpful for comorbid conditions after nutritional rehabilitation is well under-way. Oral estrogen is of no benefit for bone loss and may reinforce patients' denial by restoring menses.

For bulimia, fluoxetine at 60 mg/d is the pharmacotherapy of choice because it is approved in adults and there is a small positive trial in adolescents. Topiramate may be an alternative because it has been shown to be effective in adults and is approved for seizure disorders in children.

For binge-eating disorder, the SSRIs are effective in reducing binge eating but not weight in adults. Topiramate is effective in reducing both binge eating and weight, but tolerability has been an issue. There have been promising small trials of duloxetine and atomoxetine, which is approved for the treatment of attention-deficit/hyperactivity disorder in children aged 6 years and older. There are no clinical trials to date in children or adolescents.

Orlistat is FDA approved for the treatment of obesity in children aged 12 years and older. Most adolescents lose more than 5% of body weight, but compliance can be an issue because of gastrointestinal side effects and 3-times-daily dosing. Topiramate has been effective in adults and is approved for another indication in children (see earlier discussion). Metformin is approved for children and adolescents with diabetes and has been studied for obesity, but weight loss is modest. There are several agents in the late stages of development, many of which are new applications of currently marketed medications.

Issues associated with psychiatric comorbidity in eating disorders and obesity relate to (1) the negative impact of the eating disorder on accurate diagnosis and effective treatment, (2) implications of medical complications of eating disorders for choices of pharmacotherapeutic agents, (3) the potential for some psychotropic medications to exacerbate eating disorders and obesity, (4) the risks of medication nonadherence or misuse in patients with eating disorders, and (5) the impact of eating disorders and gastric bypass surgery on pharmacokinetics.

theoretically prolong absorption and time to peak drug concentrations. Patients who purge by self-induced vomiting are at risk for malabsorption if they purge within several hours of taking their medications, and this should be assessed when patients seem not to respond to a medication. Immediately following gastric bypass surgery, patients are at risk for decreased absorption of medications; one study of SSRIs found that the area under the concentration/time curve decreased to an average of 54% of preoperative values, and about half of the patients had depressive relapses.[129] Their drug levels returned to baseline by 6 months.

REFERENCES

1. Cali AM, Caprio S. Obesity in children and adolescents. J Clin Endocrinol Metab 2008;93:s31–6.
2. U.S. Department of Health and Human Services. Overweight and obesity: health consequences. Available at: http://www.surgeongeneral.gov/topics/obesity/calltoaction/fact_consequences.htm. Accessed February 28, 2012.
3. Hudson JI, Hiripi E, Pope HG, et al. The prevalence and correlates of eating disorders in the National Comorbidity Survey Replication. Biol Psychiatry 2007;61:348–58.
4. Nicolls DE, Lynn R, Viner RM. Childhood eating disorders: British national surveillance study. Br J Psychiatry 2011;198:295–301.
5. Peeters A, Barendregt J, Willekens F, et al. Obesity in adulthood and its consequences for life expectancy: a life-table analysis. Ann Intern Med 2003;138:24–32.
6. Reuser M, Bonneux L, Willekens F. The burden of mortality of obesity at middle and old age is small. A life table analysis of the US Health and Retirement Survey. Eur J Epidemiol 2008;23:601–7.
7. Must A, Jacques PF, Dallal GE, et al. Long-term morbidity and mortality of overweight adolescents. A follow-up of the Harvard Growth Study of 1922 to 1935. N Engl J Med 1992;327:1350–5.
8. Bender R, Jockel KH, Trautner C, et al. Effect of age on excess mortality in obesity. JAMA 1999;281:1498–504.
9. Arcelus J, Mitchell AJ, Wales J, et al. Mortality rates in patients with anorexia nervosa and other eating disorders: a meta-analysis of 36 studies. Arch Gen Psychiatry 2011;68:724–31.
10. Kuo C, Chen VC, Lee W, et al. Asthma and suicide mortality in young people: a 12-year follow-up study. Am J Psychiatry 2010;167:1092–9.
11. Feltbower RG, Bodansky HJ, Patterson CC, et al. Acute complications and drug misuse are important causes of death for children and young adults with type 1 diabetes: results from the Yorkshire Register of diabetes in children and young adults. Diabetes Care 2008;31:922–6.
12. Swanson SA, Crow SJ, Le Grange D, et al. Prevalence and correlates of eating disorders in adolescents: results from the national comorbidity survey replication adolescent supplement. Arch Gen Psychiatry 2011;68:714–23.
13. Harris EC, Barraclough B. Excess mortality of mental disorder. Br J Psychiatry 1998;173:11–53.
14. Crow SJ, Mitchell JE, Roerig JD, et al. What potential role is there for medication treatment in anorexia nervosa? Int J Eat Disord 2009;42:1–8.
15. Kaye WH, Weltzin TE, Husu LK, et al. An open trial of fluoxetine in patients with anorexia nervosa. J Clin Psychiatry 1991;52:464–71.
16. Kaye WH, Nagata T, Weltzin TE, et al. Double-blind placebo-controlled administration of fluoxetine in restricting- and restricting-purging-type anorexia nervosa. Biol Psychiatry 2001;49:644–52.

17. Attia E, Haiman C, Walsh BT, et al. Does fluoxetine augment the inpatient treatment of anorexia nervosa? Am J Psychiatry 1998;155:548–51.
18. Strober M, Pataki C, Freeman R, et al. No effect of adjunctive fluoxetine on eating behavior or weight phobia during the inpatient treatment of anorexia nervosa: an historical case-control study. J Child Adolesc Psychopharmacol 1999;9: 195–201.
19. Mischoulon D, Eddy KT, Keshaviah A, et al. Depression and eating disorders: treatment and course. J Affect Disord 2011;130:470–7.
20. Delgado PL, Miller HL, Salomon RM, et al. Tryptophan-depletion challenge in depressed patients treated with desipramine or fluoxetine: implications for the role of serotonin in the mechanism of antidepressant action. Biol Psychiatry 1999;46:212–20.
21. Powers PS, Santana CA, Bannon YS. Olanzapine in the treatment of anorexia nervosa: an open label trial. Int J Eat Disord 2002;32:146–54.
22. Powers PS, Bannon Y, Eubanks R, et al. Quetiapine in anorexia nervosa patients: an open label outpatient pilot study. Int J Eat Disord 2007;40:21–6.
23. Bissada H, Tasca G, Barber A, et al. Olanzapine in the treatment of low body weight and obsessive thinking in women with anorexia nervosa: a randomized, double-blind, placebo-controlled trial. Am J Psychiatry 2008;165:1281–8.
24. Kafantaris V, Leigh F, Hertz S, et al. A placebo-controlled pilot study of adjunctive olanzapine for adolescents with anorexia nervosa. J Child Adolesc Psychopharmacol 2011;21:207–12.
25. Norris M, Spettigue W, Buchholz A, et al. Olanzapine use for the adjunctive treatment of adolescents with anorexia nervosa. J Child Adolesc Psychopharmacol 2011;21:213–20.
26. Powers PS, Klabunde M, Kaye W. Double blind placebo-controlled trial of quetiapine in anorexia nervosa: a negative study. Eur Eat Disord Rev 2012;20:331–4.
27. Hagman J, Gralla J, Sigel E, et al. A double-blind, placebo-controlled study of risperidone for the treatment of adolescents and young adults with anorexia nervosa: a pilot study. J Am Acad Child Adolesc Psychiatry 2011;50:854–6.
28. Trunko ME, Schwartz TA, Duvvuri V, et al. Aripiprazole in anorexia nervosa and low-weight bulimia nervosa: case reports. Int J Eat Disord 2011;44:269–75.
29. Powers PS, Simpson H, McCormick KT. Anorexia nervosa and psychosis. Prim Psychiatr 2005;45:39–45.
30. Frank GK, Bailer UF, Henry SE, et al. Increased dopamine D2/D3 receptor binding after recovery from anorexia nervosa measured by positron emission tomography and [11c]raclopride. Biol Psychiatry 2005;58:908–12.
31. Kaye WH, Frank GK, McConaha C. Altered dopamine activity after recovery from restricting-type anorexia nervosa. Neuropsychopharmacology 1999;21: 503–6.
32. Kishi T, Kafantaris V, Sunday S, et al. Are antipsychotics effective for the treatment of anorexia nervosa? Results from a systematic review and meta-analysis. J Clin Psychiatry 2012;73(6):e757–66.
33. Mehler P, Clary BS, Gaudiani JL. Osteoporosis in anorexia nervosa. Eat Disord 2011;19:194–202.
34. Mehler PS, MacKenzie TD. Treatment of osteopenia and osteoporosis in anorexia nervosa: a systematic review of the literature. Int J Eat Disord 2009; 42:195–201.
35. Misra M, Katzman D, Miller KK, et al. Physiological estrogen replacement increases bone density in adolescent girls with anorexia nervosa. J Bone Miner Res 2011;26:2430–8.

36. Institute of Medicine Report Brief. Dietary reference intakes for calcium and vitamin D. 2010. Available at: http://www.iom.edu/~/media/Files/Report%20Files/2010/Dietary-Reference-Intakes-for-Calcium-and-Vitamin-D/Vitamin%20D%20and%20Calcium%202010%20Report%20Brief.pdf. Accessed March 21, 2012.
37. Abrahamsen B. Bisphosphonate adverse effects, lessons from large databases. Curr Opin Rheumatol 2010;22:404–9.
38. Czerwinski E. Atypical subtrochanteric fractures after long-term bisphosphonate therapy. Endokrynol Pol 2011;62:84–7.
39. Silverman SL. Identifying patients at risk for osteoporotic fracture: FRAX and the new NOF guidelines. Menopause Management 2009;18:14–7.
40. Zipfel S, Sammet I, Rapps R, et al. Gastrointestinal disturbances in eating disorders: clinical and neurobiological aspects. Auton Neurosci 2006;129:99–106.
41. Mehler PS. Bulimia nervosa. N Engl J Med 2003;349:875–81.
42. Work group on eating disorders. Practice guideline for the treatment of eating disorders. 3rd edition. American Psychiatric Association; 2006. Available at: http://psychiatryonline.org/data/Books/prac/EatingDisorders3ePG_04-28-06.pdf. Accessed February 25, 2012.
43. Kaye WH. Neurobiology of anorexia and bulimia nervosa. Physiol Behav 2008; 94:121–35.
44. Fluoxetine Bulimia Nervosa Study Group. Fluoxetine in the treatment of bulimia nervosa: a multi-centered, placebo-controlled, double-blind trial. Arch Gen Psychiatry 1992;49:139–47.
45. Sysko R, Sha N, Wang Y, et al. Early response to antidepressant treatment in bulimia nervosa. Psychol Med 2010;40:999–1005.
46. Goldstein DH, Wilson MG, Ashcroft RC, et al. Effectiveness of fluoxetine therapy in bulimia nervosa regardless of comorbid depression. Int J Eat Disord 1999;25: 19–27.
47. Romano SH, Halmi KA, Sarkar NP, et al. A placebo-controlled study of fluoxetine in continued treatment of bulimia nervosa after successful acute fluoxetine treatment. Am J Psychiatry 2002;159:96–102.
48. Agras WS. Pharmacotherapy of bulimia nervosa and binge eating disorder: longer-term outcomes. Psychopharmacol Bull 1997;33:433–6.
49. Kotler LA, Devlin MJ, Davies M, et al. An open trial of fluoxetine for adolescents with bulimia nervosa. J Child Adolesc Psychopharmacol 2003;13:329–35.
50. Milano W, Siano C, Petrella C, et al. Treatment of bulimia nervosa with fluvoxamine: a randomized controlled trial. Adv Ther 2005;22:278–83.
51. Milano W, Petrella C, Sabatino C, et al. Treatment of bulimia nervosa with sertraline: a randomized controlled trial. Adv Ther 2004;21:232–7.
52. Schmidt U, Cooper PJ, Essers H, et al. Fluvoxamine and graded psychotherapy in the treatment of bulimia nervosa: a randomized, double-blind, placebo-controlled, multicenter study of short-term and long-term pharmacotherapy combined with a stepped care approach to psychotherapy. J Clin Psychopharmacol 2005;24:549–52.
53. Sundblad C, Landen M, Eriksson T, et al. Effects of the androgen antagonist flutamide and the serotonin reuptake inhibitor citalopram in bulimia nervosa: a placebo-controlled pilot study. J Clin Psychopharmacol 2005;25:85–8.
54. Gibbons RD, Brown H, Hur K, et al. Suicidal thoughts and behavior with antidepressant treatment: re-analysis of the randomized placebo-controlled trials with fluoxetine and venlafaxine. Arch Gen Psychiatry 2012;69:580–7. http://dx.doi.org/10.1001/archgenpsychiatry.2011.2048.

55. U.S. Food and Drug Administration (FDA). FDA launches a multi-pronged strategy to strengthen safeguards for children treated with antidepressant medications. 2004. Available at: http://www.fda.gov/NewsEvents/Newsroom/PressAnnouncements/2004/ucm108363.htm. Accessed February 25, 2012.

56. U.S.Food and Drug Administration. FDA proposes new warnings about suicidal thinking, behavior in young adults who take antidepressant medications. 2007. Available at: http://www.fda.gov/NewsEvents/Newsroom/PressAnnouncements/2007/ucm108905.htm. Accessed February 25, 2012.

57. U.S. Food and Drug Administration. Medication guide: about using antidepressant medications in children and teenagers. 2005. Available at: http://www.fda.gov/downloads/drugs/drugsafety/informationbydrugclass/UCM161646.pdf. Accessed February 26, 2012.

58. Stanley BG, Willett VL, Donias HW, et al. Lateral hypothalamic NMDA receptors and glutamate as physiological mediators of eating and weight control. Am J Physiol 1996;270(2 Pt 2):R443–9.

59. Hoopes SP, Reimherr FW, Hedges DW, et al. Treatment of bulimia nervosa with topiramate in a randomized, double-blind, placebo-controlled trial, part 1: improvement in binge and purge measures. J Clin Psychiatry 2003;64:1335–41.

60. Nickel C, Tritt K, Muehlbacher M, et al. Topiramate treatment in bulimia nervosa patients: a randomized, double-blind, placebo-controlled trial. Int J Eat Disord 2005;38:295–300.

61. Colom F, Vieta E, Benabarre A, et al. Topiramate abuse in a bipolar patient with an eating disorder. J Clin Psychiatry 2001;62:475–6.

62. Jonas JM, Gold MS. The use of opiate antagonists in treating bulimia: a study of low-dose versus high-dose naltrexone. Psychiatry Res 1988;24:195–9.

63. Marrazzi MA, Bacon JP, Kinzie J, et al. Naltrexone use in the treatment of anorexia nervosa and bulimia nervosa. Int Clin Psychopharmacol 1995;10: 163–72.

64. Mitchell JE, Christenson G, Jennings J, et al. A placebo-controlled, double-blind crossover study of naltrexone hydrochloride in outpatients with normal weight bulimia. J Clin Psychopharmacol 1989;9:94–7.

65. Faris FL, Kim SW, Meller WH, et al. Effect of decreasing afferent vagal activity with ondansetron on symptoms of bulimia nervosa: a randomised, double-blind trial. Lancet 2000;355:792–7.

66. Guardia D, Rolland B, Karila L, et al. GABAergic and glutamatergic modulation in binge eating: therapeutic approach. Curr Pharm Des 2011;17:1396–409.

67. Brennan BP, Roberts JL, Fogarty KV, et al. Memantine in the treatment of binge eating disorder: an open-label, prospective trial. Int J Eat Disord 2008;41:520–6.

68. Grant JE, Odlaug BL, Kim SW. N-acetylcysteine, a glutamate modulator, in the treatment of trichotillomania: a double-blind, placebo-controlled study. Arch Gen Psychiatry 2009;66:756–63.

69. Braun DL, Sunday SR, Fornari VM, et al. Bright light therapy decreases winter binge frequency in women with bulimia nervosa: a double-blind, placebo-controlled study. Compr Psychiatry 1999;40:442–8.

70. Blouin AG, Blouin JH, Iversen H, et al. Light therapy in bulimia nervosa: a double-blind, placebo-controlled study. Psychiatry Res 1996;60:1–9.

71. Lam RW, Goldner EM, Solyom L, et al. A controlled study of light therapy for bulimia nervosa. Am J Psychiatry 1994;151:744–50.

72. DSM-V Work Group on Eating Disorders. Binge eating disorder proposed revision. Available at: http://www.dsm5.org/ProposedRevisions/Pages/proposedrevision.aspx?rid=372#. Accessed March 3, 2012.

73. Fairburn CG, Cooper Z, Doll HA, et al. The natural course of bulimia nervosa and binge eating disorder in young women. Arch Gen Psychiatry 2000;57: 659–65.
74. Arnold LM, McElroy SL, Hudson JI, et al. A placebo-controlled, randomized trial of fluoxetine in the treatment of binge-eating disorder. J Clin Psychiatry 2002;63: 1028–33.
75. Grilo CM, Masheb RM, Wilson GT. Efficacy of cognitive behavioral therapy and fluoxetine for the treatment of binge eating disorder: a randomized double-blind placebo-controlled comparison. Biol Psychiatry 2005;57:301–9.
76. Hudson JI, McElroy SL, Raymond NC, et al. Fluvoxamine in the treatment of binge-eating disorder: a multicenter placebo-controlled, double-blind trial. Am J Psychiatry 1998;155:1756–62.
77. Pearlstein T, Spurell E, Hohlstein LA, et al. A double-blind, placebo-controlled trial of fluvoxamine in binge eating disorder: a high placebo response. Arch Womens Ment Health 2003;6:147–51.
78. Guerdjikova AI, McElroy SL, Kotwal R, et al. High-dose escitalopram in the treatment of binge-eating disorder with obesity: a placebo-controlled monotherapy trial. Hum Psychopharmacol 2008;23:1–11.
79. McElroy SL, Hudson JI, Malhotra S, et al. Citalopram in the treatment of binge-eating disorder: a placebo-controlled trial. J Clin Psychiatry 2003;64:807–13.
80. McElroy SL, Casuto LS, Nelson EB, et al. Placebo-controlled trial of sertraline in the treatment of binge eating disorder. Am J Psychiatry 2000;157:1004–6.
81. Guerdjikova AI, McElroy SL, Winstanley ER, et al. Duloxetine in the treatment of binge eating disorder with depressive disorders: a placebo-controlled trial. Int J Eat Disord 2012;45:281–9.
82. McElroy SL, Guerdjikova A, Kotwal R, et al. Atomoxetine in the treatment of binge-eating disorder: a randomized placebo-controlled trial. J Clin Psychiatry 2007;68:390–8.
83. Claudino AM, de Oliveira IR, Appolinario JC, et al. Double-blind, randomized, placebo-controlled trial of topiramate plus cognitive-behavior therapy in binge-eating disorder. J Clin Psychiatry 2007;68:1324–32.
84. McElroy SL, Hudson JI, Capece JA, et al. Topiramate for the treatment of binge eating disorder associated with obesity: a placebo-controlled study. Biol Psychiatry 2007;61:1039–48.
85. McElroy SL, Arnold LM, Shapira NA, et al. Topiramate in the treatment of binge eating disorder associated with obesity: a randomized, placebo controlled trial. Am J Psychiatry 2003;160:255–61.
86. McElroy SL, Kotwal R, Guerdjikova AI, et al. Zonisamide in the treatment of binge eating disorder with obesity: a randomized controlled trial. J Clin Psychiatry 2006;67:1897–906.
87. Guerdjikova AI, McElroy SL, Welge JA, et al. Lamotrigine in the treatment of binge-eating disorder with obesity: a randomized, placebo-controlled monotherapy trial. Int Clin Psychopharmacol 2009;24:150–8.
88. McElroy SL, Guerdjikova AI, Winstanley EL, et al. Acamprosate in the treatment of binge eating disorder: a placebo-controlled trial. Int J Eat Disord 2011;44: 81–90.
89. Mechanick JI, Kushner RF, Sugerman HJ, et al. American Association of Clinical Endocrinologists, The Obesity Society, and American Society for Metabolic & Bariatric Surgery medical guidelines for clinical practice for the perioperative nutritional, metabolic, and nonsurgical support of the bariatric surgery patient. Obesity (Silver Spring) 2009;17(Suppl 1):S1–70.

90. Alger-Mayer S, Rosati C, Polimeni JM, et al. Preoperative binge eating status and gastric bypass surgery: a long-term outcome study. Obes Surg 2009;19: 139–45.
91. Boan J, Kolotkin RL, Westman EC, et al. Binge eating, quality of life and physical activity improve after Roux-en-Y gastric bypass for morbid obesity. Obes Surg 2004;14:341–8.
92. Kalarchian MA, Wilson GT, Brolin RE, et al. Effects of bariatric surgery on binge eating and related psychopathology. Eat Weight Disord 1999;4:1–5.
93. Wadden TA, Faulconbridge LF, Jones-Corneille LR, et al. Binge eating disorder and the outcome of bariatric surgery at one year: a prospective, observational study. Obesity (Silver Spring) 2011;19:1220–8.
94. Kersh R, Stroup DF, Taylor WC. Childhood obesity: a framework for policy approaches and ethical considerations. Prev Chronic Dis 2011;8(5):A93. Available at: http://www.cdc.gov/pcd/issues/2011/sep/10_0273.htm. Accessed March 9, 2012.
95. Barlow SE. Expert committee recommendations regarding the prevention, assessment, and treatment of child and adolescent overweight and obesity: summary report. Pediatrics 2007;120:S164.
96. McGovern L, Johnson JN, Paulo R, et al. Treatment of pediatric obesity: a systematic review and meta-analysis of randomized trials. J Clin Endocrinol Metab 2008;93:4600–5.
97. Lenard NR, Berthoud H. Central and peripheral regulation of food intake and physical activity: pathways and genes. Obesity (Silver Spring) 2008;16(Suppl 3):S11–22.
98. Cotrome L. Miracle pills for weight loss: what is the number needed to treat, number needed to harm and likelihood to be helped or harmed for naltrexone-bupropion combination? Int J Clin Pract 2010;64:1461–71.
99. McDuffie JR, Calis KA, Booth SL, et al. Effects of orlistat on fat-soluble vitamins in obese adolescents. Pharmacotherapy 2002;22:814–22.
100. Hagler RA. Orlistat misuse as purging in a patient with binge-eating disorder. Psychosomatics 2009;50:177–8.
101. Malhotra S, McElroy SL. Orlistat misuse in bulimia nervosa. Am J Psychiatry 2002;159:492–3.
102. Fernández-Aranda F, Amor A, Jiménez-Murcia S, et al. Bulimia nervosa and misuse of orlistat: two case reports. Int J Eat Disord 2001;30:458–61.
103. Diabetes Prevention Program Research Group. Reduction in the incidence of type 2 diabetes with lifestyle intervention and metformin. N Engl J Med 2002; 346:393–403.
104. Kramer CK, Leitão CB, Pinto LC, et al. Efficacy and safety of topiramate on weight loss: a meta-analysis of randomized controlled trials. Obes Rev 2011; 12:e338–47.
105. Haddock CK, Poston WS, Dill PL, et al. Pharmacotherapy for obesity: a quantitative analysis of four decades of published randomized clinical trials. Int J Obes Relat Metab Disord 2002;26:262–73.
106. Andelman MB, Jones C, Nathan S. Treatment of obesity in underprivileged adolescents. Comparison of diethylpropion hydrochloride with placebo in a double-blind study. Clin Pediatr (Phila) 1967;6:327–30.
107. Li Z, Maglione M, Tu W, et al. Meta-analysis: pharmacologic treatment of obesity. Ann Intern Med 2005;142:532–46.
108. Singh-Franco D, Perez A, Harrington C. The effect of pramlintide acetate on glycemic control and weight in patients with type 2 diabetes mellitus and in obese

patients without diabetes: a systematic review and meta-analysis. Diabetes Obes Metab 2011;13:169–80.

109. Witkamp RF. Current and future drug targets in weight management. Pharm Res 2011;28:1792–818.

110. Powell AG, Apovian CM, Aronne LJ. New drug targets for the treatment of obesity. Clin Pharmacol Ther 2011;90:40–51.

111. Järvholm K, Olbers T, Marcus C, et al. Short-term psychological outcomes in severely obese adolescents after bariatric surgery. Obesity (Silver Spring) 2012;20:318–23.

112. Aikenhead A, Lobstein T, Knai C. Review of current guidelines on adolescent bariatric surgery. Clinical Obesity 2011;1:3–11.

113. Bondada S, Jen HC, DeUgarte DA. Outcomes of bariatric surgery in adolescents. Curr Opin Pediatr 2011;23:552–6.

114. Treadwell JR, Sun F, Schoelles K. Systematic review and meta-analysis of bariatric surgery for pediatric obesity. Ann Surg 2008;248:763–6.

115. Keys A, Brozek J, Henschel A, et al. The biology of human starvation, vols. 1–2. Minneapolis (MN): University of Minnesota Press; 1950.

116. Pirke KM, Pahl J, Schweiger U, et al. Metabolic and endocrine indices of starvation in bulimia: a comparison with anorexia nervosa. Psychiatry Res 1985;15: 33–9.

117. Woodside BD, Staab R. Management of psychiatric comorbidity in anorexia nervosa and bulimia nervosa. CNS Drugs 2006;20:655–63.

118. Ricca V, Mannucci E, Paionni A, et al. Venlafaxine versus fluoxetine in the treatment of atypical anorectic outpatients: a preliminary study. Eat Weight Disord 1999;4:10–4.

119. Altman SE, Shankman SA. What is the association between obsessive-compulsive disorder and eating disorders. Clin Psychol Rev 2009;29:638–46.

120. Caserio D, Frishman WH. Cardiovascular complications of eating disorders. Cardiol Rev 2006;14:227–31.

121. Maine M, Goldberg MH. The role of third molar surgery in the exacerbation of eating disorders. J Oral Maxillofac Surg 2001;59:1297–300.

122. Zerbe KJ. Recurrent pancreatitis presenting as fever of unknown origin in a recovering bulimic. Int J Eat Disord 1992;12:337–40.

123. Powers PS, Cloak N. Medication-related weight changes: impact on treatment of eating disorder patients. In: Yager J, Powers P, editors. Clinical manual of eating disorders. Washington, DC: American Psychiatric Publishing, Inc; 2007. p. 143–61.

124. Kluge M, Schuld A, Himmerich H, et al. Clozapine and olanzapine are associated with food craving and binge eating: results from a randomized double-blind study. J Clin Psychopharmacol 2007;27:662–6.

125. Weiden PJ, Mackell JA, McDonnell DD. Obesity as a risk factor for antipsychotic noncompliance. Schizophr Res 2004;66:51–7.

126. Takii M, Uchigata Y, Tokunaga S, et al. The duration of severe insulin omission is the factor most closely associated with the microvascular complications of type 1 diabetic females with clinical eating disorders. Int J Eat Disord 2008;41: 259–64.

127. Wilcox JA. Abuse of fluoxetine by a patient with anorexia nervosa [letter]. Am J Psychiatry 1987;144:1100.

128. Benini L, Todesco T, Dalle Grave R, et al. Gastric emptying in patients with restricting and binge/purging subtypes of anorexia nervosa. Am J Gastroenterol 2004;99:1448–54.

129. Hamad GG, Helsel JC, Perel JM, et al. The effect of gastric bypass on the phar-macokinetics of selective serotonin reuptake inhibitors. Am J Psychiatry 2012; 169:256–63.

130. Lock J, Le Grange D, Agras WS, et al. Randomized clinical trial comparing fam-ily based treatment with adolescent-focused individual therapy for adolescents with anorexia nervosa. Arch Gen Psychiatry 2010;67:1025–32.

131. Agras WS, Schneider JA, Arnow B, et al. Cognitive-behavioral and response-prevention treatments for bulimia nervosa. J Consult Clin Psychol 1989;57: 215–21.

132. Fairburn CG, Jones R, Peveler RC, et al. Psychotherapy and bulimia nervosa: longer-term effects of interpersonal therapy, behavior therapy, and cognitive behavior therapy. Arch Gen Psychiatry 1993;50:419–28.

133. Carter JC, Olmsted MO, Kaplan AS, et al. Self-help for bulimia nervosa: a ran-domized controlled trial. Am J Psychiatry 2003;160:973–6.

134. Grilo CM, Masheb RM, Wilson GT, et al. Cognitive-behavioral therapy, behav-ioral weight loss, and sequential treatment for obese patients with binge-eating disorder: a randomized controlled trial. J Consult Clin Psychol 2011;79: 675–85.

135. Carter JC, Fairburn CG. Cognitive-behavioral self-help for binge eating disor-der: a controlled effectiveness study. J Consult Clin Psychol 1998;66:616–23.

136. Rosenstock J, Klaff LJ, Schwartz S, et al. Effects of exenatide and lifestyle modi-fication on body weight and glucose tolerance in obese subjects with and without pre-diabetes. Diabetes Care 2010;33:1173–5.

137. Dushay J, Gao C, Gopalakrishnan GS, et al. Short-term exenatide treatment leads to significant weight loss in a subset of obese women without diabetes. Diabetes Care 2012;35:4–11.

138. Kely AS, Metzig AM, Ridser KD, et al. Exenatide as a weight loss therapy in extreme pediatric obesity: a randomized, controlled pilot study. Obesity (Silver Spring) 2012;20:364–70.

139. Astrup A, Rössner S, Van Gaal L, et al. Effects of liraglutide in the treatment of obesity: a randomised, double-blind, placebo-controlled study. Lancet 2009; 374(9701):1606–16.

140. Smith SR, Weissman NJ, Andersen CM, et al. Multicenter, placebo-controlled trial of lorcaserin for weight management. N Engl J Med 2010;363:245–56.

141. Fidler MC, Sanchez M, Raether B, et al. A one-year randomized trial of lorca-serin for weight loss in obese and overweight adults: the BLOSSOM trial. J Clin Endocrinol Metab 2011;96:3067–77.

142. O'Neil P, Smith SR, Weissman NJ, et al. Randomized placebo-controlled clinical trial of lorcaserin for weight loss in type 2 diabetes mellitus: the BLOOM-DM study. Obesity (Silver Spring) 2012;20(7):1426–36. http://dx.doi.org/10.1038/oby2012.66.

143. NeuroSearch A/S. NeuroSearch reports on scientific advice received from the FDA and EMA concerning the clinical development programme for tesofensine. 2011. Available at: http://www.cisionwire.com/neurosearch-a-s-g/r/neurosearch-reports-on-scientific-advice-received-from-the-fda-and-ema-concerning-the-clinical-development-programme-for-tesofensine,e236452. Accessed March 17, 2012.

144. Vivus, Inc. Qnexa meets primary endpoint by demonstrating superior weight loss over components and placebo in the 28-week Equate study (OB-301). 2008. Available at: http://ir.vivus.com/releasedetail.cfm?ReleaseID=353965. Accessed March 7, 2012.

145. Allison DB, Gadde KM, Garvey WT, et al. Controlled-release phentermine/topiramate in severely obese adults: a randomized controlled trial (EQUIP). Obesity (Silver Spring) 2012;20:330–42.

146. Gadde KM, Allison DB, Ryan DH, et al. Effects of low-dose, controlled-release, phentermine plus topiramate combination on weight and associated comorbidities in overweight and obese adults (CONQUER): a randomised, placebo-controlled, phase 3 trial. Lancet 2011;377:1341–52.

147. Greenway FL, Dunayevich E, Tollefson G, et al. Comparison of combined bupropion and naltrexone therapy for obesity with monotherapy and placebo. J Clin Endocrinol Metab 2009;94:4898–906.

148. Greenway FL, Fujioka K, Plotkowski RA, et al. Effects of naltrexone plus bupropion on weight loss in overweight and obese adults (COR-I): a multicentre, randomised, double-blind, placebo-controlled, phase 3 trial. Lancet 2010;376: 595–605.

149. Wadden TA, Foreyt JP, Foster GD, et al. Weight loss with naltrexone SR/bupropion SR combination therapy as an adjunct to behavior modification: the COR-BMOD trial. Obesity (Silver Spring) 2011;19:110–20.

150. Orexigen Therapeutics Inc. Orexigen Therapeutics Phase 2b trial for Empatic meets primary efficacy endpoint demonstrating significantly greater weight loss versus comparators in obese patients. 2009. Available at: http://ir.orexigen.com/phoenix.zhtml?c=207034&p=irol-newsArticle&ID=1336796&highlight=. Accessed March 19, 2012.

Pediatric Obesity

Mark J. Holterman, MD, PhD*, Ai-Xuan Le Holterman, MD,
Allen F. Browne, MD

KEYWORDS

- Pediatric • Obesity • Diabetes • Weight management • Adolescent

KEY POINTS

- Obesity is the most common chronic disease among children.
- The cause of the increase in the incidence of obesity in children is multifactorial.
- Obesity is the root cause for many comorbidities.
- Obese children become obese adults.
- Bariatric procedures are necessary, safe, and effective components of a comprehensive weight management program for adolescents.
- Guidelines for the best bariatric surgical procedure for adolescents and preteens depends on the age and degree of obesity.
- Multi-institutional cooperative studies are necessary to develop better evidence-based guidelines.

Obesity represents the most common chronic illness of children and adolescents.
—*Sandra Gibson Hassink[1]*

Until we know how to prevent it, treating obesity is our only choice.
—*Barbara Moore & Louis Martin[2]*

Obesity is a serious life-threatening disease that affects an increasing number of children in the developed world. Obese children suffer in many physical and psychosocial ways and their burden has important consequences to our society. Although obesity prevention is the ultimate goal, currently and into the foreseeable future, there will be a significant subset of our children suffering from significant life-altering weight

This article originally appeared in Surgical Clinics of North America, Volume 92, Issue 3, June 2012.

Disclosure: The authors are involved in 2 separate Food and Drug Administration safety and efficacy trials testing the use of the Laparoscopic Adjustable Band System. One of these trials is sponsored by Allergan, Inc, makers of this device.

Division of Pediatric Surgery, Children's Hospital of Illinois, Order of St. Francis Medical Center, University of Illinois College of Medicine-Peoria, 420 Northeast Glen Oak Avenue, Suite 201, Peoria, IL 61603, USA
* Corresponding author.
E-mail address: Mark.J.Holterman@osfhealthcare.org

comorbidities. Currently, nonsurgical weight loss strategies have met with limited success, but weight management clinics that offer a surgical treatment option have been effective at achieving sustained weight loss and resolution of weight-related comorbidities. A collaborative multidisciplinary approach to the management and care of obese children is essential for success. Choosing a weight loss surgical strategy for children and adolescents should be patient specific and based on their age, severity of comorbidities, and their body mass index (BMI). The authors have developed a treatment algorithm for the care of obese adolescents and a plan for the development of aggressive treatment options for obese preteen-aged children based on the limited existing literature and their experience treating adolescents and children at The New Hope Pediatric and Adolescent Weight Management Clinic between 2005 and 2011 at the University of Illinois College of Medicine.[3] As surgeons, we must continually test our treatments, evaluate our results, and improve the care we offer our patients.

THE DISEASE OF OBESITY

It is not surprising that modern society is faced with an obesity epidemic. Our energy intake and storage mechanisms are uniquely adapted to our previously primitive diets, which often included irregularly spaced, low-caloric density foods encased in slow-to-digest cellulose. This diet required the ability to quickly ingest a large quantity of food into the stomach and upper gastrointestinal (GI) tract. A long length of small intestine was necessary to allow for digestion and nutrient absorption. Only when the food reached the distal gastrointestinal tract and there was a risk of caloric wasting via dumping and diarrhea did the brain receive signals to stop consumption. The storage of surplus energy was crucial for survival during famine. Now in modern times, our primitive GI tracts and energy homeostasis mechanisms have not been able to adapt to the improved economic infrastructure that enables and encourages a sedentary lifestyle with little energy expended on food hunting and gathering; where large quantities of high-caloric-density and easy-to-digest food are readily available; and where enhanced public sanitation and infectious disease control decreases the burden of chronic health problems. The net result is the creeping epidemic of obesity.

Obesity Throughout History

Ancient figurines from 20,000 to 25,000 years ago depicted obvious obesity, and in more recent times, obesity was seen as a sign of affluence and success. In the past 200 years, obesity has become a negative physical attribute linked to an increasing number of medical and psychosocial problems. Common-sense approaches to the treatment of obesity were aimed at limiting food intake and increasing physical activity. Such measures clearly can work for the slightly overweight to minimally obese motivated individual who has the discipline to undergo significant lifestyle change. For most seriously overweight people, diet modification and exercise have minimal success and a high recidivism rate.[4,5]

In the second half of the twentieth century, the increasing prevalence of patients with life-altering obesity prompted the development of surgical procedures for the treatment of obesity. Initial bariatric procedures, such as the jejunoileal bypass, were designed with limited understanding of the underlying physiologic mechanisms controlling hunger, satiety, caloric absorption, malnutrition, and the bystander effects on the liver and the body as a whole.[6] In the past quarter century, weight loss surgery has become more refined with combinations of intestinal bypass to interfere with caloric absorption and a variety of restrictive procedures and devices to restrict caloric ingestion. Research has been slow to unravel the puzzle of obesity and has discovered an increasingly complex array of signals that control energy homeostasis.[7] Significant work remains to be done to understand how these mechanisms increasingly fail when interacting with the social, economic, and environmental changes of our modern society. The long-term goal is to prevent and treat obesity with nonsurgical means. This goal is currently well out of reach.

Definition

Obesity is defined as a long-term positive imbalance between energy intake and expenditure, with increased adipose tissue lipid storage and number of fat cells.[8] The Centers for Disease Control and Prevention[9] (CDC) recommend using the percentile BMI-for-age and gender (BMI-for-age) charts to screen children who are overweight or obese. Children with BMI at greater than the 85th percentile are considered overweight and those with BMI greater than the 95th percentile are considered obese.[10] Those with BMI greater than the 99th percentile are considered severely obese.

Incidence

In the past 30 years, the incidence of obesity in children has increased from less than 5% to approximately 20% in the United States.[10] Childhood obesity in most developing countries is a problem of urban children of a higher socioeconomic class. In the United States, the largest increase of obesity in children is seen in the urban poor.[11]

A closer analysis of these trends reveals that between 1976 to 1980 and 2007 to 2008, obesity increased from 5.0% to 10.4% in children aged 2 to 5 years, from 6.5% to 19.6% in children aged 6 to 11 years, and from 5% to 18% in adolescents aged 12 to 19 years.[10,12] Despite these numbers, pediatric research in surgical procedures, surgical devices, and drugs has been almost exclusively performed in adolescents and not in the preteen years. Preventive dietary counseling, activity recommendations, and behavioral support for younger children have been mostly unsuccessful but may be somewhat responsible for the recent leveling off in the rate of increase of obesity among our youngsters. At present, 15% to 20% of our children are still faced with the medical, social, and economic challenges of obesity.[12]

Cause

The metabolic constitution of patients who are morbidly obese seems to disrupt the normal balance of energy inflow and energy outflow in violation of the basic law of physics and thermodynamics. How can children from the same parents in the same household with similar consumption of calories vastly differ in body compositions? There are aspects of energy homeostasis underlying the body's energy balance set-point accounting for these differences, which we do not fully understand in morbidly obese children, and which may be difficult to modify after a certain stage of postnatal development. The most visible and obvious indicator of this aberrant set-point is increased body fat mass. Intensive research is ongoing to better understand how the metabolically active fat "organ" interacts with and dynamically responds to signals from its environment, the central and peripheral nervous system, and other key organ systems in the body.[13]

Calories: Supply and Demand

When combined with increased sedentary activities (accompanied by the opportunity and expectation of snacking outside mealtime), our high caloric-density diet is a major contributor to obesity. Historically, our caloric expenditure was part of the physical activities of daily living, such as food and water procurement, manual labor, or walking. In modern society, fewer engage in heavy manual labor. Physical activity has instead become something we voluntarily perform to maintain our health in our leisure time. In addition, rather than eating because of hunger and satiety, we eat out of habit and expectation. Our current diet frequently consists of meals, fluids, and snacks that have a high-caloric density and a high glycemic index (a measure of how rapidly glucose appears in the blood after carbohydrates are ingested).

The biologic controls of caloric intake are hunger and satiety. The physiology of these sensations involves hormones, neural transmitters, and their receptors.[13,14] One such signal is mediated by leptin, which is produced by fat tissue and suppresses hunger; its level is proportional to fat mass. Patients with the rare syndrome of congenital leptin deficiency suffer from severe obesity. With leptin replacement, they stop eating and lose fat mass and weight. Obese patients are not leptin deficient but are considered to be leptin insensitive because the administration of leptin does not reverse their obesity.[13]

Ghrelin, a hormone produced in the stomach and duodenum, stimulates hunger and enhances visceral fat deposition. Ghrelin is a potent stimulator of growth hormone production.[13] Surgical procedures that bypass a large portion of the stomach (Roux-en-Y gastric bypass [RYGB]) or that excise a large portion of the stomach (sleeve gastrectomy [SG]) are associated with reduced ghrelin levels. Research scientists have developed a vaccine targeting ghrelin that interferes with ghrelin signaling in the central nervous system and that reduces weight gain in rodents and pigs.[13]

PYY and GLP-1 hormones are produced in the ileum and the colon; they suppress hunger in response to intraluminal food. Obese people have significantly longer small intestines than nonobese people and this may delay the release of these important satiety signals.[13] Procedures that increase the speed of arrival of food in the ileum may suppress hunger.

External factors, such as obesogens (eg, Tributyltin and tetrabromobisphenol A), may affect our caloric use. Obesogens, or endocrine disruptors, are functionally defined as chemicals that inappropriately alter lipid homeostasis and fat storage, change metabolic set-points, disrupt energy balance, or modify the regulation of appetite and satiety to promote fat accumulation and obesity.[15] Their increased presence in our environment parallels the increase in obesity in our society. The effects of exposure to these chemicals in childhood and the development of obesity are currently being investigated.[16,17]

Another potential obesity modulator is GI tract flora.[18] The guts of obese mice and obese people harbor an array of microbes (microbiota) that are different from that of their lean counterparts.[19] The gut microbiota and its microbiome (gene content) change with obesity and during weight loss.[20] Although intriguing, these observations may simply be associative and require further study to establish the cause-or-effect relationship and its mechanisms.

Effects of Medications

Medications are a part of our modern environment. Many medications have effects on salt and water retention and on hunger. Others may have effects on calorie utilization. Medications, such as glucocorticoids, antidiabetic drugs, antidepressants, antiepileptics, and antihistamines, are known to be associated with weight gain.[21,22] Children with a tendency toward obesity may be susceptible to weight gain with the use of these drugs. The interaction of drugs and obesity is an important consideration for all pediatric providers caring for an obese child.

Genetics

Obesity can be thought of as maladaptation of a child's physiology to genetic or epigenetic factors in our modern environment. Although the children of obese parents are much more likely to be obese themselves and identical twins raised separately are more likely to be obese if their biologic parents were obese,[23] the mother and father from the same household with similar diet and opportunities for physical activity can also have both lean and obese children.

In fact, the causes of childhood obesity may be polygenic.[24] Specific genetic mutations are involved in the rare cases of Prader-Willi syndrome and leptin deficiency. Genome-wide association studies revealed that common variants in the first intron of a gene called *FTO* and variants near the melanocortin-4 receptor gene (*MC4R*) are strongly associated with obesity and seem to be involved in energy homeostasis signals in the central nervous system. These genetic findings have identified important pathways in energy homeostasis for certain obese children and may become useful genetic markers to identify at-risk children who might benefit from earlier or more aggressive interventions.[25,26]

Comorbidities: Physical and Psychosocial

Obesity is a significant health risk. As the incidence of childhood obesity grows, pediatric clinicians now detect in childhood and adolescence many of the same chronic illnesses and risk factors that are seen in adults. Comorbidities of pediatric obesity include insulin resistance and Type 2 diabetes,[27] polycystic ovary syndrome (PCOS),[28] hypertension,[29] hypercholesterolemia,[30] dyslipidemia and cardiovascular disease,[31,32] sleep apnea,[33] asthma,[34] nonalcoholic fatty liver disease and nonalcoholic steatohepatitis (NASH),[35] orthopedic disease conditions,[36,37] and pseudotumor cerebri.[38]

Obesity is causing a rapid increase in the incidence of Type II diabetes, which historically is a disease of obese, middle-aged patients. Now a significant number of new patients with Type II diabetes are children, some presenting in the preteen years.[27] In its early stages, Type II diabetes is a problem of insulin insensitivity that can be treated with weight loss. The prolonged demand on the pancreatic beta cells to produce supraphysiologic amounts of insulin eventually results in pancreatic insufficiency, at which point significant weight loss will not reverse the need for exogenous insulin.[39] The course and development of complications of Type II diabetes in children has a similar timeline to that seen in adults. It is logical to expect that diabetes-associated comorbidities (cardiac, renal, peripheral vascular, and ocular problems) will prematurely occur in these obese children as they grow into adulthood.[40,41]

Briefly, common obesity-related medical comorbidities in children[42] include the following:

(1) Sleep apnea has a negative effect on school and work performance and is associated with premature death in young adults who developed obesity as children. (2) NASH is the second most common reason for pediatric liver transplantation. (3) PCOS is a major source of social difficulties for obese teenage girls and is associated with anemia and infertility in obese young women, many of whom became obese as children. (4) Slipped capital femoral epiphysis and Blount disease are becoming more common in obese children and frequently result in multiple orthopedic interventions with the risks for permanent disabilities. (5) Metabolic syndrome is associated with obesity and defined in adults as a combination of 3 or more of the following: elevated blood pressure, elevated fasting glucose, increased waist circumference, low high-density lipoprotein cholesterol, and elevated triglycerides. In children, there

is little agreement on the parameters of metabolic syndrome mostly because of the wide range of normal values for these metabolic measurements in childhood and adolescence. These comorbidities are preventable and, to a large extent, treatable with weight loss.

Obesity also has a major impact on an individual's mental, psychosocial, and economic health.[43] Emotional comorbidities include low self-esteem, negative body image, and depression. These comorbidities can be directly related to a child's obesity as demonstrated when his or her quality-of-life evaluation improves after successful weight loss.[44] Social comorbidities include isolation, stigmatization, negative stereotyping, discrimination, teasing, and bullying.[45] Social science analysis clearly demonstrates the prejudice against obese children by their nonobese peers, teachers, and general society. In obese children, these social comorbidities often result in poor school performance and incorrect diagnosis of learning disabilities. Frequently, these children end up in home-schooling situations.[45] Economic comorbidities take the form of wage penalties, fewer promotions, and wrongful termination.[46] As the children become wage earners, their poor school performance, their lack of advanced training, the physical limitations of their size and weight, and their absenteeism caused by their obesity-related clinical comorbidities lead to a reduction in their wage-earning potential.[46]

OBESITY: A PROBLEM FOR PATIENTS, PARENTS, HEALTH CARE SYSTEMS, AND SOCIETY

All children want to be able to fit in with their peer group and to do the things the other children do. Quality-of-life questionnaires and personal interviews with obese adolescents consistently demonstrate a sense of desperation from their inability to keep up with their peers in all physical and social activities.[44] Obese adolescents often present to the weight management clinic with a sense of resignation and helplessness brought on by years of emotional scarring and failed attempts at weight loss.

The obese child's parents In turn experience significant blame and guilt for their child's obesity. These parents are often told by others, not the least by health care professionals, that they are the cause of their child's problem for having the wrong genes, for their parenting style, and for their personal ignorance, laziness, thoughtlessness, lack of love, or selfishness.[47]

Hospitals and the health care system have a responsibility to treat the disease of obesity in children. They need to be aware of obesity-specific issues of the obese child presenting with standard medical problems,[48] including the need for specialized furniture and equipment, such as sphygmomanometers and commodes; different transfer techniques; the variability in how their body composition and physiology change the pharmacodynamics of different drugs; and the direct correlation of obesity with the increased length of hospitalization and complication rates.[49] Furthermore, hospitals and health care personnel need specific training to overcome their bias and lack of knowledge about obesity and obese children. To address these issues, obesity should be a diagnostic item in patients' problem lists to identify them at the time of admission as a special patient population and alert the personnel and health care providers to their particular needs.

From the point of view of an economist, the long-term societal effect of childhood obesity is sobering. Health care costs associated with obesity-related illnesses for children and adults are estimated at $147 billion per year.[50] The costs of caring for obese children with typical pediatric diseases, such as asthma and appendicitis, are increased by their longer hospitalizations and their higher incidence of complications.[51] Obesity comorbidities are chronic, progressive, and pediatric obesity health care costs are likely to be carried over into adulthood. On an individual basis, some progress is seen on payers' reimbursement of obesity-related services, but for the most part, coverage of recommended treatments for pediatric obesity through Medicaid or private insurance is available in only a few states.[52,53] Furthermore, it has been well established that obese people have fewer educational opportunities and, therefore, fewer and lower-paying job opportunities.[46] Their economic productivity is also compromised because of the work time lost from the high rate of associated comorbidities and disabilities.[54] National security may be adversely affected because greater than 20% of young men and 40% of young women do not qualify for the United States armed forces because of their obesity.[55] The gloomy economic outlook for obese children growing into adulthood boils down to less economic productivity and more cost to society.

OBESITY TREATMENT
Why Treat Obesity?

Society demands that health care providers aggressively treat children suffering from an illness that has serious clinical life-threatening consequences. Therefore, it is puzzling why leaders in pediatric health care, government, and third-party payers have been loath to embrace aggressive treatment of morbid obesity in children. This reluctance denies the fact that the child suffers from serious clinical, psychological, and social comorbidities directly related to obesity and that the best treatment of any of these comorbidities is for the child to achieve a healthy weight. Reluctance to effectively treat childhood obesity ignores the serious economic burden of the comorbidities of obese children, which will be carried into adulthood. Although there might be opinions that children do not need treatment of obesity because they will grow out of it, the data clearly demonstrate that adult obesity usually starts in childhood and is correlated with the duration and degree of childhood obesity.[56,57] Aggressive management strategies for children are, therefore, needed.

For obesity and bariatric interventions, many treatment recommendations are currently restricted to adolescents (aged 14 through 18 years). The inclusion of bariatric procedures in weight management protocols for children should be *need* related not *age* related.[58] The surgical and device options must be carefully considered and developed to minimize risks and anatomic rearrangements and maximize control of the comorbidities associated with obesity. The risks need to be balanced against the larger benefits of weight reduction on comorbidities.

From a philosophic standpoint, the idea of exposing a child to a bariatric surgical procedure has traditionally met with significant opposition from pediatric primary care physicians and society at large. This philosophic resistance is inconsistent with our current management approaches for other pediatric diseases. Sick children receive treatment when they have a problem, regardless of their age. A problem is first recognized and the best treatment of their problem is devised. Treatment regimens are frequently multidisciplinary and involve risks (eg, radiotherapy and chemotherapy for cancer, immunotherapy for inflammatory bowel disease, surgical reconstruction for GI tract anomalies, and cardiac surgery for cardiac anomalies). These risks are accepted because the benefits of treatment outweigh the disease. Similarly, obesity shares many of the life-threatening aspects of cancer or coronary artery disease albeit on a longer time scale because obesity currently remains a chronic and incurable disease.[59] The same issues of obesity treatment pertaining to how to work with children in different developmental stages, how to facilitate treatment adherence, how to deal with families of different capabilities, and how to provide chronic, multidisciplinary care are questions pediatric health care providers have already addressed for many other diseases.

Prevention measures may one day lead to a significant decrease in obesity. A more complete understanding of the multiple factors involved in obesity and how they interact with each other will someday lead to effective and individualized nonsurgical treatment protocols or new pharmacologic agents that curb appetite, decrease calorie absorption, or increase metabolic rates without significant side effects. Additionally, endoscopic techniques will be developed that allow for the deployment of devices that interfere with absorption or appetite without significant surgical risk. In the meantime, without bariatric treatment, a generation of obese youngsters is at risk of prolonged morbidity and early death without some form of effective intervention.

Core Treatment Program for Weight Management

There are 3 essential core elements to any adult, adolescent, or pediatric weight management program: nutrition education, activity guidance, and behavioral modification/support. Ideally, the pediatric/adolescent multidisciplinary weight management team should include pediatric specialists in the following disciplines: medicine, surgery, nursing, nutrition, activity, and mental health. Pediatric subspecialists need to be available to manage obesity-related comorbidities.

Nutritional guidance and training is a basic tool of weight management. With an increasing number of families not eating at home and not preparing their own food, families come under the influence of advertising and convenience rather than healthy nutrition. Certainly larger portions, additives in foods to improve shelf life, and sweeteners in liquids are correlated with the increase in obesity statistics, but direct physiologic pathways remain to be worked out. Instruction in portion size, reading labels for additives, and noting calories in liquids is basic education to improve everyone's nutritional health.[60] The dietician considers economic and cultural issues when developing educational materials.

Activity prescription is designed to achieve basic cardiorespiratory fitness, matching activity to the physical capabilities of each person. Obese people cannot successfully participate in activities designed for lean people. They need unique equipment, unique intensity goals, and unique duration goals. In a sense, obese people are physically handicapped and can be best served by physical therapists. Raising awareness about the economic, cultural, geographic, and seasonal obesity-potentiating aspects of our modern society, such as where to park the car, who walks the dog, the safety of the neighborhood, the availability of indoor facilities in inclement weather, and how long to walk at the mall before shopping, can be part of the activity education.[61]

Ongoing psychological/behavioral support remains the third basic component of weight management in obese children. Using the same quality-of-life assessment tool, it has been shown that obese children's rating of their quality of life was lower than that of a group of children with cancer.[62] No child wants to be obese; almost all have failed previous attempts at achieving a healthy weight. Childhood obesity is associated with emotional and behavioral problems from as young as 3 years of age, with boys being especially at risk.[63] Although obese children and their families respond when using the tools of nutrition, activity, and behavioral support,[64] the 10% loss of excess body weight[65] and the high rate of recidivism are disappointing and speak to the need for further research and efforts into the treatment of obese children.

Adjunct Therapies to the Core Treatment Program

Pharmacologic treatment

There is no pharmacologic cure for obesity. In general, drug investigations have been conducted as a single treatment but should only be considered within the context of a long-term, multidisciplinary weight management program. Specific drugs used in obesity therapy are discussed in this section.

Orlistat (Xenical) is approved for use in obese children 12 years of age and older. Orlistat inhibits pancreatic lipase production to reduce fat absorption. Its long-term applicability for a chronic disease like obesity is limited by the major side effects of liquid, fatty stools, and abdominal pain. Orlistat may be useful during the initiation phase of a multidisciplinary weight management program or for intermittent use to help maintain weight loss/control.[5]

Other drugs are related to amphetamines and suppress appetite. Sibutramine (Meridia) was recently removed from the market because of the risk of myocardial infarction and stroke. Rimonabant is a cannabinoid CB1 receptor antagonist that failed to gain Food and Drug Administration (FDA) approval because of its psychiatric side effects.[5]

Hormone analogues, such as a GLP-1 analogue and an Amylin analogue, suppress appetite and are being studied as antiobesity drugs.[66] GLP-1 is produced in the ileum and colon in the presence of food, whereas Amylin is produced in the pancreas in response to the presence of food in the proximal small bowel. Lorcaserin (a serotonergic receptor agonist-appetite suppressant) and the combination drugs Qnexa (appetite suppressant/stimulant and anticonvulsive) and Contrave (antidepressant and antiaddiction) are currently being studied.[66]

Bariatric surgical procedures in adolescents

As previously mentioned, the nonsurgical options for weight loss in morbidly obese adolescents have limited effectiveness. Surgical interventions for obesity were initially developed for morbidly obese adults and later applied to adolescents.[67] In response to concerns for the unique aspects of adolescent children, several pediatric surgeons rose to the challenge of adolescent bariatric surgery by beginning in-depth studies of the various surgical options and developing adolescent weight management programs.[68–74] Overall, there is no one perfect bariatric procedure for all obese adolescents. The ability to test these procedures in cooperative multi-institutional prospective trials should allow this field to advance rapidly. Historically, weight loss procedures were developed to minimize caloric intake (restrictive procedures), control caloric digestion (malabsorptive procedures), or to combine both effects. **Table 1** offers a detailed comparison of the more commonly performed procedures, including the laparoscopic adjustable gastric band (LAGB), SG, and RYGB.

Surgical Approaches to Weight Loss in Adolescents

The ideal bariatric procedure would result in durable and substantial weight loss, with minimal risk from short-term procedural complications and long term malnutrition, growth limitation, liver problems, malignancy or mechanical complications. These issues are crucial in the process of choosing a suitable weight loss procedure for adolescents. However, significant disagreement on the best bariatric surgical procedure for adults, much less for children, remains. Each of the procedures has advantages and disadvantages (see **Table 1**). There is no randomized clinical trial comparing the effectiveness among bariatric procedures in adolescents. Definitive comparative studies are rare and sometimes yield contradictory results.[75,76] It is, however, encouraging that individual adolescent weight management programs are increasingly reporting on their own adolescent experience.[77–85] Overall, very good weight loss response and rapid improvements in all comorbidities, including enhanced physical and psychosocial quality of life along with low morbidity, have been reported.

Table 1
Bariatric surgery comparison chart

Modality of Weight Loss	Restrictive and Malabsorptive (Stomach and Intestines)	Restrictive (Stomach Only)	
Type of Operation	**RYGB**	**SG**	**Laparoscopic Adjustable Gastric Band**
Anatomy	Small 30 cc gastric pouch Pouch connected to the small intestine Food excluded from digestive juices for 100–150 cm	Long narrow gastric sleeve (100 cc) No intestinal bypass performed Majority stomach removed	An adjustable silicone band is placed around the top part of the stomach creating a small 30–60 cc pouch
Mechanism	Food volume is restricted Mild malabsorption Negative feedback in the form of dumping syndrome when sugar or fats are consumed Faster release of GLP-1 and PYY increases early satiety	Food volume is restricted NO malabsorption NO dumping Good physiologic sense of fullness from restriction in reduced stomach Increased GLP-1 and PYY Decreased ghrelin levels curb appetite	Food volume is restricted Adjustable tightness of band delay pouch emptying and prolong sense of fullness
Weight Loss United States average statistical loss at 10 y	Excess weight loss 60%–70% Lost within 12–18 mo Initially greater weight loss, which levels off	Excess weight loss 50%–60% Lost within 12–24 mo Initially greater weight loss, which levels off	Excess weight loss 50%–60% Lost over 36 mo Weight loss gradual over first year but similar to other procedures by 2–3 y postop Requires the most effort of all bariatric procedures to be successful
Long-term Dietary Modification (Excessive carbohydrate/high calorie intake will defeat all procedures)	3 small high-protein meals per d Must avoid sugar and fats to prevent dumping syndrome Vitamin deficiency/protein deficiency usually preventable with supplements	No dumping, no diarrhea Weight regain may be more likely than in other procedures if dietary modifications not adopted for life	Certain dense foods can get stuck if not chewed well (causing pain and vomiting) No liquids with meals

Nutritional Supplements Needed (Lifetime)	Multivitamin Vitamin B12 Calcium Iron (menstruating women)	Multivitamin Calcium	Multivitamin Calcium
Potential Problems	Dumping syndrome Stricture Ulcers Bowel obstruction Anemia Vitamin/mineral deficiencies (iron, vitamin B12, folate) Anastomotic leak Weight regain Technically challenging	Nausea and vomiting Heartburn Inadequate weight loss Weight regain Staple line leak Additional procedure may be needed to obtain adequate weight loss Technically easy	Slow weight loss Slippage Erosion Infection Port problems/device malfunction Additional procedure may be needed to obtain adequate weight loss Technically easy
Hospital Stay	2–3 d	1–2 d	Overnight (<1 d)
Time out of School	2–3 wk	1–2 wk	1 wk
Operating Time	2 h	1.5 h	1 h
Insurance coverage	Most payers will cover the RYGB even in adolescents	Third-party payers have been reluctant to cover the SG, especially in children because it is considered an experimental procedure	The adjustable gastric band is not FDA approved for use in patients aged 18 years or younger. Many payers will NOT authorize this procedure. Medicaid will pay in some states

FACTORS IN EVALUATING WEIGHT LOSS PROCEDURES IN ADOLESCENTS

As previously mentioned, the current literature does not provide easy answers to the ideal operation for morbidly obese adolescents. There are no available parallel comparisons of the RYGB and LAGB in teens; limited data are now available describing the use of the SG in adolescents. Current clinical guidelines for adolescent weight loss surgical procedures are primarily based on the pros and cons analyses of the various procedures for both adults and adolescents.[86–90] To address this lack of definitive data, the Longitudinal Assessment of Bariatric Surgery (LABS) consortium was established and supported by the National Institutes of Health (NIH) in 2003 to promote collaborations between surgeons working with obesity. The adolescent version of this consortium, Teen-LABS, was started in 2007 to collect available data with the hope to develop guidelines for the optimal adolescent weight loss management strategy.[71]

At this juncture, the authors' recommendations are based on their evaluation of the more extensive adult data combined with the limited adolescent series and their own experience. A brief review of the existing bariatric procedures in use in children follows to help frame the discussion and offer standardized treatment protocols.

The LAGB is an effective procedure for 60% to 80% of patients and is especially effective for patients with a BMI of 50 or less, with an expected loss of 50% to 60% of their excess weight over a 2- to 3-year period.[91] The LAGB procedure has a short learning curve. Most complications, with incidence as high as 15%, are related to mechanical issues, such as the band's position, pouch enlargement, or mechanical port and catheter problems. In the authors' experience, these problems were primarily experienced by patients with poor weight loss who aggregate into a higher BMI (>50) group. (Holterman and colleagues, *Journal of Pediatric Surgery*. Article submitted for publication.) The authors have elected to subsequently offer SG in most of these patients or have referred them for RYGB to adult bariatric surgeons.

In comparison, the RYGB is an effective procedure that provides excellent rapid weight loss in most adolescent patients but with a slightly higher mortality rate.[92] The positive weight loss response needs to be balanced against the more serious short- and long-term surgical complications, including micronutrient and vitamin deficiencies from the aggressive anatomic rearrangement. Short- and longer-term safety concerns associated with the RYGB may limit the referral of morbidly obese patients to centers that only offer this procedure.

The SG is a technically simple procedure that has become a stand-alone, first-line weight loss procedure for many adult surgeons. After SG, patients have minimal risk of micronutrient and vitamin deficiencies and complications are infrequent and manageable. In support of the encouraging midterm data from adult patients, the American Society for Metabolic and Bariatric Surgery (ASMBS) "has accepted the SG as an approved bariatric surgical procedure primarily because of it potential value as a first-stage operation for high risk patients, with the full realization that successful long-term weight reduction in an individual patient after SG would obviate the need for a second-stage procedure."[93] The SG has also been successfully performed as a salvage operation for adolescent patients who do not respond sufficiently to or have mechanical issues with the LAGB (Dr Robert Kanard, personal communication, 2011). Short-term data of the SG as an initial operation in adolescents are encouraging.[94] Concerns for the use of SG in adolescent patients center on decreased ghrelin production and on its adverse effects on growth hormone production and growth.[95] This concern may be less relevant because adolescents should respond to supplemental growth hormone injections and most adolescents treated for weight loss surgery have already achieved growth plate fusion.

The biliopancreatic diversion/duodenal switch (BPD/DS) is an effective weight loss procedure that is technically challenging with significant short-term risks and long-term nutritional concerns.[96] This procedure is best understood as a combination of a sleeve gastrectomy and a bypass procedure in which the food that enters the duodenal bulb from the tubularized stomach is diverted into a roux limb (the new duodenum). This limb of intestine carrying the ingested food mixes with digestive enzymes carried by the native duodenum and jejunum at a downstream enteroenterostomy and limits the available time for digestion and nutrient absorption. The profound anatomic rearrangements and risk of long-term nutrient absorption problems associated with BPD/DS is unsettling to most physicians caring for adolescents and, therefore, precludes its use as a first-line bariatric procedure in this age group. The role of the BPD/DS may be as a salvage procedure after insufficient weight loss with the RYGB or SG.

DEVICES AND NEW PROCEDURES

In addition to the previously described bariatric procedures, several new devices and one new procedure are under development. Currently, the adjustable gastric band is the only weight loss device in general use. Other devices under consideration have been designed to interfere with normal gastrointestinal physiology in a reversible and adjustable fashion and may be attractive alternatives but require extensive clinical testing before they will be available for use in children.

In this section, the authors first discuss the process of FDA approval for device use in the United States and give a brief overview of the new weight loss devices under development, including various intragastric balloons, the vagal stimulator, the gastric stimulator, and the duodenojejunal bypass device, new minimally invasive procedures, including gastric imbrications, and a procedure that combines the gastric sleeve, omentectomy, and a mid–small bowel resection.

THE FDA AND BARIATRIC DEVICES

Devices for the treatment of obesity in children may be an ideal alternative to weight loss surgery because they are seen as a less-invasive treatment, may have lower morbidity, and are adjustable, reversible, and removable. These factors may make weight loss devices more acceptable as part of a multidisciplinary weight management strategy in children. It is important to appreciate that the FDA has jurisdiction over the use of medical devices (but not surgical procedures) in the United States. Medical devices for use in obesity, therefore, require extensive testing in FDA-monitored trials. These FDA-approved trials have been performed almost exclusively in adult patients.

The FDA-approved clinical indication of a device or medication frequently excludes or ignores the product's use in children, citing the lack of data or inadequate theoretical grounds. Therefore, by necessity, many pediatric health care professionals frequently resort to the use of devices and drugs that will never undergo the required clinical testing to attain FDA-approved-use-in-children status, thus exposing themselves to a potentially vulnerable medicolegal position. Indeed, the pediatric providers have traditionally used clinical judgment in their decision making to use off-label medications and devices/equipment and frequently make necessary modifications. Unfortunately, many third-party payers will not reimburse for off-label usage of a device, and hospital risk management often prevents practitioners from the use of off-label items. Furthermore, device manufacturers frequently make a business-based decision to avoid the expense of clinical trials in children for a market that is small and more prone to liability. These factors deter the development of weight loss devices for preadults and limit the available treatment options to surgical procedures that are outside the jurisdiction of the FDA. It can be argued that this lack of attention to device development and evaluation is a form of discrimination against children.

Temporary Procedures

The intragastric balloon (IB) and the Endosleeve are intraluminal devices that can be considered to be temporary because they are removed or changed on a regular basis. These procedures would be attractive in children whose bodies would revert to a more normal physiology when they achieve a healthy body fat mass. These devices could help children attain a healthy percentage body fat at which time their use might be able to be discontinued.

Intragastric balloon

The IB is designed to be inflated in the stomach and causes a continual sensation of gastric fullness and satiety. Early versions of this concept were not tolerated well because they were not adjustable and caused significant discomfort and vomiting when inflated; they also slowly deflated over time and moved into the lower GI tract, sometimes causing obstruction. Newer versions are expected to address some of these problems.[97,98]

Current IBs under development include 2 nonadjustable free-floating balloons filled either with saline (BioEnterics intragastric balloon [BIB] [Allergan Corp, Irvine, CA, USA])[98] or with air (Heliosphere [Helioscopie SA, Vienne, France])[99] and 2 adjustable systems (Endogast [Districlass Médical SA, Saint-Etienne, France][100] and Spatz, Adjustable Balloon System [Spatz FGIA, Inc, Jericho, NY, USA][101]). The Endogast is fixed in position in the proximal stomach via a transgastric catheter system that connects to a subcutaneous port and is adjusted with air insertion or removal. The Spatz is a free-floating system with a tube attached that is retrieved endoscopically for adjustments with saline. This adjustability may allow patients to adapt without vomiting and to better tolerate the presence of the device. Adjustability will also allow the balloon size to be titrated to the size of the patient and to the desired effect. The intragastric balloon systems have been used in adults and a small number of children outside the United States. Based on reports from this limited clinical experience, these devices seem to be safe and effective for temporary use.[102,103]

Endosleeve

The EndoBarrier Gastrointestinal Liner (GI Dyamics, Lexington, MA, USA) involves a sleeve of impermeable material placed inside the intestine from the proximal duodenum distally into the jejunum. Current versions extend distally for about 60 cm. The sleeve is placed and removed endoscopically. The gastrointestinal liner creates a mechanical bypass situation (as opposed to surgical) by having the food go through the inner lumen of the sleeve where it is excluded from the digestive juices outside the sleeve.[104] This separation interferes with absorption and the usual neuro-hormonal cascade of the bypassed intestine (CCK and Amylin) is not stimulated by contact with chyme. The mixing of food and digestive enzymes at a point further down the GI tract limits time for calorie absorption and prematurely initiates the satiety-inducing neuro-hormonal feedback loop when PYY and GLP-1 are released from the distal ileum. The length of sleeve necessary for an effective device has been determined in adults but a pediatric version would need to vary in diameter and length based on age. Current design and early studies on adults anticipate that the individual GI liners will have a lifespan of about 6 months, at which time they require endoscopic retrieval and possible deployment of a new EndoBarrier. A FDA-monitored trial of the Endobarrier is ongoing in adults in the United States, South America, and Europe. It is currently not FDA approved for use in the United States.

Semipermanent Procedures

The vagal-blocking devices, the gastric-stimulating devices, and the endoscopic gastroplasty techniques are designed for long-term usage without permanent anatomic change and can be removed or reversed.

Vagal-blocking devices

The vagal-blocking devices are based on the observation of the lack of appetite and weight loss frequently seen in post-vagotomy patients. Subsequent analysis has identified the existence of vagal afferent pathways to the central nervous system that control appetite. This knowledge prompted the development of electronic vagal-blocking devices that place leads around the vagus nerves in the abdomen or in the thorax with minimally invasive techniques. These leads are then connected to a subcutaneous power source/control device similar to a cardiac pacemaker or a phrenic-nerve-stimulating diaphragmatic pacing device. Of note, stimulation of the cervical portion of the vagus nerve has been used for years to control seizure activity. These devices seem to be well tolerated in the long term. The frequency, amplitude, and wave form of the stimulation can then be customized to gain maximal effect on satiety in a given individual. The current subcutaneous boxes are bulky but will decrease in size and become easier for children to tolerate. Early studies of the Maestro System (Entero-Medics Inc, St Paul, MN, USA) in adults show modest weight loss.[105] Trials are now underway in the United States.

Gastric stimulators

The use of gastric stimulation to induce weight loss is based on several possible mechanisms. The stimulation may interfere with ghrelin production or simulate the sensation of a full stomach, sending afferent messages via the vagus nerve. Trials in adults to date have been disappointing but an effect was realized in some patients.[106] Patient selection or a comprehensive weight management approach may improve its effectiveness in children. One gastric stimulation system (Tantalus, MedaCure, Orangeburg, NY, USA), has been used in Europe and is undergoing FDA trial in the United States in patients aged more than 17 years.[107]

New Procedures

Gastric imbrication

Gastric imbrication involves plicating the greater curve, fundus, and body of the stomach to leave a tube along the lesser curvature from the gastroesophageal junction to the pylorus. It mimics the SG without excision of the stomach. The mechanism is presumed to be restrictive with reduction of ghrelin production. In this procedure, gastric ghrelin production is not stimulated because the food stream is excluded from the stomach. The procedure can be performed open, laparoscopically, or endoluminally. The endoluminal approach is restricted by the size of the endoscopes necessary to do the suturing. This factor may be limiting in children. Whether the lack of stimulation on ghrelin changes the effect on growth hormone in children remains to be determined. The safety of this procedure probably lies somewhere between the devices and the other surgical procedures, and its effectiveness and durability need to be studied. Similarly to the SG, the gastric imbrication procedure should have minimal effect on micronutrient absorption.[108,109]

Combined gastric sleeve resection and mid–small bowel resection
This procedure combines a gastric sleeve resection and omentectomy with a mid–small bowel resection. The mechanism of effect for this approach is fivefold: (1) mechanical restriction; (2) reduced stimulation of appetite (lower ghrelin levels); (3) increased suppression of appetite (higher GLP-1 and PYY levels); (4) diminished surface area for caloric absorption; and (5) the inflammatory cytokines released from the omental fat are removed helping to spare the liver.[110] Theoretically, malabsorption is avoided by leaving the proximal small bowel intact and in line with the remaining GI tract to maintain fat-soluble vitamin absorption and the enterohepatic circulation of bile salts in the terminal ileum. Small series of this procedure in adults and adolescents have been reported with encouraging results but a longer follow-up will be required.[110,111] It is also not clear as to the optimal resection amount of the mid–small intestine. The sequential addition of a mid–small bowel resection to patients who do not lose adequate weight after an SG or RYGB may be a logical and safer next step rather than the BPD/DS.

SUGGESTED CLINICAL MANAGEMENT PROTOCOL FOR WEIGHT LOSS IN ADOLESCENTS AND CHILDREN

It is becoming increasingly clear to the medical community, and society at large, that better treatment strategies need to be developed for the care of morbidly obese children. Nonoperative treatments have mostly failed or have met with minimal and temporary success. Primary care physicians are frustrated with the current ineffectiveness of nonmedical weight loss for morbid obesity but remain unwilling to condone aggressive bariatric surgical procedures. In the absence of clear-cut class I evidence for the relative effectiveness of the various bariatric surgical protocols, it is challenging to set exact guidelines for the management of morbid obesity in adolescents and children. The pediatric committee for the ASMBS published their recommended guidelines in 2012, which built on earlier NIH consensus guidelines.[86] According to these guidelines, children aged 13 to 18 years with a BMI of greater than or equal to 40 or greater than or equal to 35 with significant comorbidities qualify for surgery. In addition, the children must have failed 6 months of monitored weight loss attempts and be competent to assent to their procedure. In light of the complex causes and variable extent of morbid obesity, a rational approach customizes protocols to patients' individual needs by taking into account their age, BMI, type and severity of comorbidities, and psychosocial factors. These treatment protocols would provide the structure for clinical trials to evaluate and refine treatment strategies. The authors recommend multi-institutional cooperative treatment protocols with critical long-term safety and efficacy analysis, in the same manner the Children's Oncology Group has approached childhood cancer.

It seems most prudent to offer a common-sense practical and step-wise intensification of the management options. Resolution of the medical and psychosocial comorbidities must be the primary and overarching goal, secondary to the achievement of normal or near-normal weight. Choosing a bariatric procedure based on the morbidity (frequency and severity) and the risk of mortality prioritizes these goals.

ADOLESCENTS: SUGGESTED CLINICAL MANAGEMENT PROTOCOL FOR WEIGHT LOSS

Group I: Patients aged 13 to 19 years with BMI less than or equal to 50 (**Fig. 1**)
    Because of their simplicity and low morbidity, the LAGB or SG can be a good first choice for these patients. Morbidly obese adolescents with a lower BMI respond well to the gentle progressive pattern of LAGB weight loss.

Surgical Approach to the Obese Teenagers

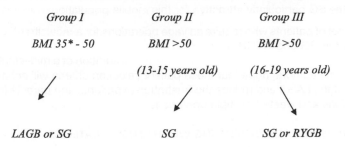

Group I	Group II	Group III
BMI 35* - 50	BMI >50	BMI >50
	(13-15 years old)	(16-19 years old)
LAGB or SG	SG	SG or RYGB

Insufficient responders to the LAGB can undergo SG or RYGB

Insufficient responders to SG can undergo RYGB, BPD/DS, or mid-small bowel resection

*= BMI 35-39 with obesity related comorbidities

BMI >35 represents a BMI that is >97 percentile for age and gender (CDC Website)

LAGB = Laparoscopic Adjustable Gastric Band

SG = Sleeve Gastrectomy

RYGB = Roux-en-Y Gastric Bypass

BPD/DS = Biliopancreatic Diversion with Duodenal Switch

Insufficient responder = insufficient weight loss or resolution of comorbidities

with LAGB or SG and/or persistent mechanical problems with the LAGB

Fig. 1. Surgical decision protocol for bariatric surgery in adolescents.

Group II: Patients aged 13 to 15 years with BMI greater than 50
From the authors' experience, adolescents with BMI greater than 50 experienced difficulties with LAGB. They lose the same net weight as their lower-BMI adolescent counterparts (Holterman A, and colleagues, *Journal of Pediatric Surgery,* article submitted for publication.), but the large amount of excess weight that remains and the slower pace of the LAGB leads to frustration and unmet expectations. Further tightening of the band to help accelerate weight loss often results in pouch enlargement, necessitating subsequent loosening of the band at the risk of regaining weight. The authors, therefore, recommend a more aggressive initial procedure, such as the SG, which would provide additional appetite suppression without the risk of micronutrient deficiencies along with an earlier and faster weight loss response.

Group III: Patients aged 16 to 19 years with BMI greater than 50
In addition to the same factors that limit the effectiveness of LAGB in group II, the age-related maturational independence of this group often leads to less-than-ideal adherence to treatment. In addition, insurance coverage changes for these adolescents can create a financial barrier to their ongoing care. The authors, therefore, recommend a more aggressive initial procedure, such as the SG or RYGB, which would provide an earlier and faster weight loss response.

The shallow learning curve for laparoscopic SG compared with the more technically challenging RYGB and its lower risk of micronutrient deficiencies may make the SG particularly attractive for this mobile population.

For the subset of patients who require salvage operations for a recalcitrant response to the LAGB, the SG and RYGB may be appropriate. A failed SG is probably best salvaged by an RYGB or BPD/DS procedure or with the addition of a mid–small bowel resection. It is the authors' hope that these patient selection criteria will enhance the success rate of the LAGB and reduce the frustration of patients and parents from unmet expectations and wasted multiple operations.

CHILDREN: GUIDELINES FOR DEVELOPING WEIGHT LOSS STRATEGIES

Although obesity can start in infancy and its comorbidities can occur in the very young, treatment outside behavior modification, activity programs, and diet training for obese children younger than 13 years is nearly nonexistent. One needs to be cognizant of many age-specific physiologic and psychological issues in the treatment of these obese children. For instance, obese children younger than 13 years old frequently have not completed their linear growth. Their BMI can improve when their weight gain is arrested while their linear growth remains. It is not clear whether this process reduces the body fat mass and resolves obesity related comorbidities. As obese children advance through the developmental stages of infancy, toddler, school age, preteen, and early teenage years (before reaching 13 years of age), the dynamics of food consumption, food choices, and activity decisions are much different from that of the adolescent. Their behavior may be more malleable and parents or health care providers may have a better chance at influencing their compliance. Any treatment program should have a multidisciplinary approach that recognizes the previously described basic tools of weight management, especially when surgical procedures and pharmacologic use are part of the therapy. Large study groups with shared protocols and databases are strongly recommended.

Of note, it has been the authors' experience that under physician and parents' guidance, younger adolescents are more accepting of the LAGB lifestyle modifications. Because of the excellent safety profile, reversibility, and adjustability of the LAGB, which allow controlled caloric ingestion and nutrition without malabsorption, the use of LAGB may be appropriate to the treatment of younger patients in their prepubertal and early puberty years (10–13 years of age with advanced obesity with or without comorbidities). Control of food ingestion in this group may allow them to undergo the longitudinal growth that leads to a normalization of their BMI without malnutrition. The adjustable gastric band can then be emptied, and if weight remains within an acceptable range, it could be easily removed.

The FDA can play a larger role in the development of drugs and devices for obesity treatment in children by supporting parallel studies in children, adolescents, and adults, taking into account their physical, physiologic, and psychological differences, and their differential responses. The traditional approach to wait for the completion of adult trials before proceeding with studies in children neglects the fact that 20% to 30% of children aged less than 13 years affected by obesity are still waiting for treatment. A new paradigm of cooperation is needed between industry, the FDA, the CDC, the NIH, and professional health care associations (American Academy of Pediatrics, National Association of Children's Hospitals and Related Institutions, American Academy of Family Physicians, American Pediatric Surgical Association, American Society for Metabolic and Bariatric Surgery, and so forth) to assist pediatric health care providers with tools and techniques to care for obese children. Rather than placing blame on parents for the lack of effective therapy and taking these children away from their families, the health care system needs to come to terms with the challenge of developing effective pediatric obesity treatment schemes.

SUMMARY

Childhood obesity is a tremendous burden for children, their families, and society. Obesity prevention remains the ultimate goal, but rapid development and deployment of effective nonsurgical treatment options is not currently achievable given the complexity of this disease. In the meantime, hundreds of thousands of our world's youth are facing discrimination, a poor quality of life, and a shortened lifespan from the burdens of this illness. Surgical options for adolescent obesity have been proven to be safe and effective and should be offered. The development of stratified protocols of increasing intensity (ie, surgical aggressiveness) should be individualized for each patient based on their disease severity and risk factors. These protocols should be offered in the context of multidisciplinary, cooperative clinical trials to critically evaluate and develop optimal treatment strategies for morbid obesity. Long-term cooperation between families, schools, communities, government, health care professionals, media, insurers, and industry is essential in addressing the prevention and treatment of childhood obesity.

REFERENCES

1. Hassink SG. A clinical guide to pediatric weight management and obesity. Philadelphia: Lippencott; 2007. p. vii.
2. Moore BJ, Martin LF. Why should obesity be treated?. In: Martin LF, editor. Obesity surgery. New York: McGraw-Hill; 2004. p. 1–15.
3. Browne AF, Browne NT. Lap-Band® in adolescents. In: Rosenthal RJ, Jones DB, editors. Weight loss surgery: a multidisciplinary approach. Edgemont (PA): Matrix Medical Communications; 2008. p. 477–88.
4. Franz MH, VanWormer JJ, Crain AL, et al. Weight-loss outcomes: a systematic review and meta-analysis of weight-loss clinical trials with a minimum 1-year follow-up. J Am Diet Assoc 2007;107:1755–67.
5. Freemark M. Pharmacotherapy of childhood obesity and pre-diabetes. In: Freemark M, editor. Pediatric obesity. New York: Springer; 2010. p. 339–56.
6. Martin LF. The evolution of surgery for morbid obesity. In: Martin LF, editor. Obesity surgery. New York: McGraw-Hill; 2004. p. 15–48.
7. Ikramudden S, Leslie D, Whitson B, et al. Energy metabolism & biochemistry of obesity. In: Rosenthal RJ, Jones DB, editors. Weight loss surgery: a multidisciplinary approach. Edgemont (PA): Matrix Medical Communications; 2008. p. 17–26.
8. Lakka HM, Bouchard C. Etiology of obesity. In: Buchwald H, Cowan G, Pories W, editors. Surgical management of obesity. Philadelphia: Saunders; 2007. p. 18–28.
9. Clinical growth charts. Centers for Disease Control and Prevention, National Center for Health Statistics; 2009. Available at: www.cdc.gov/growthcharts/clinical_charts.htm. Accessed April 10, 2012.
10. Ogden CL, Carroll MD, Curtin LR, et al. Prevalence of high body mass index in US children and adolescents, 2007–2008. JAMA 2010;303(3):242–9.
11. Popkin B. Global dynamics in childhood obesity: reflections on a life of work in the field. In: Freemark M, editor. Pediatric obesity. New York: Springer; 2010. p. 3–12.

12. National Center for Health Statistics. Health, United States, 2010: with special features on death and dying. Hyattsville (MD): U.S. Department of Health and Human Services; 2011.
13. Lustig RH. The neuroendocrine control of energy balance. In: Freemark M, editor. Pediatric obesity. New York: Springer; 2010. p. 15–32.
14. Vincent RP, Le Roux CW. Changes in gut hormones after bariatric surgery. Clin Endocrinol 2008;69(2):173–9.
15. Grün F, Blumberg B. Endocrine disrupters as obesogens. Mol Cell Endocrinol 2009;304(1–2):19–29.
16. Decherf S, Demeneix BA. The obesogen hypothesis: a shift of focus from the periphery to the hypothalamus. J Toxicol Environ Health B Crit Rev 2011; 14(5–7):423–48.
17. Grün F. Obesogens. Curr Opin Endocrinol Diabetes Obes 2010;17(5):453–9.
18. Tsai F, Coyle WJ. The microbiome and obesity: is obesity linked to our gut flora? Curr Gastroenterol Rep 2009;11(4):307–13.
19. DiBaise JK, Zhang H, Crowell MD, et al. Gut microbiota and its possible relationship with obesity. Mayo Clin Proc 2008;83(4):460–9.
20. Ley RE. Obesity and the human microbiome. Curr Opin Gastroenterol 2010; 26(1):5–11.
21. Malone M. Medications associated with weight gain. Ann Pharmacother 2005; 39(12):2046–55.
22. Leslie WS, Hankey CR, Lean ME. Weight gain as an adverse effect of some commonly prescribed drugs: a systematic review. QJM 2007;100(7):395–404.
23. Stunkard AJ, Harris JR, Pedersen NL, et al. The body-mass index of twins who have been reared apart. N Engl J Med 1990;322(21):1483–7.
24. Hinney A, Hebebrand J. Polygenic obesity. In: Freemark M, editor. Pediatric obesity. New York: Springer; 2010. p. 75–90.
25. Dina C, Meyre D, Gallina S, et al. Variation in FTO contributes to childhood obesity and severe adult obesity. Nat Genet 2007;39:724–6.
26. Loos R, Lindgren C, Li S, et al. Common variants near MC4R are associated with fat mass, weight and risk of obesity. Nat Genet 2008;40(6):1–8.
27. Weiss R, Cali A, Caprio S. Pathogenesis of insulin resistance and glucose intolerance in childhood obesity. In: Freemark M, editor. Pediatric obesity. New York: Springer; 2010. p. 163–74.
28. Glueck CJ, Morrison JA, Umar M, et al. The long-term metabolic complications of childhood obesity. In: Freemark M, editor. Pediatric obesity. New York: Springer; 2010. p. 253–64.
29. Hunley RE, Kon V. Pathogenesis of hypertension and renal disease in obesity. In: Freemark M, editor. Pediatric obesity. New York: Springer; 2010. p. 223–40.
30. McGill HC Jr, McMahan CA, Gidding SS. Childhood obesity, atherogenesis, and adult cardiovascular disease. In: Freemark M, editor. Pediatric obesity. New York: Springer; 2010. p. 265–78.
31. McCrindle BW. Pathogenesis and management of dyslipidemia in obese children. In: Freemark M, editor. Pediatric obesity. New York: Springer; 2010. p. 175–200.
32. Shah AS, Khoury PR, Dolan LM, et al. The effects of obesity and type 2 diabetes mellitus on cardiac structure and function in adolescents and young adults. Diabetologia 2011;54(4):722–30.
33. Erler T, Paditz E. Obstructive sleep apnea syndrome in children: a state-of-the-art review. Treat Respir Med 2004;3(2):107–22.
34. Verhulst S. Sleep-disordered breathing and sleep duration in childhood obesity. In: Freemark M, editor. Pediatric obesity. New York: Springer; 2010. p. 241–52.

35. Lindback SM, Gabbert C, Johnson BL, et al. Pediatric nonalcoholic fatty liver disease: a comprehensive review. Adv Pediatr 2010;57(1):85–140.
36. Montgomery CO, Young KL, Austen M, et al. Increased risk of Blount disease in obese children and adolescents with vitamin D deficiency. J Pediatr Orthop 2010;30(8):879–82.
37. Peck D. Slipped capital femoral epiphysis: diagnosis and management. Am Fam Physician 2010;82(3):258–62.
38. Wall M. Idiopathic intracranial hypertension (pseudotumor cerebri). Curr Neurol Neurosci Rep 2008;8(2):87–93.
39. Elder DA, Woo JG, D'Alessio DA. Impaired beta-cell sensitivity to glucose and maximal insulin secretory capacity in adolescents with type 2 diabetes. Pediatr Diabetes 2010;11(5):314–21.
40. Pinhas-Hamiel O, Zeitler P. Acute and chronic complications of type 2 diabetes mellitus in children and adolescents. Lancet 2007;369(9575):1823–31.
41. Shiga K, Kikuchi N. Children with type 2 diabetes mellitus are at greater risk of macrovascular complications. Pediatr Int 2009;51(4):563–7.
42. Daniels SR. Complications of obesity in children and adolescents. Int J Obes (Lond) 2009;33(Suppl 1):S60–5.
43. Washington RL. Childhood obesity: issues of weight bias. Prev Chronic Dis 2011;8(5):A94.
44. Holterman AX, Browne A, Dillard BE 3rd, et al. Short-term outcome in the first 10 morbidly obese adolescent patients in the FDA-approved trial for laparoscopic adjustable gastric banding. J Pediatr Gastroenterol Nutr 2007;45(4):465–73.
45. Puhl RM, Latner JD. Stigma, obesity, and the health of the nation's children. Psychol Bull 2007;133(4):557–80.
46. Puhl RM, Heuer CA. The stigma of obesity: a review and update. Obesity 2009; 17:941–64.
47. Edmunds LD. Parents; perceptions of health professionals' responses when seeking help for their overweight children. Fam Pract 2005;22(3):287–92.
48. Young KL, Demeule M, Stuhlsatz K, et al. Identification and treatment of obesity as a standard of care for all patients in children's hospitals. Pediatrics 2011; 128(Suppl 2):S47–50.
49. Ghobadi C, Johnson TN, Aarabi M, et al. Application of a systems approach to the bottom-up assessment of pharmacokinetics in obese patients: expected variations in clearance. Clin Pharmacokinet 2011;50(12):809–22.
50. Finkelstein EA, Trogdon JG, Cohen JW, et al. Annual medical spending attributable to obesity: payer-and service-specific estimates. Health Aff 2009;28(5): w822–31.
51. Woolford SJ, Gebremariam A, Clark SJ, et al. Incremental hospital charges associated with obesity as a secondary diagnosis in children. Obesity 2007; 15(7):1895–901.
52. Simpson LA, Cooper J. Paying for obesity: a changing landscape. Pediatrics 2009;123(Suppl 5):S301–7.
53. Lee JS, Sheer JL, Lopez N, et al. Coverage of obesity treatment: a state-by-state analysis of Medicaid and state insurance laws. Public Health Rep 2010;125(4): 596–604.
54. Finkelstein EA, DiBonaventura M, Burgess SM, et al. The costs of obesity in the workplace. J Occup Environ Med 2010;52(10):971–6.
55. Cawley J, Maclean JC. Unfit for service: the implications of rising obesity for US military recruitment. Health Econ 2011. DOI: 10.1002/hec.1794. [Epub ahead of print].

56. Lee JM, Lim S, Zoellner, et al. Don't children grow out of their obesity? Weight transitions in early childhood. Clin Pediatr (Phila) 2010;49(5):466–9.
57. Whitaker RC, Wright JA, Pepe MS, et al. Predicting obesity in young adulthood from childhood and parental obesity. N Engl J Med 1997;337:869–73.
58. Browne AF, Inge T. How young for bariatric surgery in children? Semin Pediatr Surg 2009;18(3):176–85.
59. Bray FA, Ryan DH. Medical approaches to the treatment of the obese patient. In: Mantzoros CS, editor. Obesity and diabetes. Totowa (MJ): Humana Press; 2006. p. 457–69.
60. American Dietetic Association (ADA). Position of the American Dietetic Association: individual-, family-, school-, and community-based interventions for pediatric overweight. J Am Diet Assoc 2006;106(6):925–45.
61. Bennett B, Sothern MS. Diet, exercise, behavior: the promise and limits of lifestyle change. Semin Pediatr Surg 2009;18(3):152–8.
62. Schwimmer JB, Burwinkle TM, Varni JW. Health-related quality of life of severely obese children and adolescents. JAMA 2003;289(14):1813–9.
63. Griffiths LJ, Dezateux C, Hill A. Is obesity associated with emotional and behavioural problems in children? Findings from the Millennium Cohort Study. Int J Pediatr Obes 2011;6(2–2):e423–32.
64. Epstein LF, Paluch RA, Roemmich JN, et al. Family-based obesity treatment, then and now: twenty-five years of pediatric obesity treatment. Health Psychol 2007;26(4):381–91.
65. Whitlock E, Williams S, Gold R, et al. Screening and interventions for childhood overweight: a summary of evidence for the US Preventive Services Task Force. Pediatrics 2005;116(1):e125–44.
66. Klonoff DC, Greenway F. Drugs in the pipeline for the obesity market. J Diabetes Sci Technol 2008;2(5):913–8.
67. Sugerman JH, Sugerman EL, DeMarla EJ, et al. Bariatric surgery for severely obese adolescents. J Gastrointest Surg 2003;7(1):102–7.
68. Garcia VF, Langlord L, Inge TH. Application of laparoscopy for bariatric surgery in adolescents. Curr Opin Pediatr 2003;15(3):248–55.
69. Inge TH, Garcia V, Daniels S, et al. A multidisciplinary approach to the adolescent bariatric surgical patient. J Pediatr Surg 2004;39(3):442–7.
70. Inge TH, Krebs NF, Garcia VF, et al. Bariatric surgery for severely overweight adolescents: concerns and recommendations. Pediatrics 2004;114(1):217–23.
71. Inge TH, Zeller M, Harmon C, et al. Teen-longitudinal assessment of bariatric surgery: methodological features of the first prospective multicenter study of adolescent bariatric surgery. J Pediatr Surg 2007;42(11):1969–71.
72. Nadler EP, Youn HA, Ginsburg HB, et al. Short-term results in 53 US obese pediatric patients treated with laparoscopic adjustable gastric banding. J Pediatr Surg 2007;42(1):137–41.
73. Warman J. The application of laparoscopic bariatric surgery for treatment of severe obesity in adolescents using a multidisciplinary adolescent bariatric program. Crit Care Nurs Q 2005;28(3):276–87.
74. Zitsman JL, Fennoy I, Witt MA, et al. Laparoscopic adjustable gastric banding in adolescents: short-term results. J Pediatr Surg 2011;46(1):157–62.
75. Buchwald H, Avidor Y, Braunwald E, et al. Bariatric surgery: a systematic review and met-analysis. JAMA 2004;292(14):1724–37.
76. Franco JV, Ruiz PA, Palermo M, et al. A review of studies comparing three laparoscopic procedures in bariatric surgery: sleeve gastrectomy, Roux-en-Y gastric bypass and adjustable gastric banding. Obes Surg 2011;21(9):1458–68.

77. Conroy R, Lee EJ, Jean A, et al. Effect of laparoscopic adjustable gastric banding on metabolic syndrome and its risk factors in morbidly obese adolescents. J Obes 2011;2011:906384.
78. Dillard BE 3rd, Gorodner V, Galvani C, et al. Initial experience with the adjustable gastric band in morbidly obese US adolescents and recommendations for further investigation. J Pediatr Gastroenterol Nutr 2007;45(2):240–6.
79. Holterman AX, Browne A, Tussing L, et al. A prospective trial for laparoscopic adjustable gastric banding in morbidly obese adolescents: an interim report of weight loss, metabolic and quality of life outcomes. J Pediatr Surg 2010;45(1):74–8.
80. Lawson ML, Kirk S, Mitchell T, et al. One-year outcomes of Roux-en-Y gastric bypass for morbidly obese adolescents: a multicenter study from the Pediatric Bariatric Study Group. J Pediatr Surg 2006;41(1):137–43.
81. Loux TJ, Haricharan RN, Clements RH, et al. Health-related quality of life before and after bariatric surgery in adolescents. J Pediatr Surg 2008;43(7):1275–9.
82. Nadler EP, Youn HA, Ren CJ, et al. An update on 73 US obese pediatric patients treated with laparoscopic adjustable gastric banding: comorbidity resolution and compliance data. J Pediatr Surg 2008;43(1):141–6.
83. Nadler EP, Reddy S, Isenalumhe A, et al. Laparoscopic adjustable gastric banding for morbidly obese adolescents affects android fat loss, resolution of comorbidities, and improved metabolic status. J Am Coll Surg 2009;209(5):638–44.
84. O'Brien PE, Sawyer SM, Laurie C, et al. Laparoscopic adjustable gastric banding in severely obese adolescents: a randomized trial. JAMA 2010;303(6):519–26.
85. Zitsman JL, Digiorgi MF, Marr JR, et al. Comparative outcomes of laparoscopic adjustable gastric banding in adolescents and adults. Surg Obes Relat Dis 2011;7(6):720–6.
86. Michalsky M, Reichard K, Inge T, et al. ASMBS pediatric committee best practice guidelines. Surg Obes Relat Dis 2012;8(1):1–7.
87. Michalsky M, Kramer RE, Fullmer MA, et al. Developing criteria for pediatric/adolescent bariatric surgery programs. Pediatrics 2011;128(Suppl 2):S65–70.
88. Fullmer MA, Abrams SH, Hrovat K, et al. Nutritional strategy for the adolescent patient undergoing bariatric surgery: report of a Working Group of the Nutrition Committee for the North American Society of Pediatric Gastroenterology, Hepatology and Nutrition and National Association of Children's Hospital and Related Institutions. J Pediatr Gastroenterol Nutr 2012;54(1):125–35.
89. Barnett SJ. Contemporary surgical management of the obese adolescent. Curr Opin Pediatr 2011;23(3):351–5.
90. Baur LA, Fitzgerald DA. Recommendations for bariatric surgery in adolescents in Australia and New Zealand. J Paediatr Child Health 2010;46(12):704–7.
91. Cunneen SA. Review of meta-analytic comparisons of bariatric surgery with a focus on laparoscopic adjustable gastric banding. Surg Obes Relat Dis 2008;4(Suppl 3):S47–55.
92. Xanthakos SA. Bariatric surgery for extreme adolescent obesity: indications, outcomes, and physiologic effects on the gut-brain axis. Pathophysiology 2008;15(2):135–46.
93. American Society for Metabolic and Bariatric Surgery. Updated position statement on sleeve gastrectomy as a bariatric procedure. Surg Obes Relat Dis 2010;6(1):1–5.
94. Nadler EP, Barefoot LC, Qureshi FG. Early results after laparoscopic sleeve gastrectomy in adolescents with morbid obesity. Oral presentation at the 7th Annual Academic Surgical Congress, Las Vegas (NV), February, 2012.

95. Inge RH, Xanthakos S. Sleeve gastrectomy for childhood morbid obesity: why not? Obes Surg 2010;20(1):118–20.
96. Scopinaro N, Adami FG, Marinari GM, et al. Biliopancreatic diversion. World J Surg 1998;22(9):936–46.
97. Stimac D, Majanović SK, Turk T, et al. Intragastric balloon treatment for obesity: results of a large single center prospective study. Obes Surg 2011;21(5):551–5.
98. Dumonceau JM. Evidence-based review of the Bioenterics intragastric balloon for weight loss. Obes Surg 2008;18(12):1611–7.
99. Lecumberri E, Krekshi W, Matía P, et al. Effectiveness and safety of air-filled balloon Heliosphere BAG® in 82 consecutive obese patients. Obes Surg 2011;21(10):1508–12.
100. Gaggiotti F, Tack J, Garrido AB Jr, et al. Adjustable totally implantable intragastric prosthesis (ATIIP)-Endogast for treatment of morbid obesity: one-year follow-up of a multicenter prospective clinical survey. Obes Surg 2007;17(7):949–56.
101. Machytka E, Klvana P, Kombluth A, et al. Adjustable intragastric balloons: a 12-month pilot trial in endoscopic weight loss management. Obes Surg 2011;21(10):1499–507.
102. Swidnicka-Siergiejko A, Wróblewski E, Andrezej D, et al. Endoscopic treatment of obesity. Can J Gastroenterol 2011;25(11):627–33.
103. Genco A, Bruni T, Doldi SB, et al. BioEnterics Intragastric Balloon: the Italian experience with 2,515 patients. Obes Surg 2005;15(8):1161–4.
104. Gersin KS, Torhstein RI, Tosenthal RJ, et al. Open-label, sham-controlled trial of an endoscopic duodenojejunal bypass liner for preoperative weight loss in bariatric surgery candidates. Gastrointest Endosc 2010;71(6):976–82.
105. Camilleri M, Toouli J, Herrera MF, et al. Selection of electrical algorithms to treat obesity with intermittent vagal block using an implantable medical device. Surg Obes Relat Dis 2009;5(2):224–9.
106. Shikora SA, Bergenstal R, Bessler M, et al. Implantable gastric stimulation for the treatment of clinically severe obesity: results of the SHAPE trial. Surg Obes Relat Dis 2009;5(1):31–7.
107. Sanmiguel CP, Conklin JL, Cunneen SA, et al. Gastric electrical stimulation with the TANTALUS system in obese type 2 diabetes patients: effect on weight and glycemic control. J Diabetes Sci Technol 2009;3(4):964–70.
108. Skrekas G, Antiochos K, Stafyla VK. Laparoscopic gastric greater curvature placation: results and complications in a series of 135 patients. Obes Surg 2011;21(11):1657–63.
109. Brethauer SA, Harris JL, Kroh M, et al. Laparoscopic gastric plication for treatment of severe obesity. Surg Obes Relat Dis 2011;7(1):15–22.
110. Velhote MC, Damiani D. Bariatric surgery in adolescents: preliminary 1-year results with a novel technique (Santoro III). Obes Surg 2010;20(12):1710–5.
111. Heap AJ, Cummings DE. A novel weight-reducing operation: lateral subtotal gastrectomy with Silastic ring plus small bowel reduction with omentectomy. Obes Surg 2008;18(7):819–28.

Childhood Obesity and the Media

Melanie Hingle, PhD, MPH, RD[a],*, Dale Kunkel, PhD[b]

KEYWORDS

- Childhood obesity ● Media ● Communication ● Food advertising ● Policy

KEY POINTS

- Electronic media use is significantly positively correlated with adiposity in children.
- Interventions reducing screen media use by children (eg, eliminating television from children's bedrooms; turning off the television while eating) have been associated with improvement in child weight status.
- Children's exposure to media marketing messages for unhealthy food products is well established as a significant contributor to childhood obesity.
- Food industry self-regulation initiatives have had only negligible effects in improving the nutritional quality of foods advertised to children.

An epidemic of childhood obesity afflicts American youth (**Fig. 1**). Approximately 32% of children and adolescents aged 2 to 19 years are overweight (body mass index [BMI] ≥85th percentile for children of the same age and sex), and 17% (or 12.5 million) of these children are considered obese (BMI ≥95th percentile for children of the same age and sex).[1] Adiposity poses risks for significant adverse health consequences. Obese children are more likely than normal-weight children to have hypertension and high cholesterol,[2] impaired glucose tolerance, insulin resistance, type 2 diabetes,[3] sleep apnea and asthma,[4,5] joint problems,[6] fatty liver, gallstones, gastroesophageal reflux,[3–5] as well as increased risk of social and psychological problems such as poor self-esteem and discrimination.[3,7,8] Obesity in childhood has been shown to track into adulthood, placing obese children at risk of future weight-related diseases.[9,10]

Numerous elements contribute to childhood obesity. Regular consumption of a calorie-dense, nutrient-poor diet and inadequate moderate-to-vigorous physical activity are key risk factors. Media use has also been established as a strong correlate of childhood obesity. This relationship was first identified in the 1980s[11] and has

This article originally appeared in Pediatric Clinics of North America, Volume 59, Issue 3, June 2012.

[a] Department of Nutritional Sciences, University of Arizona, 1177 East, 4th Street, Shantz Building, Room 328, Tucson, AZ 85721, USA; [b] Department of Communication, University of Arizona, 1103 East, University Boulevard, P.O. Box 210025, Tucson, AZ 85721, USA
* Corresponding author.
E-mail address: hinglem@email.arizona.edu

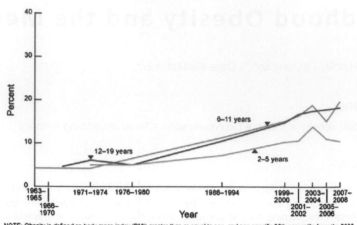

NOTE: Obesity is defined as body mass index (BMI) greater than or equal to sex- and age-specific 95th percentile from the 2000 CDC Growth Charts.
SOURCES: CDC/NCHS, National Health Examination Surveys II (ages 6–11), III (ages 12–17), and National Health and Nutrition Examination Surveys (NHANES) I–III, and NHANES 1999–2000, 2001–2002, 2003–2004, 2005–2006, and 2007–2008.

Fig. 1. Prevalence of obesity among children and adolescents, by age group, United States, 1963 to 2008. (*From* Ogden CL, Carroll M. Prevalence of obesity among children and adolescents: United States, trends 1963–1965 through 2007–2008. NCH Health E-Stats. CDC/National Center for Health Statistics; 2010. Available at http://www.cdc.gov/nchs/data/hestat/obesity_child_07_08/obesity_child_07_08.htm.)

been corroborated by dozens of studies since then.[12,13] It is often assumed that the sedentary nature of television viewing, traditionally the largest component of young people's time spent with media, is the mechanism underlying the relationship. The presumption holds that heavy media users are transformed into so-called couch potatoes who devote insufficient time to exercise because their eyes are too often glued to the screen.[14,15] Consistent with this perspective, the US Department of Health and Human Services specified a national objective of reducing television viewing to combat obesity in its *Healthy People 2010* target goals.[16]

However, more recent evidence has focused increasing attention on the role of food marketing to children as a causal factor contributing to childhood obesity.[17] Given the significant amount of time children spend watching television, they inevitably encounter large amounts of commercials for food products.[18] Televised food advertising is dominated by high-density, low-nutrient products that the public typically labels as junk food.[19,20] Advertising for unhealthy food products has also migrated to new media venues frequented by children and teens, such as the Internet.[21–23] Exposure to commercial promotions in the media wields influence on children's food product preferences, requests, diet, and ultimately their diet-related health.[24] Advertising exposure may be the principal causal mechanism that explains why screen time is significantly correlated with childhood obesity, rather than the widely presumed couch-potato hypothesis.

This review article surveys the research that documents children's patterns of media use, analyzes the evidence that shows the association between young people's screen time and weight status, considers the role of food marketing as a contributor to childhood obesity, and evaluates recent intervention efforts intended to reduce children's screen time and/or exposure to advertising messages for unhealthy food products. Overall conclusions and possible solutions to reduce the role of media as a contributor to childhood obesity are also discussed.

SCREEN TIME WITHIN THE CONTEXT OF OBESITY PREVENTION

Screen time is a term meant to represent an individual's use of electronic mass media, including television viewing, video and computer game playing, DVD viewing, Internet use, and other online activities. Media use in childhood is primarily a means of entertainment, and hence is engaged in mostly during unstructured time outside of school hours.[25] Public health researchers originally conceived of screen time as a sedentary activity, which holds obvious implications for displacing time that might otherwise be devoted to physical exercise.

Given the recent proliferation of mobile technologies and digital media, screen time can now occur from almost any geographic location via highly portable video-enabled and Internet-enabled devices such as iPads, iPods, and smartphones. The use of these mobile technologies reduces the likelihood that the user is necessarily sedentary while engaging in screen-related activities, thus rendering the construct of screen time a less precise and reliable assessment of time spent in sedentary pursuits. However, regardless of how screen time may be defined and quantified, there is little doubt that children and adolescents spend significant time with screen-based media, and that media use by youth has increased as mobile technologies have become more readily available and accessible.[26]

Screen Media Diet: Infants and Preschoolers

Survey data indicate that television viewing begins at a young age,[27] and has surged as a function of the recent expansion in programming targeted specifically at infants.[28] More than half (59%) of children less than 2 years of age watch television on an average day,[29] despite the American Academy of Pediatrics recommending no media exposure before the age of 2 years.[30] Children average 2.2 hours of viewing per day at age 1 year, increasing to 3.6 hours per day by 3 years of age.[31] By age 5 years, more than 60% have used handheld games, 81% have played console games, and 90% have used a computer.[32]

Among children less than 8 years of age, most screen time is still spent watching television (74% of media time), followed by the use of computers (13%), video games (10% of the time), and , cell phones/iPods/iPads (4%).[32] Nearly half (47%) of children aged 5 to 8 years have a television set in their bedroom, including 30% of children less than 2 years old. Overall, the average daily time that children less than 8 years old spend with television and DVDs is estimated to be about 1:40, with roughly another half hour devoted to playing video, computer, or handheld games.[16,32]

Screen Media Diet: School-aged Children and Teens

The amount of time spent with media is also increasing for older children and adolescents. From 2005 to 2010, media use for those aged 8 to 18 years increased by more than an hour a day, moving from 6:21 to 7:38 daily.[25] As with younger children, most screen time was devoted to television. Older children and teens are more likely to multitask, in terms of engaging multiple media venues simultaneously, as well as engaging in activities such as homework while also using mass media.[33] Older children and teens spend more time with media than in any other waking activity. As Rideout and colleagues[25] observed, using media comprises a full-time job for youth, accounting for 7.5 hours per day, 7 days per week.

Although there may be some benefits associated with children's screen media use, such as learning from educational programs, there is also significant risk for a range of adverse side effects. Exposure to certain types of media portrayals may increase child viewers' aggressive behavior,[34] decrease the age of first sexual intercourse,[35] and contribute to gender[36] and ethnic group stereotyping[37] in children and teens. However, regardless of the type of content viewed, heavy screen media use correlates significantly with overweight and obesity in children.

ASSOCIATION BETWEEN SCREEN TIME AND OBESITY IN CHILDREN AND ADOLESCENTS

A systematic review of the published research evidence linking television exposure with adiposity was conducted in 2006 by the Institute of Medicine (IOM).[24] The IOM identified more than 60 studies conducted over roughly the past 20 years that converged to show a small but statistically significant relationship between television exposure and child obesity. Studies were evaluated for methodological strength, and the greater the study's rigor, the greater the likelihood that it showed a significant relationship between these variables. Since the IOM review was published, numerous large-scale epidemiologic studies have emerged to further corroborate this relationship.[38–42]

Data from cross-sectional and longitudinal studies yield the same pattern of results. One review of research reported that, in 18 of 22 longitudinal studies, more hours of media exposure predicted increased weight over time.[43] Although a small minority of studies have produced nonsignificant results, the null findings are most often attributed to limitations in defining and measuring time spent with screen media,[26,44] among other confounds. One of these complications involves video game use.

Video Games

By most definitions, screen time encompasses video game play. However, studies that focused on video game play have been less consistent in showing correlations between screen time and adiposity, compared with research centered on television use.[16] Fewer studies have specifically targeted video game play, and, although some of these yield evidence of associations with obesity,[45,46] others do not.[47,48] A recent review of evidence found that there were more studies that produced no significant association between video game play and obesity than had yielded significant correlations.[49] One of the most obvious complications here is that video games are not as inherently sedentary as watching television,[50,51] especially when exercise-oriented games such as Dance Dance Revolution are considered.[52]

Possible Causal Mechanisms

The direction of causality in the relationship between screen time and obesity could potentially flow either way. That is, overweight individuals might tend to stay home and use media more than physically active people, hence accounting for the relationship between screen time and adiposity. Although plausible, this possibility is rebutted by several types of evidence. Twelve of 15 longitudinal studies that measure television use at time 1 and weight status at 1 or more subsequent points in time produced significant associations with weight gain over time.[24] In addition, an experimental intervention that reduced screen time over a 6-month period found significantly less increase in BMI and other measures of adiposity, compared with a control group.[53] The totality of evidence suggests that greater amounts of time spent with screen media lead to weight gain and the risk of obesity, rather than the other way around. What is less clear is the underlying mechanism that accounts for that relationship.

Data that merely correlate media use with childhood obesity do not clarify whether weight gain may be a function of the largely sedentary nature of the activity (ie, displacement of physically active time), or might instead be the result of some other factor/s. There are several incongruities that pose challenges for the couch-potato hypothesis. The American Academy of Pediatrics[54] has observed that, although many studies find that physical activity decreases as screen time increases,[39,55,56] many others do not.[57–59] Within child care settings, for example, 1 study found that youngsters attending day care centers with high use of electronic media had greater sedentary behavior than children in centers with low electronic media use,[60] but 2 other comparable studies found no association between these variables.[61,62]

Higher levels of screen time do not always correlate with lower levels of physical activity. An IOM review reported only 14 of 20 studies that analyzed these variables found a significant relationship (see Table 5-22 in Ref.[24]). It is common for studies to find only small proportions of children that concomitantly experience high screen time and low physical activity. For example, in one study of children aged 4 to 11 years using National Health and Nutrition Examination Survey (NHANES) data (N = 2964), less than one-quarter of boys (23.7%) and one-third of girls (29.1%) were in this category.[63] In addition, most studies that control statistically for amount of physical activity in examining the relationship between screen time and obesity still produce a significant correlation.

Perhaps the most telling evidence is provided by a study that separated time spent watching television into 2 categories, 1 with and 1 without commercial advertisements included.[42] The findings were clear. Time spent viewing commercial television was significantly correlated with BMI, whereas time watching noncommercial television was not. The overall evidence in this area clearly suggests that the role of media in contributing to childhood obesity entails more than simply displacing time that would otherwise be devoted to exercise. Another factor that may play a role involves snacking that occurs during television viewing time. However, the most likely alternative explanation for the linkage between screen time and adiposity involves the influence of advertisements for unhealthy foods that are widespread in media consumed by children.

THE ROLE OF FOOD MARKETING IN CHILDHOOD OBESITY

As indicated earlier, children engage in heavy media use, with television still dominant among an increasingly diverse range of screen media. Given that commercial messages are pervasive in most television content, it is inevitable that child viewers are exposed to large numbers of advertisements, including many for food products. According to the Federal Trade Commission, children aged 2 to 17 years see roughly 5500 televised food advertisements per year, or about 15.1 per day.[64] Commercials for food products have long been a staple in children's television programming, and the featured items are typically low-nutrient, calorie-dense fast foods, candies, snacks, and sugared cereals.[65,66]

Food Advertising to Children

Food marketers invest nearly $2 billion annually in child-targeted advertising, with the largest share devoted to television advertisements.[67] Studies of advertising content document the prevalence of obesogenic foods in television advertising targeted at youth.[66,68] For example, 2 out of every 3 cereals (66%) advertised to children fail to meet nutritional standards with regard to added sugar.[69] Nearly all (98%) food advertisements seen by children and 89% viewed by adolescents are for products high in fat, sugar, or sodium (**Fig. 2**).[19] In contrast, healthy foods that should be part of a regular diet are almost never advertised to children.[19,70,71]

As new media have evolved and attracted children's interest, advertisers have migrated to these venues along with youth audiences. Food marketers have

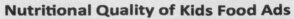

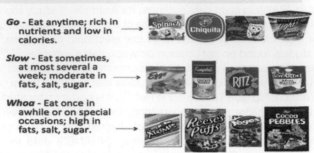

Nutritional Quality of Kids Food Ads

Go - Eat anytime; rich in nutrients and low in calories.

Slow - Eat sometimes, at most several a week; moderate in fats, salt, sugar.

Whoa - Eat once in awhile or on special occasions; high in fats, salt, sugar.

FINDING: Healthy food advertising is invisible.

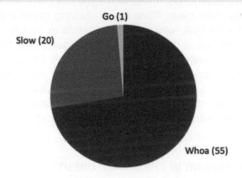

Go (1)

Slow (20)

Whoa (55)

Nutritional Quality of Food Ads in 10 Hours of Children's Programming

Fig. 2. Nutritional quality of foods advertised in children's programming. (*From* Kunkel D, McKinley C, Wright P. Assessing compliance with industry self-regulation of televised food marketing to children. Oakland (CA): Children Now; 2009; with permission.)

established Internet Web sites that offer games and other attractive entertainment options for children, creating a media experience that is a commercial promotion.[21,72,73] Product-based so-called advergames allow children to play virtual games with popular brand characters such as Chester Cheeto or Tony the Tiger,[22] blurring boundaries between commercial and entertainment content in a manner that federal regulations prohibit on television.[74] More than half of the food advertisements on children's television programs now promote such product-based Web sites.[75]

Other innovations in marketing food products to children include in-game advertising, placed within video games[76]; viral marketing, in which consumers share product-related messages with friends to receive rewards[77]; and promotional activities in schools.[78] Collectively, these efforts comprise a significant expansion of the overall commercial environment targeted at youth, which many now describe as the commercialization of childhood.[79–81]

Effects of Food Advertising on Children

Food marketing plays a significant role in shaping children's nutritional knowledge, eating habits, and weight status. Heavy exposure to televised food advertising is associated with nutritional misperceptions: the greater the exposure to food advertising, the greater the likelihood that unhealthy items will be judged as healthy and nutritious.[82–84] Numerous experiments show short-term effects on children's attitudes and product preferences for foods.[18,85] Amount of television exposure is positively correlated with children's ability to correctly identify product brands[86] and with their consumption of advertised brands.[87]

The most comprehensive review of studies examining the effects of food marketing on children was conducted by the IOM in 2006. The IOM report concluded that (1) there is strong evidence that advertising influences the short-term food consumption of children aged 2 to 11 years; (2) there is moderate evidence that advertising influences the regular diet of children 2 to 5 years of age, and weak evidence (ie, more studies are needed) that it influences children 6 to 11 years of age; and (3) there is strong evidence that exposure to advertising is associated with adiposity in children 2 to 11 years of age and teens 12 to 18 years of age. The report summarized its findings by observing that "food and beverage marketing practices geared to children and youth are out of balance with healthful diets, and contribute to an environment that puts their health at risk."[24(p374)]

The conclusion that advertising to children works as intended is clear, if unremarkable.[18] In an ideal world, parents would refuse children's purchase influence requests for unhealthy foods, negating much of the impact of advertising. In practice, parents have a high rate of yielding to children's requests.[88,89] Furthermore, most children begin to purchase snack foods with their own money as early as 8 years of age.[90] Thus, given that children's exposure to media marketing messages for unhealthy food products is now well established as a significant contributor to childhood obesity, this article reviews possible tactics and strategies that might mitigate the health risks posed in this area.

REDUCING MEDIA CONTRIBUTIONS TO CHILDHOOD OBESITY

There are 2 distinct approaches to ameliorating the role that media play in contributing to childhood obesity. The first involves individual-level interventions that seek to reduce children's screen time. The second involves institutional-level efforts to diminish children's exposure to unhealthy food advertising by limiting its presence in young people's media environment. This article addresses each of these topics in turn.

Interventions to Limit Screen Time

Since Dietz and Gortmaker's[11] influential work describing the association between television viewing and childhood obesity, a large number of intervention programs have been conducted seeking to reduce children's screen time as a means to influence adiposity. Although some of these efforts have focused on screen time reduction, most have addressed media use within the context of a healthy lifestyle intervention that also included strategies to improve diet and physical activity. Given our focus on the role of media in childhood obesity, discussion of the intervention literature in this article is limited to media use issues only.

One of the first noteworthy experiments to focus on the effects of reducing screen time on obesity was conducted by Thomas Robinson[53] in the late 1990s. This randomized controlled trial consisted of a series of 18 lessons (30–50 minutes in length) taught by trained third and fourth grade classroom teachers over a period of 6 months, along with the use of an electronic device to assist participants in monitoring their media time. The intervention group achieved significant reductions in time devoted to media, an outcome that was linked to reductions in several measures of adiposity. The reduction in adiposity was achieved without any significant change in moderate-to-vigorous physical activity levels by the treatment group.

Subsequent studies have corroborated the finding that interventions that prove successful at reducing screen time typically achieve significant improvements in weight status.[91–95] Like the initial Robinson[53] trial, most observe that this outcome occurs despite the lack of any increase in strenuous physical exercise among participants. This pattern is confirmed by a recent meta-analysis,[96] and thus seems robust.

Based on this body of evidence, an expert panel convened by the US Centers for Disease Control and Prevention[97] recommended the following intervention tactics as the most likely to be effective:

1. Eliminate television from children's bedrooms
2. Reduce spontaneous media use in favor of planned media activities
3. Turn off the television while eating
4. Use school-based curricula to reduce children's screen time.

In the future, it will be important for research to better explicate the reasons why reductions in screen time lead to weight loss. Scholars have suggested that changes in energy intake, such as reduced snacking opportunities, as well as increases in low-level physical activity (eg, visiting friends outside the house instead of watching television at home), may underlie the effect. However, despite the lack of clarity about why reducing screen time helps to combat adiposity, it is clear that one way to reduce the obesity epidemic is to limit young people's time spent with media.

Limiting Unhealthy Food Advertising to Children

Although the first intervention strategy seeks to limit children's time spent with media, the second takes a different approach, seeking to reduce the amount of advertising for unhealthy foods that children encounter during their media use. The issue of unhealthy food marketing to children combines 2 distinct concerns: (1) the fairness of advertising to children, which applies to all merchandise; and (2) the propriety of promoting products to children that cannot be consumed safely in abundance. Youngsters do not comprehend the selling intent of commercials until at least 8 years of age, and they do not comprehend the persuasive bias inherent in advertising messages until several years later.[18,98,99] Before such recognition develops, children understand commercial claims and appeals as accurate, balanced, and truthful, failing to apply the skeptical eye of a more mature perspective. Based on this evidence, the American Psychological Association has concluded that all advertising targeted at young children is unfair because they lack the cognitive ability to defend against commercial persuasion.[100] Add in the consideration that most child-targeted food advertisements promote unhealthy products and it becomes obvious that food marketing to children is a serious public health issue.

Responding to public concern, the food industry established a self-regulatory effort known as the Children's Food and Beverage Advertising Initiative (CFBAI) in 2006.[101] With participation from more than a dozen of the nation's leading food conglomerates, the CFBAI is a pledge program in which each company commits to advertise foods to children only if they meet specified nutritional criteria for defining healthful products. For example, varying limits are placed on the amount of added fat, salt, and sugar allowed for a product to qualify as healthy, thus making it permissible to advertise

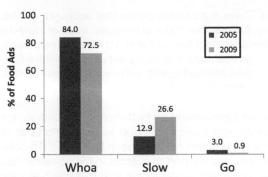

Fig. 3. Nutritional quality of foods advertised to children, before and after industry self-regulation. (*From* Kunkel D, McKinley C, Wright P. Assessing compliance with industry self-regulation of televised food marketing to children. Oakland (CA): Children Now; 2009; with permission.)

to children. Although the industry reports consistent evidence that companies generally fulfill their pledges,[101] independent research shows that the initiative has had only negligible effects in improving the nutritional quality of foods advertised to children.

In 2005, before industry self-regulation, 84% of all foods advertised on children's television programs were classified in the poorest nutritional category, according to standards used by the Department of Health and Human Services.[75] In 2009, several years following adoption of the CFBAI, that percentage had decreased only to 72.5%; nearly 3 out of 4 of the food products that met the industry's self-regulatory criteria for a healthy item were still nutritionally deficient (**Fig. 3**).

This result occurred for several reasons. Each participating company was allowed to use different nutritional standards to qualify their products as healthy for the purposes of the CFBAI, and many of their criteria were too lenient and self-serving.[102] In addition, more than one-quarter (28.7%) of food advertising to children originated with companies that chose not to participate in the CFBAI and hence were free to market whatever items they chose.[75] Industry self-regulation has achieved little in terms of addressing concerns about children's exposure to unhealthy food marketing, a finding confirmed by numerous studies using a broad range of nutritional measures.[103–105]

In 2011, the American Academy of Pediatrics issued a policy recommendation calling for a federal ban on junk food advertising during television programming viewed predominantly by young children.[30(p204)] Meanwhile, the food industry spent $51 million lobbying against regulation in the same year.[106] Although the industry asserts that First Amendment free speech protections prohibit any governmental restrictions on food advertising to children,[107] public health legal scholars have aggressively rebutted this position,[108,109] suggesting that a policy battle on this front may soon be on the horizon. One economics study[110] estimates that the impact of banning food advertisements on television would reduce the baseline rate of childhood obesity in the United States from 17% to somewhere in the range of 10.5% to 14.5%.

SUMMARY

Childhood obesity is viewed by many as the principal threat to the nation's public health. The malady currently afflicts more than 1 of every 6 American youth between the ages of 2 and 19 years,[111] each of whom faces a high probability of remaining obese into adulthood. The disease affects everyone in the country, given the tens of billions of dollars in obesity-related health care costs that are borne annually by the federal government. There is no single cause that accounts for the epidemic; it is a confluence of many factors that have converged to alter contemporary lifestyles, with media a prominent factor in this problem. To reverse the prevalence of childhood obesity will require significant shifts in many aspects of children's everyday environments. Reducing the time children spend with media, as well as reducing the number of advertisements for unhealthy food products in child-targeted media, are key goals in the battle.

Progress to date has been limited on both fronts. Population norms for children's media use continue at high levels.[25,27] Food industry efforts at reform have been tepid,[112] and governmental action has also been lacking.[113] To obtain sufficient societal awareness, concern, and support to overcome the epidemic requires changes on the scale of a social movement similar to the shift that has been accomplished in attitudes and regulations toward smoking and tobacco.[114] Although that challenge is daunting, it is nonetheless critical for maintaining the health of future generations.

REFERENCES

1. Ogden CL, Carroll MD, Curtin LR, et al. Prevalence of high body mass index in US children and adolescents, 2007-2008. JAMA 2010;303(3):242–9.
2. Freedman DS, Mei Z, Srinivasan SR, et al. Cardiovascular risk factors and excess adiposity among overweight children and adolescents: the Bogalusa Heart Study. J Pediatr 2007;150(1):12–17, e2.
3. Whitlock EP, Williams SB, Gold R, et al. Screening and interventions for childhood overweight: a summary of evidence for the US Preventive Services Task Force. Pediatrics 2005;116(1):e125–44.
4. Han JC, Lawlor DA, Kimm SY. Childhood obesity. Lancet 2010;375(9727): 1737–48.
5. Sutherland ER. Obesity and asthma. Immunol Allergy Clin North Am 2008;28(3): 589–602.
6. Taylor ED, Theim KR, Mirch MC, et al. Orthopedic complications of overweight in children and adolescents. Pediatrics 2006;117(6):2167–74.
7. Dietz W. Health consequences of obesity in youth: childhood predictors of adult disease. Pediatrics 1998;101:518–25.
8. Swartz MB, Puhl R. Childhood obesity: a societal problem to solve. Obes Rev 2003;4(1):57–71.
9. Whitaker RC, Wright JA, Pepe MS, et al. Predicting obesity in young adulthood from childhood and parental obesity. N Engl J Med 1997;37(13):869–73.
10. Serdula MK, Ivery D, Coates RJ, et al. Do obese children become obese adults? A review of the literature. Prev Med 1993;22:167–77.
11. Dietz WH Jr, Gortmaker SL. Do we fatten our children at the television set? Obesity and television viewing in children and adolescents. Pediatrics 1985; 75(5):807–12.
12. Gortmaker SL, Must A, Sobol AM, et al. Television viewing as a cause of increasing obesity among children in the United States, 1986-1990. Arch Pediatr Adolesc Med 1996;150(4):356–62.
13. Lobstein T, Baur L, Uauy R. Obesity in children and young people: a crisis in public health. Obs Rev 2004;5(s1):4–85.
14. Bar-Or O, Foreyt J, Bouchard C, et al. Physical activity, genetic and nutritional consideration in childhood weight management. Med Sci Sports Exerc 1998;30:2–10.
15. Chen J, Kennedy C. Television viewing and children's health. J Soc Pediatr Nurs 2001;1:35–6.

16. Vandewater E, Cummings H. Media use and childhood obesity. In: Calvert S, Wilson B, editors. The handbook of children, media, and development. West Sussex (United Kingdom): Blackwell Publishing; 2008. p. 355–80.
17. Lobstein T, Dibb S. Evidence of a possible link between obesogenic food advertising and child overweight. Obes Rev 2005;6:203–8.
18. Kunkel D, Castonguay J. Children and advertising: content, comprehension, and consequences. In: Singer DG, Singer JL, editors. Handbook of children and the media. 2nd edition. Thousand Oaks (CA): Sage Publications; 2012. p. 95–418.
19. Powell LM, Schermbeck RM, Szczypka G, et al. Trends in the nutritional content of television food advertisements seen by children in the United States. Arch Pediatr Adolesc Med 2011;165(12):1078–86.
20. Rudd Center for Food Policy and Obesity. Trends in television food advertising to you people: 2010 update. New Haven (CT): Yale University; 2011.
21. Chester J, Montgomery KC. Interactive food & beverage marketing: targeting children and youth in the digital age. The Berkeley Media Studies Group web site. Available at: http://digitalads.org/documents/digiMarketingFull.pdf. 2007. Accessed February 1, 2012.
22. Culp J, Bell R, Cassaday D. Characteristics of food industry websites and advergames targeting children. J Nutr Educ Behav 2010;42(3):197–201.
23. Jain A. Temptations in cyberspace: new battlefields in childhood obesity. Health Aff 2010;29(3):425–9.
24. Institute of Medicine (IOM). Food marketing to children and youth: threat or opportunity? Washington, DC: National Academies Press; 2006.
25. Rideout VJ, Foehr UG, Roberts DF. Generation M2: media in the lives of 8- to 18-year-olds. Menlo Park (CA): The Henry J Kaiser Family Foundation; 2010.
26. Vandewater E, Lee S. Measuring children's media use in the digital age: issues and challenges. Am Behav Sci 2009;52(8):1152–76.
27. Vandewater E, Rideout V, Wartella E, et al. Digital childhood: electronic media and technology use among infants, toddlers, and preschoolers. Pediatrics 2007;199:1006–15.
28. Birch L, Parker L, Burns A. Early childhood obesity prevention policies. Washington, DC: The National Academies Press; 2011.
29. Rideout VJ, Vandewater E, Wartella E. Zero to six: electronic media in the lives of infants, toddlers and preschoolers. Menlo Park (CA): The Henry J Kaiser Family Foundation; 2003.
30. American Academy of Pediatrics, Council on Communications and Media. Media use by children younger than two years. Pediatrics 2011;128:1040–5.
31. Christakis D, Zimmerman F, DiGiuseppe D, et al. Early television exposure and subsequent attentional problems in children. Pediatrics 2004;113(4):708–13.
32. Common sense media. Zero to eight: children's media use in America; common sense media Web site. Available at: http://www.commonsensemedia.org/sites/default/files/research/zerotoeightfinal2011.pdf. 2011. Accessed February 1, 2012.
33. Foehr U. Media multitasking among American youth: prevalence, predictors, and pairings. Menlo Park (CA): The Henry J Kaiser Family Foundation; 2006.
34. Bushman B, Huesmann L. Effects of violent media on aggression. In: Singer D, Singer J, editors. Handbook of children and the media. 2nd edition. Thousand Oaks (CA): Sage Publications; 2012. p. 249–72.
35. Collins R, Elliott M, Berry S, et al. Watching sex on TV affects adolescent initiation of sexual intercourse. Pediatrics 2004;114(3):e280–9.

36. Signorielli N. Television's gender role images and contribution to stereotyping: past present future. In: Singer D, Singer J, editors. Handbook of children and the media. 2nd edition. Thousand Oaks (CA): Sage Publications; 2012. p. 321–40.
37. Asamen J, Berry G. Television, children, and multicultural awareness: comprehending the medium in a complex multimedia society. In: Singer D, Singer J, editors. Handbook of children and the media. 2nd edition. Thousand Oaks (CA): Sage Publications; 2012. p. 363–78.
38. Gable S, Chang Y, Krull J. Television watching and frequency of family meals are predictive of overweight onset and persistence in a national sample of school-aged children. J Am Diet Assoc 2007;107(1):53–61.
39. Sisson SB, Broyles ST, Baker BL, et al. Screen time, physical activity, and overweight in U.S. youth: National Survey of Children's Health 2003. J Adolesc Health 2010;47(3):309–11.
40. te Velde S, De Bourdeaudhuij I, Thorsdottir I, et al. Patterns in sedentary and exercise behaviors and associations with overweight in 9–14-year-old boys and girls - a cross-sectional study. BMC Public Health 2007;7(16):1–9.
41. Utter J, Scragg R, Schaaf D. Associations between television viewing and consumption of commonly advertised foods among New Zealand children and young adolescents. Public Health Nutr 2006;9(5):606–12.
42. Zimmerman FJ, Bell JF. Associations of television content type and obesity in children. Am J Public Health 2010;100:334–40.
43. Nunez-Smith M, Wolf E, Huang H, et al. Media and child and adolescent health: a systematic review. San Francisco (CA): Common Sense Media; 2008.
44. Salmon J, Jorna M, Hume C, et al. A translational research intervention to reduce screen behaviours and promote physical activity among children: Switch-2-Activity. Health Promot Int 2011;26(3):311–21.
45. McMurray RG, Harrel JS, Deng S, et al. The influence of physical activity, socio-economic status, and ethnicity on the weight status of adolescents. Obes Res 2000;8(2):130–9.
46. Vandewater E, Shim M, Caplovitz A. Linking obesity and activity level with children's television and video game use. J Adolesc 2004;27(1):71–85.
47. Wake M, Hesketh K, Waters E. Television, computer use and body mass index in Australian primary school children. J Paediatr Child Health 2003;39(2):130–4.
48. Kautiainen S, Koivusilta L, Lintonen T, et al. Use of information and communication technology and prevalence of overweight and obesity among adolescents. Int J Obes (Lond) 2005;29(8):925–33.
49. Rey-Lopez JP, Vicente-Rodriguez G, Biosca M, et al. Sedentary behaviour and obesity development in children and adolescents. Nutr Metab Cardiovasc Dis 2008;18(3):242–51.
50. Pate RR. Physically active video gaming: an effective strategy for obesity prevention? Arch Pediatr Adolesc Med 2008;162(9):895–6.
51. Graf DL, Pratt LV, Hester CN, et al. Playing active video games increases energy expenditure in children. Pediatrics 2009;124(2):534–40.
52. Daley A. Can exergaming contribute to improving physical activity levels and health outcomes in children? Pediatrics 2009;124:763–74.
53. Robinson TN. Reducing children's television viewing to prevent obesity: a randomized controlled trial. J Am Med Assoc 1999;282(16):1561–7.
54. Council on Communications and Media. Children, adolescents, obesity and the media. Elk Grove Village (IL): American Academy of Pediatrics; 2011.

55. Nelson MC, Neumark-Sztainer D, Hannan PJ, et al. Longitudinal and secular trends in physical activity and sedentary behavior during adolescence. Pediatrics 2006;118(6):e1627–34.
56. Hardy LL, Bass SL, Booth ML. Changes in sedentary behavior among adolescent girls: a 2.5-year prospective cohort study. J Adolesc Health 2007;40(2):158–65.
57. Burdette HL, Whitaker RC. A national study of neighborhood safety, outdoor play, television viewing, and obesity in preschool children. Pediatrics 2005; 116(3):657–62.
58. Taveras EM, Field AE, Berkey CS, et al. Longitudinal relationship between television viewing and leisure-time physical activity during adolescence. Pediatrics 2007;119(2):e314–25.
59. Melkevik O, Torsheim T, Iannotti RJ, et al. Is spending time in screen-based sedentary behaviors associated with less physical activity: a cross national investigation. Int J Behav Nutr Phys Act 2010;7:46–56.
60. Dowda M, Brown W, McIver K, et al. Policies and characteristics of the preschool environment and physical activity of young children. Pediatrics 2009; 123(2):e261–6.
61. Bower J, Hales D, Tate D, et al. The childcare environment and children's physical activity. Am J Prev Med 2008;34(1):23–9.
62. Dowda M, Pate R, Trost S, et al. Influences of preschool policies and practices on children's physical activity. J Community Health 2004;29(3):183–96.
63. Anderson S, Economos C, Must A. Active play and screen time in US children aged 4 to 11 years in relation to sociodemographic and weight status characteristics: a nationally representative cross-sectional analysis. BMC Public Health 2008;8:366–79.
64. Holt D, Ippolito P, Desrochers D, et al. Children's exposure to TV advertising in 1977 and 2004: information for the obesity debate. Federal Trade Commission Web site. Available at: http://www.ftc.gov/os/2007/06/cabecolor.pdf. 2007. Accessed February 12, 2012.
65. Kunkel D, McIlrath M. Message content in advertising to children. In: Palmer EL, Young BM, editors. The faces of televisual media: teaching violence, selling to children. Mahwah (NJ): Lawrence Erlbaum; 2003. p. 287–300.
66. Palmer E, Carpenter CF. Food and beverage marketing to children and youth: trends and issues. Media Psychol 2006;8(2):165–90.
67. Federal Trade Commission. Marketing food to children and adolescents: a review of industry expenditures, activities, and self-regulation. Federal Trade Commission web site. Available at: http://www.ftc.gov/opa/2008/07/foodmkting.shtm. Accessed February 11, 2012.
68. Story M, French S. Food advertising and marketing directed at children and adolescents in the US. Int J Behav Nutr Phys Act 2004;1(3):1–17.
69. Schwartz MB, Vartanian LR, Wharton CM, et al. Examining the nutritional quality of breakfast cereals marketed to children. J Am Diet Assoc 2008;108(4):702–5.
70. Gantz W, Schwartz N, Angelini J, et al. Food for thought: television food advertising to children in the United States. Menlo Park (CA): The Henry J Kaiser Family Foundation; 2007.
71. Stitt C, Kunkel D. Food advertising during children's television programming on broadcast and cable channels. Health Commun 2008;23:573–84.
72. Alvy LM, Calvert SL. Food marketing on popular children's websites: a content analysis. J Am Diet Assoc 2008;108(4):710–3.
73. Lingas E, Dorfman L, Bukofzer E. Nutrition content of food and beverage products on web sites popular with children. Am J Public Health 2009;99(7):1–10.

74. Kunkel D, Wilcox B. Children and media policy: historical perspectives and current practices. In: Singer DG, Singer JL, editors. Handbook of children and the media. 2nd edition. Thousand Oaks (CA): Sage Publications; 2012. p. 569–94.
75. Kunkel D, McKinley C, Wright P. Assessing compliance with industry self-regulation of televised food marketing to children. Oakland (CA): Children Now; 2009.
76. Simply Zesty. Trends in in-game advertising. Simply Zesty Web site. Available at: http://www.simplyzesty.com/advertising-and-marketing/advertising/trends-ingame-advertising/. 2010. Accessed February 13, 2012.
77. Montgomery KC, Chester J. Interactive food and beverage marketing: targeting adolescents in the digital age. J Adolesc Health 2009;45:S18–29.
78. Public Citizen. School commercialism: high costs, low revenues. Public Citizen Web site. Available at: www.citizen.org; 2012. Accessed February 12, 2012.
79. Linn S. Consuming kids: the hostile takeover of childhood. New York: The New Press; 2004.
80. Schor JB. Born to buy: the commercialized child and the new consumer culture. New York: Scribner; 2004.
81. Thomas SG. Buy, buy baby: how consumer culture manipulates parents and harms young minds. New York: Houghton Mifflin; 2007.
82. Harrison K. Is "fat free" good for me? A panel study of television viewing and children's nutritional knowledge and reasoning. Health Commun 2005;17:117–32.
83. Signorielli N, Lears M. Television and children's conceptions of nutrition: unhealthy messages. Health Commun 1997;4:245–57.
84. Signorielli N, Staples J. Television and children's conceptions of nutrition. Health Commun 1997;9:289–301.
85. Gunter B, Oates C, Blades M. Advertising to children on TV: content, impact, and regulation. Mahwah (NJ): Lawrence Erlbaum Associates; 2005.
86. Valkenburg PM, Buijzen M. Identifying determinants of young children's brand awareness: television, parents, and peers. Appl Dev Psychol 2005;26:456–68.
87. Buijzen M, Schuurman J, Bomhof E. Associations between children's television advertising exposure and their food consumption patterns: a household diary survey study. Appetite 2008;50(2):231–9.
88. O'Dougherty M, Story M, Stang J. Observations of parent-child co-shoppers in supermarkets: children's involvement in food selections, parental yielding, and refusal strategies. J Nutr Educ Behav 2006;38:183–8.
89. Wilson G, Wood K. The influence of children on parental purchases during supermarket shopping. Int J Consum Stud 2004;28(4):329–36.
90. Dotson MJ, Hyatt EM. Major influence factors in children's consumer socialization. J Consum Market 2005;22(1):35–43.
91. Dennison B, Russo T, Burdick P, et al. An intervention to reduce television viewing by preschool children. Arch Pediatr Adolesc Med 2004;158(2):170–6.
92. Epstein L, Roemmich J, Robinson J, et al. A randomized trial of the effects of reducing television viewing and computer use on body mass index in young children. Arch Pediatr Adolesc Med 2008;162(3):239–45.
93. Epstein L, Paluch R, Gordy C, et al. Decreasing sedentary behaviors in treating pediatric obesity. Arch Pediatr Adolesc Med 2000;154(3):220–6.
94. Gortmaker SL, Peterson K, Wiecha J, et al. Reducing obesity via a school-based interdisciplinary intervention among youth: planet health. Arch Pediatr Adolesc Med 1999;153:409–18.
95. Robinson T, Borzekowski D. Effects of the smart classroom curriculum to reduce child and family screen time. J Comm 2006;56(1):1–26.

96. Wahi G, Parkin P, Beyene J, et al. A systematic review and meta-analysis of randomized controlled trials. Arch Pediatr Adolesc Med 2011;165(11): 979–86.
97. Jordan A, Robinson T. Children, television viewing, and weight status: summary and recommendations from an expert panel meeting. Ann Am Acad Pol Soc Sci 2008;615:119–32.
98. Kunkel D. Mismeasurement of children's understanding of the persuasive intent of advertising. J Child Media 2010;4:109–17.
99. Wright P, Friestad M, Boush D. The development of marketplace persuasion knowledge in children, adolescents, and young adults. J Public Policy Mark 2005;24(2):222–33.
100. Kunkel D, Wilcox BL, Cantor J, et al. Report of the APA task force on advertising and children. American Psychological Association Web site. Available at: http://www.apa.org/pi/families/resources/advertising-children.pdf. 2004. Accessed February 13, 2012.
101. Kolish E, Hernandez M, Blanchard K. The Children's Food and Beverage Advertising Initiative in action: a report on compliance and implementation during 2010 and a five year retrospective: 2006-2011. Arlington (VA): Council of Better Business Bureaus; 2011.
102. Wootan M, Batada A, Balkus O. Report card on food-marketing policies. Center for Science in the Public Interest Web site. Available at: http://cspinet.org/new/pdf/marketingreportcard.pdf. Accessed February 13, 2012.
103. Batada A, Seitz M, Wootan M, et al. Nine out of 10 food advertisements shown during Saturday morning children's programming are for foods high in fat, sodium, or added sugars, or low in nutrients. J Am Diet Assoc 2008; 108:673–8.
104. Harris J, Weinberg M, Schwartz M, et al. Trends in television food advertising: progress in reducing unhealthy marketing to young people? Rudd Center for Food Policy and Obesity Web site. Available at: http://www.yaleruddcenter.org/resources/upload/docs/what/reports/RuddReport_TVFoodAdvertising_2.10.pdf. 2010. Accessed February 13, 2012.
105. Powell L, Szczypka G, Chaloupka F. Trends in exposure to television food advertisements among children and adolescents in the United States. Arch Pediatr Adolesc Med 2011;164(9):1–9.
106. Sunlight Foundation. Food and media companies lobby to weaken guidelines on marketing food to children. Sunlight Foundation Web site. Available at: http://reporting.sunlightfoundation.com/2011/Food_and_media_companies_lobby/. 2011. Accessed February 13. 2012.
107. Jaffe DL. Food marketing: can "voluntary" government restrictions improve children's health? Testimony on behalf of the Association of National Advertisers for the Subcommittee on Commerce, Manufacturing and Trade and the Subcommittee on Health House Energy and Commerce Committee. Washington, DC: House Energy and Commerce Committee; 2011. Available at: http://energycommerce.house.gov/hearings/hearingdetail.aspx?NewsID=8973. Accessed February 13, 2012.
108. Graff S, Kunkel D, Mermin S. Government can regulate food advertising to children because cognitive research shows that it is inherently misleading. Health Aff 2012;31(2):392–8.
109. Harris J, Graff S. Protecting young people from junk food advertising: implications of psychological research for First Amendment law. Am J Public Health 2012;102:214–22.

110. Veerman JL, Van Beeck E, Barendregt J, et al. By how much would limiting TV food advertising reduce childhood obesity? Eur J Public Health 2009;19(4): 365–9.
111. Ogden CL, Carroll MD, Kit BK, et al. Prevalence of obesity and trends in body mass index among US children and adolescents, 1999-2010. JAMA 2012; 307(5):E1–8.
112. Kraak V, Story M, Wartella E, et al. Industry progress to market a healthful diet to American children and adolescents. Am J Prev Med 2011;41(3):322–33.
113. Brescoll VL, Kersh R, Brownell KD. Assessing the feasibility and impact of federal childhood obesity policies. Ann Am Acad Pol Soc Sci 2008;615:178–94.
114. Klein JD, Dietz W. Childhood obesity: the new tobacco. Health Aff 2010;29(3): 388–92.

Obesity-Associated Nonalcoholic Fatty Liver Disease

Yusuf Yilmaz, MD[a,b], Zobair M. Younossi, MD, MPH, AGAF[c,*]

KEYWORDS

- Obesity • Nonalcoholic fatty liver disease • Epidemiology • Pathophysiology

KEY POINTS

- Obesity is strongly associated with the prevalence of nonalcoholic fatty liver disease (NAFLD) in both adult and pediatric populations.
- NAFLD is not invariably associated with obesity; in particular, there is evidence suggesting that NAFLD associated with the carriage of the high-risk rs738409 C>G single-nucleotide polymorphism in PNPLA3 is characterized by an increase in liver fat but no insulin resistance or adipose tissue inflammation.
- Nutrition, physical activity, and behavioral modifications are a critical component of the treatment regimen for all obese patients with NAFLD.
- Bariatric surgeries that affect or restrict the flow or absorption of food through the gastrointestinal tract may improve liver histology in morbidly obese patients with nonalcoholic steatohepatitis (NASH), although randomized clinical trials and quasi-randomized clinical studies are lacking.
- Although primary prevention is the long-term goal for diminishing obesity, early detection of both NASH and hepatic fibrosis using noninvasive biochemical and imaging markers that may replace liver biopsy is the current challenge.

INTRODUCTION

In past decades, the prevalence of obesity and overweight has been largely on the rise and this condition is on the brink of replacing smoking as the leading cause of preventable death.[1,2] Because of its association with an increased risk of suffering from

This article originally appeared in Clinics in Liver Disease, Volume 18, Issue 1, February 2014.

Conflicts of Interest: The authors have nothing to disclose.

[a] Department of Gastroenterology, School of Medicine, Marmara University, Fevzi Cakmak Mah, Mimar Sinan Cad. No. 41 Ust Kaynarca, Pendik, Istanbul 34899, Turkey; [b] Institute of Gastroenterology, Marmara University, Karaciger Arastirmalari Birimi, Basibuyuk, Maltepe, Istanbul 34840, Turkey; [c] Department of Medicine, Betty and Guy Beatty Center for Integrated Research, Center for Liver Diseases, Inova Health System, Inova Fairfax Hospital, Claude Moore Health Education and Research Building, 3rd Floor, 3300 Gallows Road, Falls Church, VA 22042, USA

* Corresponding author. Betty and Guy Beatty Center for Integrated Research, Claude Moore Health Education and Research Building, 3rd Floor, 3300 Gallows Road, Falls Church, VA.

E-mail address: zobair.younossi@inova.org

multiple diseases, obesity takes enormous health and personal tolls on modern societies (**Box 1**).[3–17] In fact, recently, the American Medical Association classified obesity as a disease. The obesity pandemic is likely the result of dramatic changes in the health, financial, and cultural environment over the past century.[18,19] Historically, in the years before the development of medical advancements that prevented debilitating diseases that caused their victims to become dreadfully feeble as they slowly died, being heavy was considered a sign of strength.[20] Indeed, at times when food was scarce, having a rotund physique was regarded as a status symbol and an indicator of prosperity and good health. But as times changed, the detrimental effects that overweight and obesity had on health were discovered and the conditions became so prevalent that they are currently recognized as leading risk factors for morbidity and mortality worldwide.[20] Although the fundamental cause of obesity is a positive imbalance between energy intake and energy expenditure, the etiology of obesity is multifactorial and involves a complex interaction among genetic, environmental, psychosocial, and behavioral factors.[21,22] From a pathophysiological standpoint, the development of obesity is associated with adipose tissue remodeling,[23] which leads to adipocyte dysfunction, abnormal cytokine secretion, and chronic low-grade inflammation.[24] Obesity also contributes to fat deposition in nonadipose tissues as ectopic fat, and it is a major risk factor for nonalcoholic fatty liver disease (NAFLD).[8]

NAFLD is a clinicopathological condition characterized by lipid accumulation in the liver causing liver damage similar to alcohol, but occurring in individuals without a history of chronic alcohol consumption.[25–30] NAFLD represents a wide spectrum of liver diseases ranging from simple steatosis to nonalcoholic steatohepatitis (NASH) and fibrosis to irreversible cirrhosis. Simple steatosis is defined histologically as greater than 5% hepatic lipid accumulation that rarely progresses to advanced liver diseases, whereas NASH constitutes an inflammation and hepatocellular damage having a

---

Box 1
Main obesity-associated diseases

Disease

Type 2 diabetes

Malignancies

Ischemic heart disease and heart failure

Venous thrombosis

Gastroesophageal reflux disease

Nonalcoholic fatty liver disease

Erectile dysfunction

Stroke

Hypertension

Osteoarthritis

Gout

Gallbladder disease

Obstructive sleep apnea

Asthma

Depression

strong potential to progress into cirrhosis, end-stage liver failure, and hepatocellular carcinoma (HCC).[31,32] Although NAFLD is an independent risk for cardiovascular disease and mortality, only NASH is associated with advanced liver disease. Therefore, treatment strategies to address NAFLD will be important, primarily, from a cardiovascular disease standpoint. On the other hand, clinical trials focused on liver disease must focus on patients with established diagnosis of NASH.

Concomitant with obesity, NAFLD is an increasingly recognized condition; up to 30% of adults in Western countries have NAFLD.[33] Insulin resistance is the key pathogenic abnormality associated with obesity-associated NAFLD.[34] A fatty liver is insulin resistant and overproduces glucose and very low density lipoprotein, and also other proinflammatory molecules, such as C-reactive protein and interleukin-6, which lead to hyperglycemia, hyperinsulinemia, and lipid disorders.[34] Due to those metabolic consequences, NAFLD is closely linked to the metabolic syndrome and is considered its hepatic expression.[25,35] However, not all obese persons deposit fat in the liver[35] and liver fat content is recognized to be independent of age, sex, and body mass index.[36] The deviation in liver fat accumulation between individuals is thought to explain, at least in part, why some obese and even lean individuals develop metabolic syndrome and insulin resistance, whereas others equally obese do not.[37] Similarly, not all patients with NAFLD have a diagnosis of metabolic syndrome.[38]

Over the past several years, epidemiologic studies have informed the public health impact of obesity-associated NAFLD. The aim of the present review is to give an overview of the epidemiology and the possible mechanisms underlying the observed association between obesity and NAFLD.

PREVALENCE AND INCIDENCE OF OBESITY-ASSOCIATED NAFLD

The prevalence of obesity has increased dramatically worldwide (**Fig. 1**), and the rate of obesity has more than doubled since 1980.[39] At least 1.46 billion adults were overweight or obese and 170 million of the world's children were overweight or obese in 2008.[40] In future prospects this number will only increase further.[41] In

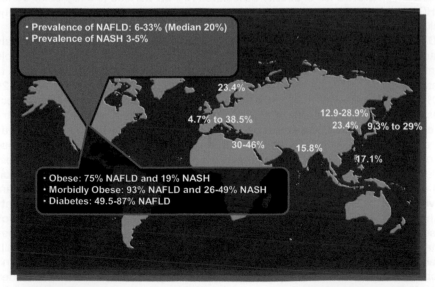

Fig. 1. Worldwide prevalence of NAFLD.

Europe, obesity has increased 10% to 40% in the past 10 years, and 10% to 25% of men and 10% to 30% of women are obese depending on the European country.[42] In the United States, 64% and 50% of the population are currently estimated to be overweight or obese, respectively.[43] The trend of the obesity epidemics is not only true for adults, but has also trickled down to affect children of all ages.[44] For children between the ages of 2 and 5, the prevalence of overweight and obesity increased from 5.0% to almost 14.0%, from 6.5% to almost 19.0% for children aged 6 to 11 years, and from 5.0% to 17.5% for adolescents between the ages of 12 and 19.[45]

Owing largely to the obesity epidemic, NAFLD is now the most common chronic liver condition worldwide. Based on the available data, NAFLD is estimated to occur in one-third of the general population in the United States.[46] In adults, women are most frequently diagnosed with NAFLD,[47] but this likely to represent a bias because men traditionally drink more alcohol than women and therefore may get excluded from a diagnosis based on alcohol intake. Concerning ethnicity, the lowest rates of NAFLD are seen in African American individuals and the highest in Asian and Hispanic individuals, with White in between.[48,49] Differently from NAFLD that can be screened by ultrasound and liver enzymes, determining the true prevalence of NASH is complicated.[28,29] Liver biopsy provides the only definitive diagnosis of NASH,[32] but its invasiveness and cost complicate its use as a diagnostic tool in the general population.[33] However, NASH seems to occur in approximately 3% of the lean population, 19% of the obese population, and the almost half of morbidly obese persons.[50,51] Importantly, the increasing burden of obesity-associated NAFLD will be transposed in the future to an increased need for hepatic transplantation for NASH. In fact, currently, NASH ranks as the third most common indication for liver transplantation (2001: 1.2%; 2009: 9.7%).[52] Another important future consequence of the epidemic of obesity-associated NAFLD will likely be a higher incidence of HCC. In a recent study conducted in 6 European countries, a total of 160 cases of HCC were detected during a 22-month follow-up; of note, 43% of the cases occurred in the absence of any other risk factor, such as alcohol abuse, cirrhosis, or infection with hepatitis B or C.[53] Therefore, the high prevalence of obesity-associated NAFLD will lead to a higher incidence of HCC in the general population with a concomitant burden on treatment availability, including liver transplantation.

Data on the incidence, predictive factors, and remission rates of NAFLD remain scanty. In particular, it is still difficult to draw firm conclusions regarding people from the general population who do not drink alcohol. A recent study conducted in a sample of the 147 patients who did not have NAFLD at baseline showed that 28 (19%) developed NAFLD at a 7-year follow-up.[54] Baseline body mass index, homeostasis model assessment of insulin resistance (HOMA-IR) score, blood cholesterol, triglycerides, leptin levels, and weight gain were significantly higher and adiponectin was lower among those who developed NAFLD at 7-year follow-up, compared with those who remained NAFLD-free. However, only weight gain and baseline HOMA-IR were independent predictors for the development of NAFLD.[54] Collectively, these longitudinal results suggest that obesity (and associated insulin resistance) is an important driving force behind the development of NAFLD. Conversely, one-third of patients with NAFLD showed improvement of their disease within the 7-year follow-up; such cases were chiefly dependent on modest weight reduction. Taken together, these data indicate that weight gain is an independent predictor of incident NAFLD in initially healthy subjects. Therefore, weight loss interventions represent the optimal (and probably the only effective) population-based strategy to reduce the future burden of NAFLD.

WORLDWIDE DIFFERENCES IN OBESITY-ASSOCIATED NAFLD

Although obesity and NAFLD are major health concerns worldwide, there are significant geographic differences in the prevalence of these conditions. In the United States, obesity is particularly associated with a heavy reliance on high-fat, high-calorie meals ("junk food"), which is more common among people of low socioeconomic position.[55] However, the opposite phenomenon can be found in developing countries, where it is the better-educated population that has the highest prevalence of obesity.[56] In general, robust comparisons of obesity prevalence between countries are difficult because of different methodological approaches in data collection.[57] The most important of these differences is probably that between measured and self-reported measures, with self-reported data more likely to underestimate the presence of obesity compared with actual measurements.[58-60] The worldwide prevalence of obesity is monitored by the World Health Organization through the Global Database on body mass index.[61,62] Although methodological caveats limit the reliability of comparisons between countries, Asia has the lowest and the Pacific Islands have the highest estimates of obesity prevalence.[62] Overall, most countries have rising trends of obesity. However, decreasing trends in the prevalence of obesity have been noted in men from Denmark and Saudi Arabia, as well as among women living in Denmark, Ireland, Saudi Arabia, Finland, and Spain.[62]

In parallel with the obesity epidemics, NAFLD has become the most common form of liver disease in the United States and most countries worldwide. Importantly, estimates in the US general population suggest that approximately 6 million individuals have progressed to NASH and about 600,000 to NASH-related cirrhosis.[63] NAFLD is also considered a major health issue in Japan, Australia, Europe, and the Middle East.[64-68] Studies conducted in the United States have suggested the presence of racial and ethnic variations in NAFLD, which result in a nonuniform distribution, with the disorder being most common among Latino individuals and least prevalent among African American individuals.[48,69-72] In general, Hispanic individuals have the highest prevalence of NAFLD, followed by non-Hispanic white individuals, whereas African American individuals have the lowest rates.[73] Such differences do not seem to be entirely explained by variations in the prevalence of the stereotypical metabolic risk factors and the effect of HOMA-IR on the risk of NASH is modified by ethnicity.[74] In particular, HOMA-IR does not seem to be a significant risk factor for NASH among Latinos, but it is significant among non-Latino whites.[75] Therefore, ethnicity may act as an important modifier of the association between obesity and NAFLD. It is also possible that these ethnic variations may reflect differences in genetic susceptibility to visceral adiposity, including hepatic involvement.[70] In general, the ongoing search for relevant genetic variants should result in a better understanding of energy metabolism and hopefully clarify the molecular mechanisms underlying the association between obesity and NAFLD. For example, Lallukka and colleagues[75] recently showed that NAFLD associated with the carriage of the high-risk rs738409 C>G single-nucleotide polymorphism in PNPLA3 is characterized by an increase in liver fat but no insulin resistance or adipose tissue inflammation, whereas obesity-associated NAFLD has all 3 of these features. Moreover, the Genetics of Obesity-Related Liver Disease (GOLD) Consortium has shown that NAFLD is about 26% to 27% heritable with 5 single-nucleotide polymorphisms in the PNPLA3, NCAN, GCKR, LYPLAL1, and PPP1R3B genes found to be associated with hepatic steatosis as measured using computed tomography in individuals of European ancestry.[76] In the future, it will be necessary to understand how specific combinations of environmental and genetic factors can give rise to ethnic differences in obesity-associated NAFLD. In this context, eliminating ethnic disparities in health should be an international priority, and obesity and NAFLD are prime targets.

CLINICAL CORRELATIONS

As discussed previously, NAFLD is a complex phenotype that arises from numerous genetic, environmental, behavioral, and even social origins.[34,63] The lifestyle factors contributing to the rising epidemic of obesity, and hence obesity-related NAFLD, are embedded in changes in society worldwide, mainly increased sedentary or inactive lifestyles[77] and consumption of calorie-rich foods in the form of soft drinks,[78] fast foods,[79] and sugar-enriched products.[80] Importantly, the clustering of unhealthy behaviors in obese children, such as poor nutritional habits, low levels of physical activity, and "junk-food" consumption dictate the need for multifaceted global programs to tackle global NAFLD risk at an early stage.[81,82] However, further research is needed to identify culturally sensitive strategies for obesity prevention and their impact not only on body weight, but also on NAFLD morbidity and mortality.

The importance of lifestyle management in the treatment of patients with obesity-related NAFLD cannot be overemphasized.[82] Adoption of a healthy lifestyle facilitates weight loss and decreases insulin resistance, and produces independent beneficial effects on the liver.[83–86] It is noteworthy that obesity-related metabolic abnormalities and fatty infiltration of the liver may be present even at a young age, and progress asymptomatically for decades before clinical manifestations set in.[87,88] In this scenario, nutrition, physical activity, and behavioral modifications aimed at weight loss are a critical component of the treatment regimen for all obese patients with NAFLD, even at a young age. Besides exercise and dieting, many therapeutic targets have been recently identified, on both the intake and the expenditure side of the energy balance equation, thereby providing hope that new agents may become available in the future.[89] For obese patients with NAFLD who do not respond to a trial of diet, exercise, and behavioral therapy, pharmacotherapy can be tried.[90] The use of drugs should be individualized, taking into account the severity of liver disease, comorbidities, and practical considerations related to cost, side effects, and frequency of dosing. Randomized trials and carefully constructed observational studies are needed to optimize effectiveness of nonsurgical weight loss interventions in obese patients and determine if the small weight losses they produce can have an impact on NAFLD incidence and clinical course. Moreover, intensive counseling and behavioral treatments need to be implemented to support long-term weight loss maintenance.

Among weight loss interventions, bariatric surgery results in the most dramatic weight loss, and, thus, studies of obese patients are the most likely to show reduced risk of NAFLD. Restrictive surgical procedures are indeed capable of inducing earlier satiety by decreasing the volume of the stomach (laparoscopic-adjustable gastric banding) or restricting the stomach and bypassing the small bowel (Roux-en-Y gastric bypass). Bariatric surgeries that affect or restrict the flow of food through the gastrointestinal tract have been shown to be an important therapeutic option that may result in a histologic improvement of NASH in morbidly obese patients (body mass index $\geq$35 kg/m^2).[91] Although long-term weight loss and resolution of obesity-associated NAFLD have been reported in most patients,[92] the lack of randomized clinical trials and quasi-randomized clinical studies still does not allow assessment of the benefits and harms of bariatric surgery as a therapeutic approach for patients with NASH.[93] Taken together, these data indicate that preventing and managing obesity-related NAFLD requires multiple, parallel efforts.

Table 1
Example of therapeutic interventions for NASH

Therapy	Histologic Improvement	Liver Enzymes	Impact on Hepatic Fibrosis	Use Recommended
Metformin	Not consistently	Not consistently improved	Unknown	Not recommended
Rosiglitazone	Not consistently	Improvement noted	Unknown	Not recommended
Pioglitazone	Not consistently	Not consistently	No	Considered to treat diabetes but not solely for NASH
Vitamin E	Improvement	Improvement	No	Recommended for nondiabetic individuals with biopsy-proven NASH
Statins	Unknown	Unknown	Unknown	Not recommended for treatment of NASH but can be used to treat hyperlipidemia in patients with NAFLD
Orlistat	No	Possible improvement with weight loss	Unknown	Not recommended solely for NASH
Ursodeoxycholic acid	No improvement	Not consistently	No	Not recommended

In addition to weight reduction strategies to address obesity-related NAFLD, there have been a number of medical therapies designed to treat histologic NASH. These include antioxidants, such as vitamin E, insulin sensitizers, such as pioglitazone and metformin, lipid-lowering agents, such as statins, and cytoprotective agents, such as ursodeoxycholic acid (**Table 1**).[94,95] Despite decades of clinical trials, current evidence suggests that only vitamin E may be beneficial for treatment of nondiabetic patients with NASH, but no single treatment can be recommended to all patients with NASH.[94,95]

SUMMARY

The main conclusions from this review are the following: (1) obesity is strongly associated with the prevalence of NAFLD in both adult and pediatric populations[95,96]; (2) obesity is an independent predictor of incident NAFLD in initially healthy subjects; (3) NAFLD is not invariably associated with obesity, in particular there is evidence suggesting that NAFLD associated with high-risk rs738409 C>G single-nucleotide polymorphism in PNPLA3 is characterized by an increase in liver fat but no insulin resistance or adipose tissue inflammation; (4) there are significant ethnic variations in the prevalence of obesity-related NAFLD, which may be explained by both environmental and genetic factors; (5) nutrition, physical activity, and behavior modifications aimed at weight loss are a critical component of the treatment regimen for all obese patients with NAFLD; (6) bariatric surgeries that affect or restrict the flow of food through the gastrointestinal tract may improve liver histology in morbidly obese patients with NASH, although randomized clinical trials and quasi-randomized clinical studies are lacking; (7) because only patients with histologically proven NASH are shown to have progressive liver disease, clinical trials must focus on this subtype of NAFLD; and (8) although vitamin E is recommended for nondiabetic individuals with NASH, no single treatment could be recommended to all patients with NASH.

In general, obesity-associated NAFLD should be considered an important and often underrecognized public health problem. As the prevalence of obesity increases, the prevalence of NAFLD with its associated morbidity and mortality will increase as well. Although primary prevention is the long-term goal for diminishing the prevalence of obesity, early detection of both NASH and hepatic fibrosis using noninvasive biochemical and imaging markers that may replace liver biopsy is the overriding current challenge.[97–102] From a clinical standpoint, treating NAFLD in the obese requires addressing obesity as part of the therapeutic plan. Lifestyle management is required in every case, with a focus on weight loss and risk reduction. In most patients, additional therapies, including medications, aggressive diet counseling, behavioral techniques, and sometimes bariatric surgery in morbidly obese subjects, will be required. Data showing improved liver histology among individuals who lose weight and maintain the loss strengthen confidence in the obesity-NAFLD link, and also provide a note of hope that weight loss in obese individuals may help them prevent end-stage liver disease. Research on the biologic mechanisms underlying the obesity-NAFLD link is still in early stages, but may lead to potential treatments and preventive agents.

REFERENCES

1. Flegal KM, Williamson DF, Pamuk ER, et al. Estimating deaths attributable to obesity in the United States. Am J Public Health 2004;94:1486–9.
2. Hurt RT, Frazier TH, McClave SA, et al. Obesity epidemic: overview, pathophysiology, and the intensive care unit conundrum. JPEN J Parenter Enteral Nutr 2011;35:4S–13S.
3. Kautzky-Willer A, Lemmens-Gruber R. Obesity and diabetes. Handb Exp Pharmacol 2012;214:307–40.
4. Vucenik I, Stains JP. Obesity and cancer risk: evidence, mechanisms, and recommendations. Ann N Y Acad Sci 2012;1271:37–43.
5. Nikolopoulou A, Kadoglou NP. Obesity and metabolic syndrome as related to cardiovascular disease. Expert Rev Cardiovasc Ther 2012;10:933–9.
6. Braekkan SK, Siegerink B, Lijfering WM, et al. Role of obesity in the etiology of deep vein thrombosis and pulmonary embolism: current epidemiological insights. Semin Thromb Hemost 2013;39:533–40.
7. Nocon M, Labenz J, Jaspersen D, et al. Association of body mass index with heartburn, regurgitation and esophagitis: results of the progression of gastroesophageal reflux disease study. J Gastroenterol Hepatol 2007;22:1728–31.
8. Fabbrini E, Sullivan S, Klein S. Obesity and nonalcoholic fatty liver disease: biochemical, metabolic, and clinical implications. Hepatology 2010;51:679–89.
9. Diaz-Arjonilla M, Schwarcz M, Swerdloff RS, et al. Obesity, low testosterone levels and erectile dysfunction. Int J Impot Res 2009;21:89–98.
10. Kernan WN, Inzucchi SE, Sawan C, et al. Obesity: a stubbornly obvious target for stroke prevention. Stroke 2013;44:278–86.

11. Aghamohammadzadeh R, Heagerty AM. Obesity-related hypertension: epidemiology, pathophysiology, treatments, and the contribution of perivascular adipose tissue. Ann Med 2012;44(Suppl 1):S74–84.
12. Berenbaum F, Eymard F, Houard X. Osteoarthritis, inflammation and obesity. Curr Opin Rheumatol 2013;25:114–8.
13. Juraschek SP, Miller ER 3rd, Gelber AC. Body mass index, obesity, and prevalent gout in the United States in 1988–1994 and 2007–2010. Arthritis Care Res (Hoboken) 2013;65:127–32.
14. Dittrick GW, Thompson JS, Campos D, et al. Gallbladder pathology in morbid obesity. Obes Surg 2005;15:238–42.
15. Drager LF, Togeiro SM, Polotsky VY, et al. Obstructive sleep apnea: a cardiometabolic risk in obesity and metabolic syndrome. J Am Coll Cardiol 2013. http://dx.doi.org/10.1016/j.jacc.2013.05.045.
16. Boulet LP. Asthma and obesity. Clin Exp Allergy 2013;43:8–21.
17. Luppino FS, de Wit LM, Bouvy PF, et al. Overweight, obesity, and depression: a systematic review and meta-analysis of longitudinal studies. Arch Gen Psychiatry 2010;67:220–9.
18. Novak NL, Brownell KD. Role of policy and government in the obesity epidemic. Circulation 2012;126:2345–52.
19. Matthews CM. Exploring the obesity epidemic. Proc (Bayl Univ Med Cent) 2012; 25:276–7.
20. Eknoyan G. A history of obesity, or how what was good became ugly and then bad. Adv Chronic Kidney Dis 2006;13:421–7.
21. Nammi S, Koka S, Chinnala KM, et al. Obesity: an overview on its current perspectives and treatment options. Nutr J 2004;3:3.
22. Lee YS. The role of genes in the current obesity epidemic. Ann Acad Med Singapore 2009;38:45–53.
23. Sun K, Kusminski CM, Scherer PE. Adipose tissue remodeling and obesity. J Clin Invest 2011;121:2094–101.
24. Lee MJ, Wu Y, Fried SK. Adipose tissue remodeling in pathophysiology of obesity. Curr Opin Clin Nutr Metab Care 2010;13:371–6.
25. Kim CH, Younossi ZM. Nonalcoholic fatty liver disease: a manifestation of the metabolic syndrome. Cleve Clin J Med 2008;75:721–8.
26. Younossi ZM. Review article: current management of non-alcoholic fatty liver disease and non-alcoholic steatohepatitis. Aliment Pharmacol Ther 2008;28:2–12.
27. Nugent C, Younossi ZM. Evaluation and management of obesity-related nonalcoholic fatty liver disease. Nat Clin Pract Gastroenterol Hepatol 2007;4:432–41.
28. Ong JP, Younossi ZM. Epidemiology and natural history of NAFLD and NASH. Clin Liver Dis 2007;11:1–16.
29. Milić S, Stimac D. Nonalcoholic fatty liver disease/steatohepatitis: epidemiology, pathogenesis, clinical presentation and treatment. Dig Dis 2012;30:158–62.
30. Paredes AH, Torres DM, Harrison SA. Nonalcoholic fatty liver disease. Clin Liver Dis 2012;16:397–419.
31. Kleiner DE, Brunt EM. Nonalcoholic fatty liver disease: pathologic patterns and biopsy evaluation in clinical research. Semin Liver Dis 2012;32:3–13.
32. Brunt EM, Tiniakos DG. Histopathology of nonalcoholic fatty liver disease. World J Gastroenterol 2010;16:5286–96.
33. Bellentani S, Scaglioni F, Marino M, et al. Epidemiology of non-alcoholic fatty liver disease. Dig Dis 2010;28:155–61.
34. Tuyama AC, Chang CY. Non-alcoholic fatty liver disease. J Diabetes 2012;4: 266–80.

35. Liu CJ. Prevalence and risk factors for non-alcoholic fatty liver disease in Asian people who are not obese. J Gastroenterol Hepatol 2012;27:1555–60.
36. Jakobsen MU, Berentzen T, Sørensen TI, et al. Abdominal obesity and fatty liver. Epidemiol Rev 2007;29:77–87.
37. Kotronen A, Yki-Järvinen H. Fatty liver: a novel component of the metabolic syndrome. Arterioscler Thromb Vasc Biol 2008;28:27–38.
38. Yilmaz Y. NAFLD in the absence of metabolic syndrome: different epidemiology, pathogenetic mechanisms, risk factors for disease progression? Semin Liver Dis 2012;32:14–21.
39. Flegal KM, Carroll MD, Ogden CL, et al. Prevalence and trends in obesity among US adults, 1999–2008. JAMA 2010;303:235–41.
40. Swinburn BA, Sacks G, Hall KD, et al. The global obesity pandemic: shaped by global drivers and local environments. Lancet 2011;378:804–14.
41. Shamseddeen H, Getty JZ, Hamdallah IN, et al. Epidemiology and economic impact of obesity and type 2 diabetes. Surg Clin North Am 2011;91:1163–72.
42. Tsigos C, Hainer V, Basdevant A, et al. Management of obesity in adults: European clinical practice guidelines. Obes Facts 2008;1:106–16.
43. Ogden CL, Carroll MD. Prevalence of overweight, obesity, and extreme obesity among adults: United States, trends 1960–1962 through 2007–2008. Hyattsville, MD: National Center for Health Statistics; 2010.
44. Skelton JA, Irby MB, Grzywacz JG, et al. Etiologies of obesity in children: nature and nurture. Pediatr Clin North Am 2011;58:1333–54.
45. Ben-Sefer E, Ben-Natan M, Ehrenfeld M. Childhood obesity: current literature, policy and implications for practice. Int Nurs Rev 2009;56:166–73.
46. Sanyal AJ. NASH: a global health problem. Hepatol Res 2011;41:670–4.
47. Sheth SG, Gordan FD, Chopra S. Nonalcoholic steatohepatitis. Ann Intern Med 1997;126:137–45.
48. Browning JD, Szczepaniak LS, Dobbins R, et al. Prevalence of hepatic steatosis in an urban population in the United States: impact of ethnicity. Hepatology 2004;40:1387–95.
49. Petersen KF, Dufour S, Feng J, et al. Increased prevalence of insulin resistance and nonalcoholic fatty liver disease in Asian-Indian men. Proc Natl Acad Sci U S A 2006;103:18273–7.
50. Silverman JF, O'Brien KF, Long S, et al. Liver pathology in morbidly obese patients with and without diabetes. Am J Gastroenterol 1990;85:1349–55.
51. Wanless IR, Lentz JS. Fatty liver hepatitis (steatohepatitis) and obesity: an autopsy study with analysis of risk factors. Hepatology 1990;12:1106–10.
52. Charlton MR, Burns JM, Pedersen RA, et al. Frequency and outcomes of liver transplantation for nonalcoholic steatohepatitis in the United States. Gastroenterology 2011;141:1249–53.
53. Reeves H, Villa E, Bellentani S, et al. The emerging impact of hepatocellular carcinoma arising on a background of NAFLD. J Hepatol 2012;56(Suppl 2):S3.
54. Zelber-Sagi S, Lotan R, Shlomai A, et al. Predictors for incidence and remission of NAFLD in the general population during a seven-year prospective follow-up. J Hepatol 2012;56:1145–51.
55. Jeffery RW, French SA. Epidemic obesity in the United States: are fast foods and television viewing contributing? Am J Public Health 1998;88:277–80.
56. Drewnowski A, Specter SE. Poverty and obesity: the role of energy density and energy costs. Am J Clin Nutr 2004;79:6–16.
57. Ford ES, Mokdad AH, Giles WH, et al. Geographic variation in the prevalence of obesity, diabetes, and obesity-related behaviors. Obes Res 2005;13:118–22.

58. Shields M, Connor Gorber S, Janssen I, et al. Bias in self-reported estimates of obesity in Canadian health surveys: an update on correction equations for adults. Health Rep 2011;22:35–45.

59. Dauphinot V, Wolff H, Naudin F, et al. New obesity body mass index threshold for self-reported data. J Epidemiol Community Health 2009;63:128–32.

60. Bolton-Smith C, Woodward M, Tunstall-Pedoe H, et al. Accuracy of the estimated prevalence of obesity from self reported height and weight in an adult Scottish population. J Epidemiol Community Health 2000;54:143–8.

61. Nguyen DM, El-Serag HB. The epidemiology of obesity. Gastroenterol Clin North Am 2010;39:1–7.

62. Nishida C, Mucavele P. Monitoring the rapidly emerging public health problem of overweight and obesity: the WHO global database on body mass index. SCN News 2005;29:5–12.

63. Erickson SK. Nonalcoholic fatty liver disease. J Lipid Res 2009;50(Suppl): S412–6.

64. Bacon BR, Farahvash MJ, Janney CG, et al. Nonalcoholic steatohepatitis: an expanded clinical entity. Gastroenterology 1994;107:1103–9.

65. Matteoni CA, Younossi ZM, Gramlich T, et al. Nonalcoholic fatty liver disease: a spectrum of clinical and pathological severity. Gastroenterology 1999;116: 1413–9.

66. Powell EE, Cooksley WG, Hanson R, et al. The natural history of nonalcoholic steatohepatitis: a follow-up study of forty-two patients for up to 21 years. Hepatology 1990;11:74–80.

67. Nonomura A, Mizukami Y, Unoura M, et al. Clinicopathologic study of alcohol-like liver disease in non-alcoholics; non-alcoholic steatohepatitis and fibrosis. Gastroenterol Jpn 1992;27:521–8.

68. el Hassan AY, Ibrahim EM, al Mulhim FA, et al. Fatty infiltration of the liver: analysis of prevalence, radiological and clinical features and influence on patient management. Br J Radiol 1992;65:774–8.

69. Clark JM, Brancati FL, Diehl AM. The prevalence and etiology of elevated aminotransferase levels in the United States. Am J Gastroenterol 2003;98: 960–7.

70. Weston SR, Leyden W, Murphy R, et al. Racial and ethnic distribution of nonalcoholic fatty liver in persons with newly diagnosed chronic liver disease. Hepatology 2005;41:372–9.

71. Caldwell SH, Harris DM, Patrie JT, et al. Is NASH underdiagnosed among African Americans? Am J Gastroenterol 2002;97:1496–500.

72. Mohanty SR, Troy TN, Huo D, et al. Influence of ethnicity on histological differences in non-alcoholic fatty liver disease. J Hepatol 2009;50:797–804.

73. Attar BM, Van Thiel DH. Current concepts and management approaches in nonalcoholic fatty liver disease. ScientificWorldJournal 2013;2013:481893.

74. Bambha K, Belt P, Abraham M, et al. Ethnicity and nonalcoholic fatty liver disease. Hepatology 2012;55:769–80.

75. Lallukka S, Sevastianova K, Perttilä J, et al. Adipose tissue is inflamed in NAFLD due to obesity but not in NAFLD due to genetic variation in PNPLA3. Diabetologia 2013;56:886–92.

76. Speliotes EK, Yerges-Armstrong LM, Wu J, et al. Genome-wide association analysis identifies variants associated with nonalcoholic fatty liver disease that have distinct effects on metabolic traits. PLoS Genet 2011;7:e1001324.

77. Rector RS, Thyfault JP. Does physical inactivity cause nonalcoholic fatty liver disease? J Appl Physiol 2011;111:1828–35.

78. Zelber-Sagi S, Nitzan-Kaluski D, Goldsmith R, et al. Long term nutritional intake and the risk for non-alcoholic fatty liver disease (NAFLD): a population based study. J Hepatol 2007;47:711–7.
79. Zelber-Sagi S, Ratziu V, Oren R. Nutrition and physical activity in NAFLD: an overview of the epidemiological evidence. World J Gastroenterol 2011;17: 3377–89.
80. Yilmaz Y. Review article: fructose in non-alcoholic fatty liver disease. Aliment Pharmacol Ther 2012;35:1135–44.
81. Caporaso N, Morisco F, Camera S, et al. Dietary approach in the prevention and treatment of NAFLD. Front Biosci 2012;17:2259–68.
82. Centis E, Marzocchi R, Suppini A, et al. The role of lifestyle change in the prevention and treatment of NAFLD. Curr Pharm Des 2013;19(29):5270–9.
83. Rodriguez B, Torres DM, Harrison SA. Physical activity: an essential component of lifestyle modification in NAFLD. Nat Rev Gastroenterol Hepatol 2012;9: 726–31.
84. Thoma C, Day CP, Trenell MI. Lifestyle interventions for the treatment of non-alcoholic fatty liver disease in adults: a systematic review. J Hepatol 2012;56: 255–66.
85. Patel AA, Torres DM, Harrison SA. Effect of weight loss on nonalcoholic fatty liver disease. J Clin Gastroenterol 2009;43:970–4.
86. Harrison SA, Day CP. Benefits of lifestyle modification in NAFLD. Gut 2007;56: 1760–9.
87. Pacifico L, Anania C, Martino F, et al. Management of metabolic syndrome in children and adolescents. Nutr Metab Cardiovasc Dis 2011;21:455–66.
88. Nobili V, Svegliati-Baroni G, Alisi A, et al. A 360-degree overview of paediatric NAFLD: recent insights. J Hepatol 2013;58:1218–29.
89. Malinowski SS, Byrd JS, Bell AM, et al. Pharmacologic therapy for nonalcoholic fatty liver disease in adults. Pharmacotherapy 2013;33:223–42.
90. Nakajima K. Multidisciplinary pharmacotherapeutic options for nonalcoholic fatty liver disease. Int J Hepatol 2012;2012:950693.
91. Rabl C, Campos GM. The impact of bariatric surgery on nonalcoholic steatohepatitis. Semin Liver Dis 2012;32:80–91.
92. Pillai AA, Rinella ME. Non-alcoholic fatty liver disease: is bariatric surgery the answer? Clin Liver Dis 2009;13:689–710.
93. Chavez-Tapia NC, Tellez-Avila FI, Barrientos-Gutierrez T, et al. Bariatric surgery for non-alcoholic steatohepatitis in obese patients. Cochrane Database Syst Rev 2010;(1):CD007340.
94. Sanyal AJ, Chalasani N, Kowdley KV, et al, NASH CRN. Pioglitazone, vitamin E, or placebo for nonalcoholic steatohepatitis. N Engl J Med 2010;362(18): 1675–85.
95. Chalasani N, Younossi Z, Lavine JE, et al. The diagnosis and management of non-alcoholic fatty liver disease: practice guideline by the American Gastroenterological Association, American Association for the Study of Liver Diseases, and American College of Gastroenterology. Gastroenterology 2012; 143(2):503.
96. Younossi ZM, Stepanova M, Afendy M, et al. Changes in the prevalence of the most common causes of chronic liver diseases in the United States from 1988 to 2008. Clin Gastroenterol Hepatol 2011;9(6):524–30.
97. Yilmaz Y, Ulukaya E. Toward a biochemical diagnosis of NASH: insights from pathophysiology for distinguishing simple steatosis from steatohepatitis. Curr Med Chem 2011;18:725–32.

98. Wieckowska A, Feldstein AE. Diagnosis of nonalcoholic fatty liver disease: invasive versus noninvasive. Semin Liver Dis 2008;28:386–95.
99. Wieckowska A, McCullough AJ, Feldstein AE. Noninvasive diagnosis and monitoring of nonalcoholic steatohepatitis: present and future. Hepatology 2007;46: 582–9.
100. Miele L, Forgione A, Gasbarrini G, et al. Noninvasive assessment of fibrosis in non-alcoholic fatty liver disease (NAFLD) and non-alcoholic steatohepatitis (NASH). Transl Res 2007;149:114–25.
101. Younossi ZM, Page S, Rafiq N, et al. A biomarker panel for non-alcoholic steatohepatitis (NASH) and NASH-related fibrosis. Obes Surg 2011;21:431–9.
102. Younossi ZM, Jarrar M, Nugent C, et al. A novel diagnostic biomarker panel for obesity-related nonalcoholic steatohepatitis (NASH). Obes Surg 2008;18: 1430–7.

Obesity and GERD

Paul Chang, MD, Frank Friedenberg, MD, MS (Epi)*

KEYWORDS

- Obesity • Gastroesophageal reflux disease • Barrett esophagus • Waist-to-hip ratio
- Adiponectin • Leptin

KEY POINTS

- The prevalence of obesity and gastroesophageal reflux disease (GERD) has increased substantially in the past 30 years.
- Central adiposity, measured as the waist-to-hip ratio, is more closely associated with GERD complications than measures of overall obesity such as body mass index.
- Visceral adipose tissue is metabolically active and secretes adipokines along with inflammatory cytokines that may predispose to complications of GERD such as Barrett esophagus and esophageal carcinoma.

INTRODUCTION
Disease Description

The typical manifestations of gastroesophageal reflux disease (GERD) are heartburn and/or regurgitation. GERD can be further classified into erosive GERD and nonerosive GERD based on endoscopic appearance of esophageal mucosa. The term "atypical GERD" is used in situations where the predominant symptoms are extraesophageal such as cough, laryngitis, and asthma.[1] GERD is a common disorder with a prevalence of approximately 20% in the United States.[2] The recognized sequelae of GERD include Barrett esophagus (BE) and esophageal adenocarcinoma. Obesity, defined as a body mass index (BMI) greater than or equal to 30, is common in the Western world and is increasing in other parts of the world, particularly Asia. Epidemiologic data demonstrate that overall obesity (typically measured as BMI kg/m^2) is a risk factor for both GERD and esophageal adenocarcinoma.[3] There is evidence that central abdominal obesity, as opposed to an elevated BMI, is the most important factor associated with BE (**Table 1**).[4]

PREVALENCE/INCIDENCE

A systematic review estimated the prevalence of GERD in the United States at 18.1% to 27.8%.[2] El-Serag and others in their systematic review divided studies on the

This article originally appeared in Gastroenterology Clinics of North America, Volume 43, Issue 1, March 2014.

Section of Gastroenterology, Temple University School of Medicine, Philadelphia, PA, USA

* Corresponding author. Temple University Hospital, Parkinson Pavilion, 8th Floor, 3401 North Broad Street, Philadelphia, PA 19140.

E-mail address: friedfk@tuhs.temple.edu

2352-7986/14/$ – see front matter © 2014 Elsevier Inc. All rights reserved.

Table 1
Risk factors for GERD
Obesity
Caffeine intake
Spicy foods
Tobacco
Pregnancy
Alcohol
Recumbent position
Connective tissue disorders
Hiatal hernia
Decreased LES tone
Zollinger-Ellison syndrome
Post-prandial supination

prevalence of GERD into 4 temporal categories. Relative to pre-1995, the rate ratio for GERD prevalence was 1.45 for the period 1995 to 1999, 1.46 for 2000 to 2004, and 1.51 for 2005 to 2009. Obesity is an even more common health issue in the United States. Data from the 2009–2010 National Health and Examination Survey estimate a prevalence of 35.5% for men and 35.8% for women, which is not significantly changed compared with the period 2003 to 2008.[5] Previous trends showed that the prevalence of obesity was increasing in America but the trend may be beginning to level.

Cross-sectional epidemiologic studies have demonstrated a higher prevalence of GERD in obese individuals compared with the nonobese. Jacobsen and colleagues[6] used a supplemental GERD questionnaire added to the Nurses' Health Study to show that subjects who reported at least weekly symptoms had a near linear increase in the adjusted odds ratio (OR) for reflux symptoms for each BMI strata. A similar link was seen in the results from the 80,110 insurance members from the Kaiser Permanente Multi-Phasic Health Check-Up cohort.[7] The association between BMI and GERD was stronger among whites compared with black members, with ORs of 1.58 and 1.33, respectively. When controlling for abdominal diameter the ORs were 1.39 and 1.15, respectively.

Smaller studies have confirmed the link between obesity and GERD. El-Serag and others interviewed 453 hospital employees and found that 26% had weekly heartburn or regurgitation symptoms.[8] Subjects were offered endoscopy and 196 agreed, and they found that increasing levels of obesity were associated with a greater likelihood of GERD and esophagitis. The proportion of subjects with GERD symptoms were 23.3%, 26.7%, and 50% for BMI groups <25, 25–30, and >30, respectively. Prevalence rates for erosive esophagitis (EE) were 12.5%, 29.8%, and 26.9%. Two small cohort studies from Olmstead County, MN have also evaluated the relationship between obesity and GERD. The first study identified obesity as a risk factor for the initial development of GERD as well as the persistence of symptoms.[9] The second study found that BMI was associated with GERD (OR = 1.9) independent of diet and energy expenditure.[10]

The effect of weight change on GERD symptoms has been studied. Jacobson and colleagues[6] studied select individuals from the Nurses' Health Study and found that an increase of BMI by more than 3.5 kg/m^2 when compared with no weight change was associated with an increase risk of frequent symptoms of reflux.

WORLD-WIDE INCIDENCE RATES

The prevalence of obesity is somewhat lower outside of the United States. The European Prospective Investigation into Cancer and Nutrition study estimated the prevalence of obesity was 17% in 2005, which increased from 13% in 1998.[11] Based on a systematic review, the prevalence rate of GERD in Europe was estimated to be 15% for the period 2005 to 2009. Similar to the trend seen in the United States, this prevalence rate is significantly higher than the rate before 1995.[2] The epidemiologic relationship between obesity and GERD has been observed in Europe as well. The German National Health Interview and Examination Survey found the OR for GERD to be 1.8 for overweight and 2.6 for obese individuals.[12] In England, the Bristol Helicobacter Project found that obese individuals had an OR of 2.91 for heartburn and an OR of 2.23 for regurgitation.[13] A telephone survey in Spain of 2500 subjects revealed that obese individuals had an OR of 1.74 for GERD symptoms. It was also noted that patients with GERD symptoms for more than 10 years were more likely to be obese (OR = 1.92).[14] This group also found that a weight gain of more than 5 kg in the past year demonstrated a 2.7-fold higher risk of new GERD symptoms.[15] In Norway, Nilsson and colleagues[16] conducted nationwide surveys during the periods 1984 to 1986 (N = 74,599) and 1995 to 1997 (N = 65,363). They found that for severely obese men (BMI>35 kg/m^2) the OR for GERD was 3.3, whereas the OR for severely obese women was 6.3. A link showing an association between estrogen levels and GERD was observed. Premenopausal women and those who were post-menopausal but taking hormone replacement therapy were at an increased risk for GERD relative to untreated post-menopausal women.

A relationship between obesity and GERD has been seen in Asia. Kang and colleagues[17] studied 2457 subjects who underwent upper endoscopy in Korea. They found a relationship between higher strata of BMI and the presence of EE. In Shanghai, a nested case-control study found an association between obesity and dwelling in an urban environment with GERD.[18]

Studies that have failed to identify a relationship between GERD and obesity have also been reported. A study of 820 subjects from Sweden showed that those who had been overweight or obese had an adjusted OR of 0.99 for GERD. They also found no association between obesity and severity of reflux symptoms.[19] Similarly, a prospective cohort study in Olmsted, MN of 607 individuals surveyed more than 10.5 years did not find an association with GERD symptoms and weight loss of greater than 10 pounds.[9]

In summary, the preponderance of population-based studies supports the association between obesity and GERD reflux. The association has been demonstrated in the United States where obesity rates are the highest and has also been seen in Europe and Eastern Asia (**Fig. 1**). Shortcomings of these studies are that they primarily relied on self-reported height and weight to calculate BMI and did not look specifically at abdominal obesity. There appears to be a dose response as well with increasing levels of obesity associated with higher prevalence rates. Weight loss has not been consistently associated with amelioration of symptoms at a population level.

CLINICAL CORRELATION
Complications of GERD

Long-term complications of GERD such as EE, BE, and esophageal adenocarcinoma have been associated with obesity. In a large endoscopic study, El-Serag reported that relative to those with no erosions, those with EE were more likely to be overweight or obese.[8] A similar association was seen in Korea where Lee and colleagues[29] did an endoscopy study in Korea studying 3000 participants. They found that obese individuals compared to normal weight subjects had an OR of 3.3 for EE. A meta-analysis by Hampel and colleagues[30] confirmed the association with increasing levels of obesity and esophageal mucosal injury.

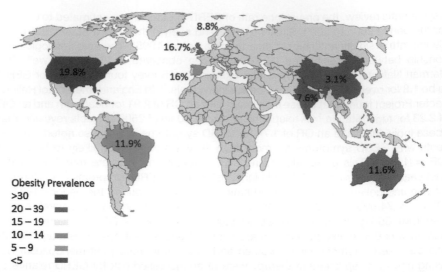

Fig. 1. World map of obesity and GERD prevalence in select countries. The obesity prevalence coded by the color key. The percentages indicate the GERD prevalence. (*Data from* Refs.[2,5,20–28])

Associations of BE and obesity have been demonstrated by Stein and colleagues[31] who established that for each 5-unit increase in BMI, the risk of BE increased by 35%. Abdominal obesity ("central obesity") has been shown to be a more specific risk factor for BE. Corley and colleagues,[32] using data from the Kaiser Permanente database, found that a larger abdominal circumference (measured at the iliac crest with the abdomen relaxed), independent of BMI, was associated with BE. Edelstein and colleagues[33] found that for individuals in the highest category of waist-to-hip ratio the adjusted OR for BE was 1.9 and 4.1 for long-segment BE. Rubenstein and colleagues[34] found that abdominal obesity as measured by waist circumference increased the risk of EE and BE, whereas gluteofemoral obesity was protective. Finally, El-Serag used abdominal computed tomographic imaging to demonstrate that greater amounts of visceral adipose tissue but not subcutaneous adipose tissue conferred a significantly increased risk for BE.[4]

Not all studies have demonstrated an association between obesity and BE. An Australian study found that BMI was not an independent risk factor for BE.[35] A study in Canada by Veugelers and colleagues[36] also did not show an association between obesity and BE. They did, however, find an association of BMI with esophageal adenocarcinoma.

The incidence of esophageal adenocarcinoma has been rising in the United States.[37] From 1975 to 2001, the incidence of esophageal adenocarcinoma has increased approximately 6-fold. There are several studies that have examined the relationship between obesity and esophageal adenocarcinoma. In 1998, a National Cancer Institute study by Chow and colleagues[38] found an association between increasing strata of BMI and esophageal cancer, specifically among younger nonsmoking individuals. A Swedish study identified obesity with an OR of 16.2 for the development of adenocarcinoma compared with the leanest individuals (BMI<22 kg/m^2). A recently pooled analysis from 12 world-wide epidemiologic studies showed that patients with a BMI greater than or equal to 40 compared with nonoverweight patients had an OR of 4.76 for esophageal adenocarcinoma.[39] Engel and colleagues[40] found that the population attributable risk (proportion of occurrences in the population that may be preventable if a factor were totally eliminated) for body weight (using BMI<23.1 as the control group) increased steadily from 5.4% (BMI = 23.2–25.1) to 21.3% (BMI = 27.3–40.1).

Pathophysiology

Several physiologic abnormalities that could lead to prolonged esophageal acid exposure have been found to occur more frequently in obese compared with normal weight individuals. Many of these disturbances have been identified in the severely obese (BMI>35) before bariatric surgery and may not apply to those with lesser degrees of obesity. For example, esophageal manometry before bariatric surgery has revealed that many patients have a motility disorder. In a study of 345 patients, 25.6% of patients had abnormal manometry. The most common abnormal findings were nutcracker esophagus and nonspecific motility disorder.[41] Other studies in severely obese subjects revealed similar findings, with nonspecific motility disorder, nutcracker esophagus, and hypotensive lower esophageal sphincter (LES) as the most common manometric abnormalities.[42,43] Interestingly, most of these patients were asymptomatic.

Studies looking specifically at prebariatric surgical patients with symptoms of GERD excluding asymptomatic patients have also been reported. Hong and colleagues[44] studied 61 patients and 32.8% had abnormal manometry, most commonly nonspecific esophageal motor disorder. Another study using manometry, 24-hour pH measurement, and impedance grouped patients into 3 groups. Group 1 (control group) had 10 normal-weight asymptomatic subjects, group 2 had 22 nonobese GERD patients, and group 3 consisted of 22 obese GERD patients. All group 1 patients had normal esophageal acid exposure, motility, and bolus transit. From group 2 there were 5 patients with abnormal manometry, 2 with ineffective esophageal motility, 2 with nutcracker esophagus, and 1 with hypertensive LES (>50 mm Hg). Group 3 also had 5 patients with abnormal manometry, including 2 with ineffective esophageal motility, 2 with nutcracker esophagus, and 1 with diffuse esophageal spasm. The only difference between the obese and nonobese GERD subjects was that obese patients had fewer episodes of complete bolus transit (as measured by impedance) compared with the nonobese, 66% versus 88% $P = .01$.[45]

A hypotensive LES, defined as basal pressure less than 10 mm Hg, is clearly a predisposing factor for GERD. Studies examining the relationship between LES pressure and BMI have been performed, although the results are inconsistent. One study examined 64 consecutive patients and divided subjects into 3 groups. Group A had 23 subjects with a BMI less than 25, group B had 25 subjects with a BMI between 25 and 30, and group C had 16 subjects with a BMI >30. The investigators observed a strong inverse relationship between BMI and LES pressure ($P<.001$).[46]

Transient relaxations of the lower esophageal sphincter (TRLES) have been observed to be more common in patients with obesity. The main stimulus for TRLES is gastric distension, particularly in the fundus.[47,48] A study by Wu and colleagues[49] divided subjects into 3 groups, 28 obese, 28 overweight, and 28 normal subjects. These individuals were studied with upper endoscopy, manometry, and pH recordings. The overweight and obese groups were found to have significantly higher rates of TRLES during the 2-hour postprandial period (obese group 17.3, overweight 3.8, normal 2.1 episodes per hour; $P<.001$). Total distal esophageal acid exposure as well as the proportion of TRLES accompanied by acid reflux was also greater in the obese and overweight groups.

The presence of a hiatal hernia has also been associated with obesity. Suter and colleagues[41] studied morbidly obese patients with history of reflux symptoms with upper endoscopy, 24-hour pH monitoring, and manometry. They observed that of

345 subjects approximately half had a hiatal hernia. Furthermore, patients with a hiatal hernia were more likely to have esophagitis compared with those without a hiatal hernia. Pandolfino and colleagues[50] subsequently reported that obese patients have a pressure gradient along the esophagogastric junction that supported the development of a hiatal hernia.

Abdominal obesity likely increases intra-abdominal pressure due to transmission of gravitational force of the adipose tissue to the abdominal cavity. Lambert and colleagues[51] studied morbidly obese patients with a urinary catheter as a surrogate for intra-abdominal pressure and found that obese patients compared with nonobese patients had higher intra-abdominal pressures. This relationship between obesity and elevated intra-abdominal/intragastric pressures has been confirmed by others with use of intragastric manometry.[52,53]

Gastric volume and motor abnormalities have been proposed as other mechanisms for GERD in obese individuals. Multiple studies have found that the capacitance of gastric contents in obese subjects is larger compared with lean individuals.[54,55] Whether the greater volume of contents leads to increased GERD is not known. It has also been theorized that obese individuals may have delayed gastric emptying due to neuronal or humoral mechanisms.[56–58] Buchholz and colleagues[59] using standardized scintigraphic gastric emptying studies showed no difference in gastric emptying in obese and nonobese patients. Retention percentages at 1 hour and 4 hours were 48% and 47% and 1.7% and 1.1%, respectively.

The link between obesity and esophageal neoplasia may be via altered secretion of adipokines such as adiponectin and leptin. Adiponectin is a protein that has antiinflammatory and immunomodulatory functions and stimulates apoptosis.[60] Secretion of adiponectin decreases with obesity. Rubenstein and colleagues[61] found an inverse association between plasma adiponectin levels and the presence of BE in a case-control study. In a separate study, this group found that levels of the low molecular weight subtype of adiponectin were inversely associated with the risk of BE.[62] In contrast to the inverse relationship seen between obesity and adiponectin, leptin levels correlate directly with obesity.[63] Leptin is secreted by adipocytes and gastric chief cells and has been shown to have mitogenic properties and induce proliferation in several human cell lines including esophageal cancer cells.[64] Kendall and colleagues[65] found that male subjects with BE had higher levels of plasma leptin relative to healthy controls. Those with a leptin level in the highest quartile had an OR of 3.3 for the presence of BE. The link between BE and central obesity (rather than BMI) may be partially explained by the fact that leptin reaches very high values in central obesity (**Figs. 2** and **3**).

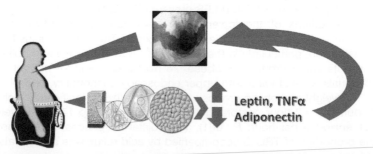

Leptin, TNFα
Adiponectin

Fig. 2. Mechanism of increased abdominal obesity leading to BE. The increased adipose tissue leads to increases in leptin and tumor necrosis factor α, which have been linked to a higher risk of BE. Increased adipose tissue has also been inversely linked with adiponectin levels, which are protective for the development of BE.

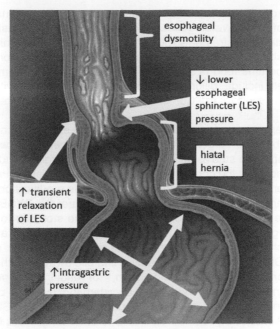

Fig. 3. Summary of potential pathogenic mechanisms in the obese leading to GERD.

Weight Loss and GERD

In Norway, the HUNT 3 study surveyed 44,997 subjects from 2006 to 2009 and found that weight loss was dose-dependently associated with a reduction of symptoms.[66] A prospective cohort study of 332 obese adults enrolled in a structured weight loss program was performed by Singh and colleagues.[67] Mean weight loss was 13 kg and the prevalence of GERD decreased from 37% to 15% with 81% of subjects experiencing a reduction in symptom scores. Fraser-Moodie and colleagues[68] observed 34 patients who had GERD and a BMI greater than 23. Patients were given dietary advice (not a structured weight loss protocol) and lost an average of 4 kg. For the 27 patients (79.4%) who lost weight, they experienced a decrease in symptoms by 75% compared with baseline using a modified DeMeester questionnaire.

Conversely, Kjellin and colleagues[69] randomized 20 obese patients with GERD to a very low-caloric diet (VLCD, approximately 800 Kcal/d) or no change in diet. Patients in the VLCD group lost an average of 10.8 kg, and the control group gained 0.6 kg. Those on the VLCD did not have significant changes in reflux symptoms. The control group was then given the VLCD and lost weight but again no change in symptoms were observed. Frederiksen and colleagues[70] studied 34 morbidly obese patients who were prescribed liquid VLCD pre- and post-vertical banded gastroplasty and found no change in acid exposure time from baseline compared with 10 to 14 days after the start of VLCD or 3 weeks after surgery.

Bariatric Surgery and GERD

The use of bariatric surgery has increased over the past 2 decades as it has proved to be an effective treatment of obesity. In 2006, the number of bariatric operations in the United States was reported as 112,999.[71] Bariatric surgeries can be classified as restrictive, malabsorptive, or both. In restrictive surgeries, the gastric anatomy is altered to reduce gastric volume to induce early satiety, which in turn leads to weight loss. Examples of restrictive surgeries include vertical banded gastroplasty, intragastric balloon, sleeve gastrectomy (SG) and laparoscopic adjustable gastric banding (LAGB). Malabsorptive surgeries induce malabsorption by shortening the gut, and/or altering the time food is subjected to digestive juices. Examples of malabsorptive surgeries include biliopancreatic diversion with and without duodenal switch and jejunoileal bypass. Combined techniques include Roux-en-Y gastric bypass (RYGB).

There have been several studies published that have examined changes in GERD symptoms after bariatric surgery. These studies have generally been prospective cohort and retrospective studies and not randomized controlled studies. Analysis of results is confounded by the common practice of repairing hiatal hernias during surgery and the heterogeneity in post-bariatric diet, lifestyle modification, and PPI use.

The most common bariatric surgeries performed are the RYGB, LAGB,[71] and more recently the SG.[72] RYGB involves stapling of the stomach to create a small ($\leq$30 mL) upper gastric pouch.[73] A roux limb of jejunum is then anastomosed to the gastric pouch bypassing absorptive surface area. Potential mechanism for RYGB reducing GERD symptoms include diverting bile away from the esophagus,[74] eliminating acid production in the gastric pouch,[75] or reducing volume of acid refluxate.[76] De Groot and colleagues[77] performed a systematic review on bariatric surgery and the effects on GERD. They identified 8 studies that evaluated GERD symptoms after RYGB and 3 studies that compared RYGB to other weight loss techniques with respect to GERD symptoms. All studies showed an improvement in GERD symptoms after RYGB except one by Korenkov and colleagues.[78] Most of the studies included in the systematic review used questionnaires (QUEST) and only 4 of the 11 studies used objective measurements (ie, endoscopy, 24-h pH monitoring) to define GERD.

In LAGB, a band device is placed around the fundus of the stomach immediately below the esophagogastric junction, and a subcutaneous reservoir is used to adjust the band size.[77] In the same systematic review by De Groot and colleagues,[77] the effects of LAGB on GERD were analyzed. Of 12 studies identified, 4 reported a positive effect on GERD, 2 studies found a positive effect so long as there was no pouch dilatation and/or a prior esophageal motility disorder was not present, 2 studies showed an increase in symptoms based on pH metry, manometry, and/or endoscopic findings, and 4 studies showed conflicting data in different domains of the diagnostic tests. Because of the conflicting data it is difficult to come to a conclusion on the effects of LAGB on GERD symptoms.

In SG the stomach is vertically divided reducing the volume to about 25% of the original size. In a recent systematic review by Chiu and colleagues,[72] which included 15 studies of SG, 4 found a post-operative increase in GERD prevalence, 7 showed reduced prevalence, and in 4 studies the prevalence before and after surgery could not be determined. As with most studies examining the effects of bariatric surgery on GERD, there was significant heterogeneity between studies including differences in follow-up time ranging from 6 months to 5 years, differences in the case definition of GERD, and lack of control groups. Therefore, similar to LAGB, it is difficult to come to conclusively determine the effects of SG on GERD.

In summary, surgical management is an effective approach to weight loss, and the data has generally shown that this weight loss can have positive effects on GERD. RYGB studies have provided the most consistent evidence for reducing GERD after surgery. Thus, in patients with severe GERD preoperatively, preferential consideration should be given to performing RYGB as the bariatric procedure of choice.

SUMMARY

Epidemiologic studies strongly suggest that the prevalence of GERD is increasing, and the major contributing factor to this trend is the rising prevalence of obesity. This trend has been observed in the United States as well as in Europe and Eastern Asia. Central obesity as opposed to BMI appears to be a better marker for the risks of metaplastic and neoplastic complications of GERD. Visceral adipose tissue secretes hormonal mediators, which may increase the risk of BE and esophageal adenocarcinoma. Studies have preliminarily shown that leptin levels have a direct relationship with the development of BE, and adiponectin levels are inversely related. Other factors that may play a role in the pathophysiology of GERD due to obesity include the increased prevalence of esophageal motor disorders, higher number of transient relaxations of the lower esophageal sphincter, and increased intra-abdominal pressure. The benefit of weight loss through diet as a means to decrease GERD symptoms is not yet established. However, gastric bypass surgery leads to substantial weight loss and the data have consistently shown a decrease in GERD symptoms. Unfortunately, only a few studies have included pH data to confirm improvement after surgery.

REFERENCES

1. Hom C, Vaezi MF. Extraesophageal manifestations of gastroesophageal reflux disease. Gastroenterol Clin North Am 2013;42(1):71–91.
2. El-Serag HB, Sweet S, Winchester CC, et al. Update on the epidemiology of gastro-oesophageal reflux disease: a systematic review. Gut 2013. [Epub ahead of print].
3. El-Serag H. The association between obesity and GERD: a review of the epidemiological evidence. Dig Dis Sci 2008;53(9):2307–12.
4. El-Serag HB, Hashmi A, Garcia J, et al. Visceral abdominal obesity measured by CT scan is associated with an increased risk of Barrett's oesophagus: a case-control study. Gut 2013. [Epub ahead of print].
5. Flegal KM, Carroll MD, Kit BK, et al. Prevalence of obesity and trends in the distribution of body mass index among US adults, 1999-2010. JAMA 2012;307(5):491–7.
6. Jacobson BC, Somers SC, Fuchs CS, et al. Body-mass index and symptoms of gastroesophageal reflux in women. N Engl J Med 2006;354(22):2340–8.
7. Corley DA, Kubo A, Zhao W. Abdominal obesity, ethnicity and gastro-oesophageal reflux symptoms. Gut 2007;56(6):756–62.
8. El-Serag HB, Graham DY, Satia JA, et al. Obesity is an independent risk factor for GERD symptoms and erosive esophagitis. Am J Gastroenterol 2005;100(6):1243–50.
9. Cremonini F, Locke GR 3rd, Schleck CD, et al. Relationship between upper gastrointestinal symptoms and changes in body weight in a population-based cohort. Neurogastroenterol Motil 2006;18(11):987–94.
10. Nandurkar S, Locke GR 3rd, Fett S, et al. Relationship between body mass index, diet, exercise and gastro-oesophageal reflux symptoms in a community. Aliment Pharmacol Ther 2004;20(5):497–505.
11. von Ruesten A, Steffen A, Floegel A, et al. Trend in obesity prevalence in European adult cohort populations during follow-up since 1996 and their predictions to 2015. PLoS One 2011;6(11):e27455.
12. Nocon M, Labenz J, Willich SN. Lifestyle factors and symptoms of gastro-oesophageal reflux – a population-based study. Aliment Pharmacol Ther 2006;23(1):169–74.

13. Murray L, Johnston B, Lane A, et al. Relationship between body mass and gastro-oesophageal reflux symptoms: the Bristol Helicobacter Project. Int J Epidemiol 2003;32(4):645–50.
14. Diaz-Rubio M, Moreno-Elola-Olaso C, Rey E, et al. Symptoms of gastro-oesophageal reflux: prevalence, severity, duration and associated factors in a Spanish population. Aliment Pharmacol Ther 2004;19(1):95–105.
15. Rey E, Moreno-Elola-Olaso C, Artalejo FR, et al. Association between weight gain and symptoms of gastroesophageal reflux in the general population. Am J Gastroenterol 2006;101(2):229–33.
16. Nilsson M, Johnsen R, Ye W, et al. Obesity and estrogen as risk factors for gastro-esophageal reflux symptoms. JAMA 2003;290(1):66–72.
17. Kang MS, Park DI, Oh SY, et al. Abdominal obesity is an independent risk factor for erosive esophagitis in a Korean population. J Gastroenterol Hepatol 2007; 22(10):1656–61.
18. Ma XQ, Cao Y, Wang R, et al. Prevalence of, and factors associated with, gastro-esophageal reflux disease: a population-based study in Shanghai, China. Dis Esophagus 2009;22(4):317–22.
19. Lagergren J, Bergstrom R, Nyren O. No relation between body mass and gastro-oesophageal reflux symptoms in a Swedish population based study. Gut 2000; 47(1):26–9.
20. Martinez JA, Moreno B, Martinez-Gonzalez MA. Prevalence of obesity in Spain. Obes Rev 2004;5(3):171–2.
21. Ponce J, Vegazo O, Beltran B, et al. Prevalence of gastro-oesophageal reflux disease in Spain and associated factors. Aliment Pharmacol Ther 2006;23(1): 175–84.
22. Thorburn AW. Prevalence of obesity in Australia. Obes Rev 2005;6(3):187–9.
23. Moraes-Filho JP, Chinzon D, Eisig JN, et al. Prevalence of heartburn and gastro-esophageal reflux disease in the urban Brazilian population. Arq Gastroenterol 2005;42(2):122–7.
24. Rtveladze K, Marsh T, Webber L, et al. Health and economic burden of obesity in Brazil. PLoS One 2013;8(7):e68785.
25. He J, Ma X, Zhao Y, et al. A population-based survey of the epidemiology of symptom-defined gastroesophageal reflux disease: the Systematic Investigation of Gastrointestinal Diseases in China. BMC Gastroenterol 2010;10:94.
26. Wang Y, Mi J, Shan XY, et al. Is China facing an obesity epidemic and the consequences? The trends in obesity and chronic disease in China. Int J Obes (Lond) 2007;31(1):177–88.
27. Bhatia SJ, Reddy DN, Ghoshal UC, et al. Epidemiology and symptom profile of gastroesophageal reflux in the Indian population: report of the Indian Society of Gastroenterology Task Force. Indian J Gastroenterol 2011;30(3):118–27.
28. Griffiths PL, Bentley ME. The nutrition transition is underway in India. J Nutr 2001; 131(10):2692–700.
29. Lee HL, Eun CS, Lee OY, et al. Association between GERD-related erosive esophagitis and obesity. J Clin Gastroenterol 2008;42(6):672–5.
30. Hampel H, Abraham NS, El-Serag HB. Meta-analysis: obesity and the risk for gastroesophageal reflux disease and its complications. Ann Intern Med 2005; 143(3):199–211.
31. Stein DJ, El-Serag HB, Kuczynski J, et al. The association of body mass index with Barrett's oesophagus. Aliment Pharmacol Ther 2005;22(10):1005–10.
32. Corley DA, Kubo A, Levin TR, et al. Abdominal obesity and body mass index as risk factors for Barrett's esophagus. Gastroenterology 2007;133(1):34–41 [quiz: 311].

33. Edelstein ZR, Bronner MP, Rosen SN, et al. Risk factors for Barrett's esophagus among patients with gastroesophageal reflux disease: a community clinic-based case-control study. Am J Gastroenterol 2009;104(4):834–42.
34. Rubenstein JH, Morgenstern H, Chey WD, et al. Protective role of gluteofemoral obesity in erosive oesophagitis and Barrett's oesophagus. Gut 2013. [Epub ahead of print].
35. Smith KJ, O'Brien SM, Smithers BM, et al. Interactions among smoking, obesity, and symptoms of acid reflux in Barrett's esophagus. Cancer Epidemiol Biomarkers Prev 2005;14(11 Pt 1):2481–6.
36. Veugelers PJ, Porter GA, Guernsey DL, et al. Obesity and lifestyle risk factors for gastroesophageal reflux disease, Barrett esophagus and esophageal adenocarcinoma. Dis Esophagus 2006;19(5):321–8.
37. Pohl H, Welch HG. The role of overdiagnosis and reclassification in the marked increase of esophageal adenocarcinoma incidence. J Natl Cancer Inst 2005; 97(2):142–6.
38. Chow WH, Blot WJ, Vaughan TL, et al. Body mass index and risk of adenocarcinomas of the esophagus and gastric cardia. J Natl Cancer Inst 1998;90(2): 150–5.
39. Hoyo C, Cook MB, Kamangar F, et al. Body mass index in relation to oesophageal and oesophagogastric junction adenocarcinomas: a pooled analysis from the International BEACON Consortium. Int J Epidemiol 2012;41(6): 1706–18.
40. Engel LS, Chow WH, Vaughan TL, et al. Population attributable risks of esophageal and gastric cancers. J Natl Cancer Inst 2003;95(18):1404–13.
41. Suter M, Dorta G, Giusti V, et al. Gastro-esophageal reflux and esophageal motility disorders in morbidly obese patients. Obes Surg 2004;14(7):959–66.
42. Koppman JS, Poggi L, Szomstein S, et al. Esophageal motility disorders in the morbidly obese population. Surg Endosc 2007;21(5):761–4.
43. Jaffin BW, Knoepflmacher P, Greenstein R. High prevalence of asymptomatic esophageal motility disorders among morbidly obese patients. Obes Surg 1999;9(4):390–5.
44. Hong D, Khajanchee YS, Pereira N, et al. Manometric abnormalities and gastro esophageal reflux disease in the morbidly obese. Obes Surg 2004;14:744–9.
45. Quiroga E, Cuenca-Abente F, Flum D, et al. Impaired esophageal function in morbidly obese patients with gastroesophageal reflux disease: evaluation with multichannel intraluminal impedance. Surg Endosc 2006;20(5):739–43.
46. Kouklakis G, Moschos J, Kountouras J, et al. Relationship between obesity and gastroesophageal reflux disease as recorded by 3-hour esophageal pH monitoring. Rom J Gastroenterol 2005;14(2):117–21.
47. Kahrilas PJ, Shi G, Manka M, et al. Increased frequency of transient lower esophageal sphincter relaxation induced by gastric distention in reflux patients with hiatal hernia. Gastroenterology 2000;118(4):688–95.
48. Fisher BL, Pennathur A, Mutnick JL, et al. Obesity correlates with gastroesophageal reflux. Dig Dis Sci 1999;44(11):2290–4.
49. Wu JC, Mui LM, Cheung CM, et al. Obesity is associated with increased transient lower esophageal sphincter relaxation. Gastroenterology 2007;132(3): 883–9.
50. Pandolfino JE, El-Serag HB, Zhang Q, et al. Obesity: a challenge to esophagogastric junction integrity. Gastroenterology 2006;130(3):639–49.
51. Lambert DM, Marceau S, Forse RA. Intra-abdominal pressure in the morbidly obese. Obes Surg 2005;15(9):1225–32.

52. Varela JE, Hinojosa M, Nguyen N. Correlations between intra-abdominal pressure and obesity-related co-morbidities. Surg Obes Relat Dis 2009;5(5):524–8.
53. El-Serag HB, Tran T, Richardson P, et al. Anthropometric correlates of intragastric pressure. Scand J Gastroenterol 2006;41(8):887–91.
54. Geliebter A, Hashim SA. Gastric capacity in normal, obese, and bulimic women. Physiol Behav 2001;74(4–5):743–6.
55. Granstrom L, Backman L. Stomach distension in extremely obese and in normal subjects. Acta Chir Scand 1985;151(4):367–70.
56. Zahorska-Markiewicz B, Jonderko K, Lelek A, et al. Gastric emptying and obesity. Hum Nutr Clin Nutr 1986;40(4):309–13.
57. Wright RA, Krinksy S, Fleeman C, et al. Gastric emptying and obesity. Gastroenterology 1983;84(4):747–51.
58. Tosetti C, Corinaldesi R, Stangellini V, et al. Gastric emptying of solids in morbid obesity. Int J Obes Relat Metab Disord 1996;20(3):200–5.
59. Buchholz V, Berkenstadt H, Goitein D, et al. Gastric emptying is not prolonged in obese patients. Surg Obes Relat Dis 2013;9(5):714–7.
60. Kelesidis I, Kelesidis T, Mantzoros CS. Adiponectin and cancer: a systematic review. Br J Cancer 2006;94(9):1221–5.
61. Rubenstein JH, Dahlkemper A, Kao JY, et al. A pilot study of the association of low plasma adiponectin and Barrett's esophagus. Am J Gastroenterol 2008; 103(6):1358–64.
62. Rubenstein JH, Kao JY, Madanick RD, et al. Association of adiponectin multimers with Barrett's oesophagus. Gut 2009;58(12):1583–9.
63. Weigle DS. Leptin and other secretory products of adipocytes modulate multiple physiological functions. Ann Endocrinol (Paris) 1997;58(2):132–6.
64. Ogunwobi O, Mutungi G, Beales IL. Leptin stimulates proliferation and inhibits apoptosis in Barrett's esophageal adenocarcinoma cells by cyclooxygenase-2-dependent, prostaglandin-E2-mediated transactivation of the epidermal growth factor receptor and c-Jun NH2-terminal kinase activation. Endocrinology 2006; 147(9):4505–16.
65. Kendall BJ, Macdonald GA, Hayward NK, et al. Leptin and the risk of Barrett's oesophagus. Gut 2008;57(4):448–54.
66. Ness-Jensen E, Lindam A, Lagergren J, et al. Weight loss and reduction in gastroesophageal reflux. A prospective population-based cohort study: the HUNT study. Am J Gastroenterol 2013;108(3):376–82.
67. Singh M, Lee J, Gupta N, et al. Weight loss can lead to resolution of gastroesophageal reflux disease symptoms: a prospective intervention trial. Obesity (Silver Spring) 2013;21(2):284–90.
68. Fraser-Moodie CA, Norton B, Gornall C, et al. Weight loss has an independent beneficial effect on symptoms of gastro-oesophageal reflux in patients who are overweight. Scand J Gastroenterol 1999;34(4):337–40.
69. Kjellin A, Ramel S, Rossner S, et al. Gastroesophageal reflux in obese patients is not reduced by weight reduction. Scand J Gastroenterol 1996;31(11): 1047–51.
70. Frederiksen SG, Johansson J, Johnsson F, et al. Neither low-calorie diet nor vertical banded gastroplasty influence gastro-oesophageal reflux in morbidly obese patients. Eur J Surg 2000;166(4):296–300.
71. Livingston EH. The incidence of bariatric surgery has plateaued in the U.S. Am J Surg 2010;200(3):378–85.
72. Chiu S, Birch DW, Shi X, et al. Effect of sleeve gastrectomy on gastroesophageal reflux disease: a systematic review. Surg Obes Relat Dis 2011;7(4):510–5.

73. DeMaria EJ. Bariatric surgery for morbid obesity. N Engl J Med 2007;356(21): 2176–83.
74. Frezza EE, Ikramuddin S, Gourash W, et al. Symptomatic improvement in gastro-esophageal reflux disease (GERD) following laparoscopic Roux-en-Y gastric bypass. Surg Endosc 2002;16(7):1027–31.
75. Cobey F, Oelschlager B. Complete regression of Barrett's esophagus after Roux-en-Y gastric bypass. Obes Surg 2005;15(5):710–2.
76. Smith SC, Edwards CB, Goodman GN. Symptomatic and clinical improvement in morbidly obese patients with gastroesophageal reflux disease following Roux-en-Y gastric bypass. Obes Surg 1997;7(6):479–84.
77. De Groot NL, Burgerhart JS, Van De Meeberg PC, et al. Systematic review: the effects of conservative and surgical treatment for obesity on gastro-oesophageal reflux disease. Aliment Pharmacol Ther 2009;30(11–12):1091–102.
78. Korenkov M, Kohler L, Yucel N, et al. Esophageal motility and reflux symptoms before and after bariatric surgery. Obes Surg 2002;12(1):72–6.

Sleep Disorders and the Development of Insulin Resistance and Obesity

Omar Mesarwi, MD, Jan Polak, MD, PhD, Jonathan Jun, MD, Vsevolod Y. Polotsky, MD, PhD*

KEYWORDS

- Obstructive sleep apnea • Metabolism • Diabetes • Sleep duration
- Glucose homeostasis

KEY POINTS

- Sleep is a physiologic state of decreased metabolism and likely serves a reparative role. Normal sleep is characterized by reduced glucose turnover by the brain and other metabolically active tissues. Circadian and sleep-related changes in glucose tolerance occur in normal subjects.
- Sleep duration has decreased over the past several decades. Cross-sectional and longitudinal data suggest a link between short sleep duration and type 2 diabetes. Forced decreased sleep duration in healthy individuals has also been linked to impaired glucose homeostasis.
- Obstructive sleep apnea is a disorder of sleep characterized by diminished or abrogated airflow, which results in intermittent hypoxia and sleep fragmentation. A large body of evidence suggests an association between this disorder and impaired glucose tolerance.
- The quality and quantity of sleep may have a profound effect on obesity and type 2 diabetes, and therefore should be routinely assessed in endocrine clinic.

METABOLIC CHANGES IN SLEEP

Sleep is a physiologic recurring state of reduced consciousness, absence of voluntary activity, and suspension of sensory activity. Approximately one-third of the human life-span is spent asleep, yet its fundamental purpose remains a mystery.[1] However, it has been recognized for decades that sleep is necessary for optimal cognitive, motor, and

This article originally appeared in Endocrinology and Metabolism Clinics of North America, Volume 42, Issue 3, September 2013.

Funded by: NIH; Grant number(s): HL080105; HL109475.

The authors disclose no financial relationships relevant to the authorship of this article.

Division of Pulmonary and Critical Care Medicine, Johns Hopkins University School of Medicine, 5501 Hopkins Bayview Circle, Baltimore, MD 21224, USA

* Corresponding author.

E-mail address: vpolots1@jhmi.edu

http://dx.doi.org/10.1016/j.ccol.2014.09.035
2352-7986/14/$ – see front matter © 2014 Elsevier Inc. All rights reserved.

metabolic function.[2,3] The drive to sleep is controlled by homeostatic regulation, whereby sleep propensity increases with time awake, and circadian regulation, where sleep propensity waxes and wanes according to the time of day.[4]

According to a standardized scoring system by the American Academy of Sleep Medicine,[5] adult sleep is divided into two electroencephalographic stages: non–rapid eye movement (NREM) and rapid-eye movement (REM) sleep. NREM sleep is further subdivided into progressively deeper sleep stages referred to as N1, N2, and N3 (or slow-wave) sleep. During sleep, sympathetic tone, blood pressure, heart rate, and metabolic rate decrease, with a more marked suppression of these parameters in NREM compared with REM stages.[6] In fact, REM is often described as "active" sleep, as neural activity during REM bears a resemblance to wakefulness. Respiratory, hemodynamic, and metabolic changes are also more erratic during REM sleep. A typical sleep period in adults consists mostly of NREM sleep with REM periods occurring at 60-minute to 90-minute intervals. Slow-wave sleep usually occurs in the first few hours of sleep, whereas periods of REM lengthen toward the latter hours of sleep.

One of the functions ascribed to sleep is that of energy conservation and cellular repair. Sleep induces a fall in core body temperature, and oxygen consumption decreases by approximately 10%. These changes were first described in the mid-twentieth century[7] and were reaffirmed by subsequent studies,[8] some of which showed trends of progressively lower metabolic rate from REM to N3 sleep.[9,10] Glycogen stores,[11] ATP levels,[12] and peptide synthesis[13] increase in the brain during mammalian sleep. Several hormonal changes that foster growth and repair also occur during NREM sleep. For example, growth hormone (GH) is secreted in the first few hours of a usual sleep period, coinciding with slow-wave sleep.[14–16] This surge in GH induces peripheral lipolysis and insulin resistance, which may serve to spare the catabolism of protein and glucose stores.[17] Conversely, most hypothalamic-pituitary-adrenocortical hormones are suppressed during NREM sleep.[18]

In parallel with decreased metabolic demand, glucose turnover decreases during sleep. The changes in energy requirements during sleep are driven by a decrease in the high glucose demands of the brain.[19–21] During NREM sleep, the uptake of glucose in the brain falls progressively, while hepatic glucose output decreases, commensurate with reductions in cerebral blood flow.[22,23] Other metabolically active tissues, such as skeletal muscle, exhibit reduced blood flow and glucose uptake.[24,25] The underlying mechanisms involved in lowered glucose turnover during sleep are not known. Patterns of insulin, cortisol, and glucagon secretion make these hormones unlikely mediators.[26] Substrate availability does not limit brain metabolism, as glucose levels are usually unchanged during sleep.[22,26]

Increases in glucose during sleep have been reported, but in the setting of specialized research or clinical conditions. Frank and colleagues[27] infused glucose continuously in volunteers as they slept, either at night or during the day. This protocol revealed a rise in evening glucose and a superimposed glucose elevation during sleep, regardless of the time of day that sleep occurred. Thus, circadian and sleep-related changes in glucose tolerance occur in healthy subjects. This physiologic glucose intolerance may play a role in the "dawn phenomenon," which describes hyperglycemia in the early morning in diabetic subjects.[28] This phenomenon was also later reported to a lesser degree in individuals who did not have diabetes.[29] The pathogenesis of the dawn phenomenon is not known, but it is associated with increased catecholamines[29,30] and GH,[31–33] both of which induce insulin resistance.

Lipid metabolism during sleep has received comparatively less scrutiny. Glycerol and free fatty acids (FFA) decreased progressively during sleep in one study,[26] and the investigators speculated that reduced adipose tissue lipolysis may signal a reduction in hepatic gluconeogenesis. However, another study showed that lipid turnover decreases during early sleep, then subsequently rises in a GH-dependent manner.[34] Discrepancies between these studies may relate to the extent and distribution of slow-wave sleep, when GH is primarily secreted. In fact, a "rebound" in slow-wave sleep that occurs after sleep deprivation is accompanied by significant elevations of GH, plasma glycerol, and FFA.[35]

Circadian rhythms, independent of sleep, also affect hormone profiles and metabolism. For example, cortisol levels peak early in the morning, regardless of sleep-wake state.[36,37] Ghrelin, a peptide synthesized in multiple tissues and which stimulates appetite, is secreted in a pulsatile fashion in anticipation of daily meals.[25] However, ghrelin is also secreted in early sleep, suggesting a correlation with GH.[38] Closer analysis of the interacting influences of sleep and circadian rhythm require protocols that disrupt the timing of cues that ordinarily serve to delineate a 24-hour day. Scheer and colleagues[39] subjected volunteers to a week of 28-hour "days" to parse the effects of sleep and circadian rhythm on glucose metabolism. This study showed that, independent of the time of day, glucose and insulin increased following meals, and both decreased during sleep. Mild diurnal fluctuations in glucose also occurred, without changes in insulin. More striking, they found that circadian misalignment caused significant insulin resistance and elevations of blood pressure.[40] In the sections that follow, we examine how altered quantity, timing, or quality of sleep can affect glucose metabolism and obesity.

Key points:

- Sleep, particularly NREM sleep, is a physiologic state of decreased global metabolism that likely serves a reparative role.
- Normal NREM sleep is characterized by decreased glucose turnover, but there are conflicting data regarding lipid metabolism during sleep.
- Brain metabolism in REM sleep is similar to wakefulness.

THE METABOLIC EFFECTS OF SLEEP DURATION

Today's "around-the-clock" society, characterized by demands for high work performance, prolonged daily commutes, and leisure activity, has significantly compromised sleep duration. Self-reported sleep times have decreased from more than 8 hours in the 1960s to approximately 6.5 hours in 2012. Up to 30% of middle-aged Americans sleep fewer than 6 hours a night.[41–46] Similar results were reported in other countries[47,48] and were confirmed in population-based cohorts in which sleep duration was objectively measured.[49,50] Sleep duration is also compromised by sleep disorders, such as insomnia and obstructive sleep apnea (OSA). Whether it is voluntarily or involuntarily compromised, sleep loss has significant health consequences. These consequences range from impaired cognitive function[51,52] to increased all-cause morbidity and mortality.[53–56] Derangements in sleep also affect glucose homeostasis and appetite control. Impaired sleep thus might contribute to the rising prevalence of type 2 diabetes (T2DM) and obesity in modern society. In the following section we examine evidence linking short sleep duration to decreased glucose tolerance, insulin sensitivity, and insulin secretion. Of note, excessive sleep has also been associated with metabolic dysfunction[57,58]; however, this association has not been adequately explored, and may be confounded by medical comorbidities (eg, sleep apnea, depression) that can lengthen sleep time.

Cross-sectional studies suggest that short sleep duration is associated with an increased prevalence of T2DM or impaired glucose homeostasis. Data from large cohorts (Sleep Heart Health Study, Finnish Type 2 Diabetes Study, Quebec Family study,

Behavioral Risk Factor Surveillance System, National Health Interview Study, and Isfahan Healthy Heart Program) have demonstrated that middle-aged to elderly subjects with self-reported short sleep duration are approximately twice as likely to be diagnosed with T2DM, and are at higher risk for impaired glucose tolerance. These results were independent of common T2DM risk factors in all studies[58–62] but one.[63] Similar associations between short sleep and T2DM have been observed in patients in a hypertension clinic,[64] young subjects with a family history of T2DM,[65] obese adolescents,[66] and pregnant women.[67,68] Interestingly, the association may be statistically stronger in women than men.[59,60] However, a smaller study conducted in middle-aged adults observed no association between sleep duration and diabetes.[69] Self-perceived insufficient, poor, or short sleep is also associated with prediabetic metabolic impairments, such as elevated glucose and insulin levels, HbA1c, or whole-body insulin resistance.[61,67,69–77] Moreover, inadequate sleep has been shown to worsen glucose control in patients with preexisting T2DM.[78,79] Despite various definitions of short sleep time among cross-sectional studies, outcomes of these studies are rather uniform, suggesting a significant association between short sleep duration and worsened glucose homeostasis. However, cross-sectional studies cannot establish causality. In fact, it has been reported that T2DM negatively impacts sleep architecture, making an inverse or bi-directional relationship between sleep and glucose regulation plausible.[80–82]

Stronger evidence for a causal link between short sleep duration and diabetes is provided by prospective studies following diabetes-free individuals with various sleep durations over time. Twelve published studies have been conducted in the United States, Japan, Germany, Sweden, and South Korea, investigating 661 to 70,026 adult subjects for incident diabetes over a 4-year to 32-year follow-up period.[83–94] All of these studies, except the two most recent,[93,94] were included in a meta-analysis of 90,623 subjects,[57] which showed an increased relative risk (RR) of developing diabetes in subjects with short (RR = 1.28) as well as long sleep duration (RR = 1.48), compared with subjects with normal sleep duration (typically 7–8 hours), after adjusting for known confounding variables. Similarly, more recent studies confirmed short sleep as a risk factor for newly developed diabetes[79,93]; however, this association became insignificant in one study after adjusting for multiple confounding variables.[93] Limitations of these prospective studies include differing definitions of short sleep duration, reliance on self-reported data, and the potential for residual confounding bias. Nonetheless, prospective and cross-sectional studies provide strong circumstantial evidence for the independent role of short sleep in the development of T2DM.

Experiments in human volunteers demonstrate how short-term changes in sleep duration can directly impact glucose homeostasis. After total sleep deprivation lasting from 24 hours to 5 days, studies report decreased insulin sensitivity[95–97] and impaired fasting or postprandial glucose levels.[98–102] Additionally, sleep deprivation reduced postprandial insulin secretion,[98] suggesting impaired pancreatic β-cell function. However, not all parameters of glucose metabolism were affected equally across studies and some investigators did not find impairments in glucose homeostasis after total sleep deprivation,[103] probably due to methodological differences and interindividual variability. Still, no study to date has reported improved glucose metabolism after sleep loss. Some studies have restricted sleep to 4 to 5 hours per night, more closely modeling the sleep habits of today's society. Although a few studies have not observed impairments in glucose metabolism,[104,105] most studies show that glucose tolerance and/or insulin sensitivity are substantially impaired when sleep is restricted for a few days to several weeks in a laboratory or in the home environment.[106–113] The metabolic phenotype induced by partial sleep deprivation is characterized by features typically observed in T2DM, such as diminished muscle glucose uptake, enhanced hepatic glucose output, and inadequate glucose-induced insulin secretion.[106,108,109,114]

Mechanisms inducing impairments in insulin sensitivity and glucose metabolism during acute sleep deprivation are complex and poorly understood. The suggested endocrine and molecular mediators are typically supported by limited and often indirect evidence. For example, sleep deprivation increases circulating levels of cortisol (elevated evening cortisol and 24-hour profile)[102,106–108,115–117] and induces sympathetic activation,[107] accompanied by elevated catecholamine levels.[111] However, metabolic impairments were also reported in studies in which cortisol or catecholamine levels remained unchanged.[108–110,114] Moreover, sleep restriction was reported to reduce thyroid-stimulating hormone and testosterone levels,[107,118] disrupt the pattern of GH secretion,[119] and elevate levels of proinflammatory cytokines.[120] These complex endocrine changes might contribute to impaired insulin signaling in peripheral tissues. In adipocytes, changes in production of circulating adipokines occurred after short sleep duration.[97,121,122] Although mechanisms are not fully understood, metabolic impairments induced by experimental sleep deprivation are reversible after sleep recovery in young and older individuals.[109]

Sleep loss also affects appetite and food intake, thereby promoting obesity. Following partial sleep deprivation, subjects increase caloric intake by approximately 20%,[104,123–126] with a preference for foods rich in carbohydrates and fat.[124,126–130] Additionally, a meta-analysis of several studies confirmed that short sleep increases appetite.[131] Among many factors that regulate food intake,[132] leptin (which suppresses appetite) and ghrelin (which stimulates appetite) have been investigated extensively under conditions of sleep restriction. Considering the numerous interacting factors that affect food intake, it is not surprising that results are mixed. Decreased leptin and increased ghrelin levels were observed in some studies following sleep deprivation[107,127,133–136] and in some cross-sectional studies,[137,138] but opposite results or no changes have also been reported elsewhere.[102,104,112,117,125,135,139,140] Although methodological differences might be responsible for inconsistent results, it is also possible that other mechanisms, such as decreased levels of satiety promoting peptide YY,[141] might contribute to increased food intake. If these appetite-stimulating effects of acute sleep loss are extrapolated to chronic sleep loss, one might expect obesity to develop in those with reduced sleep time. Indeed, cross-sectional and prospective studies have linked short sleep with weight gain and abdominal fat accumulation.[142,143] Interestingly, short sleep was associated with lower fat loss during caloric restriction in overweight subjects.[135] Some mechanistic studies of sleep loss and energy regulation have been attempted in animals. In rodents, sleep deprivation appears to lead to weight loss and energy catabolism, culminating in death. However, dramatic metabolic differences between species and stressful sleep deprivation protocols have limited the clinical applicability of these findings.[144]

There is evidence that the timing of sleep, in addition to the duration, may be a critical factor for metabolic health. Approximately 20% of workers in the United States perform their jobs under flexible or shift schedules,[145,146] which misaligns sleep timing with circadian rhythms. Shift work induces profound and sustained misalignment between circadian and homeostatic or behavioral rhythms.[39,147,148] As previously noted, an acute circadian misalignment is associated with impaired glucose tolerance and pancreatic β-cell dysfunction, leading to elevated postprandial glucose excursions,[39] independent of sleep duration. Furthermore, decreased leptin levels and an inverted cortisol profile across sleep and wake might further deteriorate glucose regulation and food intake. Thus, adequate and properly timed sleep may be important for normal glucose and weight regulation.

Key points:
- Pressures of modern society have resulted in decreased sleep duration over the past several decades.
- Cross-sectional studies suggest a link between short sleep duration and the prevalence of T2DM. These results are echoed by longitudinal studies that have even described a worsening of preexisting glucose intolerance.
- Short-term studies in healthy volunteers also demonstrate a variety of measures of impaired glucose homeostasis with short sleep time.
- Decreased sleep duration is associated with the development of obesity, although the mechanisms that underlie this are not clear.

EFFECTS OF OSA ON INSULIN RESISTANCE AND OBESITY

One sleep disorder with a potential impact on metabolic health is OSA. OSA is a common sleep disorder with an estimated prevalence of 4% to 5% in the general population. It is about twice as common in men as in women.[149] OSA is characterized by repeated collapse of the upper airway during sleep, causing intermittent oxygen desaturations and arousals from sleep. During sleep, a patient or bed partner may recall snoring, gasping, or witnessed pauses in breathing. While awake, the patient may complain of excessive daytime sleepiness, fatigue, or morning headaches. A patient may also describe poor workplace performance or impaired vigilance during driving or other monotonous activity. When OSA is suspected, a polysomnogram (PSG) should be performed, a test that monitors a patient's sleep architecture, breathing patterns, and gas exchange during sleep. A diagnosis of OSA is made by an examination of airflow and breathing effort during sleep. Obstructive *apneas* are noted when oronasal airflow ceases for more than 10 seconds despite continued breathing effort. Obstructive *hypopneas* are noted when airflow decreases significantly (but does not completely cease), leading to a fall in oxygen level or an arousal from sleep. The combined rate of apneas and hypopneas per hour, or the apnea-hypopnea index (AHI), is used to classify OSA severity. An AHI of 5 to 15, 15 to 30, or more than 30 events per hour describes mild, moderate, or severe OSA, respectively. The first-line treatment for OSA is a nasal mask which delivers continuous positive airway pressure (CPAP), thereby splinting the airway open. This often results in much more restful sleep, markedly reduced daytime symptoms, and improved gas exchange. Besides its more obvious impact on quality of life,[150,151] OSA is associated with significant long-term health consequences. Sleep apnea is a risk factor for cardiovascular disease,[152,153] and more recently an association has also been shown between OSA and a variety of metabolic disorders, including hypertension, dyslipidemia, nonalcoholic fatty liver disease, glucose intolerance, and T2DM. In this section, we briefly examine the evidence supporting links between OSA and insulin resistance and obesity.

Theoretically, OSA is a plausible cause of insulin resistance and T2DM, as it can induce sleep loss and hypoxia, each of which can impact glucose metabolism. The nature of sleep loss in OSA is best described as "sleep fragmentation," whereby deeper stages of sleep are replaced by less restful, lighter stages of sleep. When healthy volunteers are frequently awakened from sleep with acoustic and mechanical stimulation, they exhibit decreased morning insulin sensitivity, and increased morning cortisol levels and sympathetic activity.[154] Tasali and colleagues[155] showed qualitatively similar results when slow-wave sleep was specifically interrupted, and that the effect was "dose dependent"; that is, the magnitude of the disruption correlated with the magnitude of the blunting of insulin sensitivity. Acute hypoxia also causes glucose intolerance,[156–159] and one study showed that intermittent hypoxia in healthy volunteers decreased insulin sensitivity and increased sympathetic tone.[160] Mouse models of OSA that involve exposures to intermittent hypoxia have further implicated reactive oxygen species,[161] increased sympathetic tone,[161,162] inflammation,[163] and pancreatic beta cell apoptosis[164,165] as possible causes of glucose intolerance and impaired insulin secretion. Additionally, intermittent hypoxia induced arousals in mice,[166] which demonstrates the interconnectedness between the two defining characteristics of OSA.

Biologic plausibility itself is insufficient proof that sleep apnea *causes* worsened insulin resistance, however, so we must examine the clinical evidence as well. Cross-sectional studies have provided some of the support for an association between the two. In diabetic individuals, the average prevalence of OSA has been reported at 71%[167] and as high as 86% among obese diabetic patients in one recent study, with most having moderate to severe OSA.[168] This suggests that considerably more diabetic patients have OSA than are diagnosed. Twenty years ago, Levinson and colleagues[169] showed that men with OSA had twofold the expected prevalence of impaired glucose tolerance compared with published data from a control population. Subsequent studies attempted to account for the confounding influence of obesity, which is an obvious shared risk factor for OSA and T2DM. Ip and colleagues[170] showed that OSA was associated with a higher degree of insulin resistance as measured by HOMA-IR, even after correction for body mass index (BMI). Similar results were shown in another study that examined oral glucose tolerance among apneic individuals after adjusting for BMI and body fat, and hypoxia appeared to drive the association between OSA and impaired glucose tolerance.[171] McArdle and colleagues[172] showed that men with OSA had a significantly higher HOMA-IR when compared with controls matched for age, BMI, and smoking status. Numerous other cross-sectional studies support a robust association between OSA and insulin resistance.[167,173]

Longitudinal studies have the potential to provide stronger evidence for a causal association between OSA and T2DM. Reichmuth and colleagues[174] examined the baseline prevalence and incidence of T2DM in a cohort of 1387 patients from Wisconsin, some with OSA. OSA was associated with a higher prevalence of T2DM, but the incidence of T2DM over 4 years was not increased by OSA when adjusted for waist girth. A Swedish study found that OSA (defined only by nocturnal intermittent hypoxia) was associated with increased incidence of T2DM over 16 years in women, but not men, although this increase was not statistically significant.[175] However, the Busselton Health Study found that subjects with moderate to severe OSA were more likely to develop T2DM over 4 years after adjusting for age, gender, waist circumference, and BMI, but only 9 of the subjects developed T2DM during the study, resulting in wide confidence intervals.[176] A larger study of Veterans Affairs patients identified OSA as an independent risk factor for incident diabetes over 2.7 years, and CPAP appeared to attenuate this risk in those with more severe OSA.[177] A recent longitudinal study of 141 men over 11 years showed a fourfold increased risk of T2DM in those with nocturnal hypoxia.[178] Collectively, these studies point to an impact of OSA on glucose metabolism, but they are limited by sample size, and difficulties in accounting for effects of CPAP treatment during the trail periods.

Does CPAP treatment improve glucose metabolism in OSA? This finding would provide the strongest degree of evidence for a causal link between OSA and T2DM. To date, 9 randomized controlled trials have examined the effect of CPAP (compared with sham CPAP) on glucose metabolism.[167] The studies ranged in duration from 1 week to 3 months and examined various markers of insulin sensitivity, including fasting glucose, HOMA, HbA1c, and hyperinsulinemic euglycemic clamp testing. Four studies showed a beneficial effect of therapeutic CPAP, whereas the other five did not. The largest study randomized 86 patients with OSA to 3 months of CPAP or sham, and then crossed patients over to the other treatment group after a 1-month washout period. Several components of the metabolic syndrome were improved after CPAP, including a significant but modest absolute reduction in HbA1c (0.2%). However, CPAP did not alter fasting glucose, insulin, or HOMA.[179] It appears that most studies showing a benefit of CPAP were characterized by subjects with more severe OSA,[180] or who were more adherent to CPAP.[181] Hence, although some studies show improvements in markers of insulin sensitivity with CPAP use, no firm conclusions can be drawn from the available evidence. Moreover, even if CPAP attenuates diabetes risks, poor adherence to this therapy remains a significant clinical problem.

Much clearer is the relationship between obesity and the development of OSA. Approximately 70% of patients with OSA are obese,[182] whereas 60% of obese patients have OSA; this figure is nearly 100% of the morbidly obese (BMI $\geq$40).[183] Young and colleagues[184] examined a cohort of 600 patients who underwent PSG and determined that a single standard deviation higher of any measure of body habitus was associated with a threefold increased risk of having an AHI of 5 or higher. Moreover, weight loss has been shown both to decrease the AHI in patients with OSA,[185] and to decrease the collapsibility of the upper airway.[186] However, one study found that some patients who lose weight and subsequently achieve a cure of their sleep apnea may later develop an increased AHI on repeat PSG after long-term follow-up, despite maintaining their weight loss.[187] This suggests that although obesity clearly contributes to the development of OSA, it is indeed a complex, multifactorial illness.

Because of mounting evidence linking OSA to the development of other facets of the metabolic syndrome, there has also been speculation that OSA itself can cause obesity; however, the data supporting this reciprocal relationship are scant. A small study by Loube and colleagues[188] showed that patients who were compliant with CPAP use (>4 hours per night) were more likely than noncompliant patients to have significant weight loss (10 pounds or greater) on follow-up after 6 months; in fact, none of the 11 patients who were nonadherent to CPAP achieved this degree of weight loss. However, other studies have not replicated this finding, and at least one study has demonstrated no weight loss, and some weight gain in a subset of patients compliant with CPAP.[189] Intriguingly, there is evidence that CPAP may reduce visceral body fat even if overall weight is not significantly altered.[190] Therefore, no clear conclusion can be drawn about the possibility of OSA causing obesity based on the currently available evidence.

Key points:

- A growing body of evidence, including data from cross-sectional and longitudinal studies, links OSA with the development of insulin resistance.
- The effect of CPAP on insulin resistance and type 2 diabetes has not been consistent in several randomized clinical trials; large randomized clinical trials should be conducted to better assess this effect.
- Though a multifactorial illness, obesity clearly is a major risk factor for the development of OSA. The effect of OSA on obesity is not well defined.

In conclusion, sleep is a necessary human activity, and although the exact functions are unclear, it is associated with a state of decreased metabolism and energy conservation. Impairments in the timing and particularly the duration of sleep seem to be associated with worsened glucose tolerance and perhaps the development of T2DM. Sleep disorders, such as OSA, may predispose to the development and the progression of T2DM. Because of disturbing worldwide trends in sleep habits, obesity, and T2DM, it will be critical for clinicians and researchers to recognize and address the potential impact of sleep disorders on metabolic health.

REFERENCES

1. Rechtschaffen A. Current perspectives on the function of sleep. Perspect Biol Med 1998;41(3):359–90.
2. Siegel JM. The REM sleep-memory consolidation hypothesis. Science 2001; 294(5544):1058–63.
3. Siegel JM. Clues to the functions of mammalian sleep. Nature 2005;437(7063): 1264–71.
4. Daan S, Beersma DG, Borbely AA. Timing of human sleep: recover process gated by a circadian pacemaker. Am J Physiol 1984;246:R161–83.
5. Berry R, Brooks R, Gamaldo C, et al. AASM Manual for the scoring of sleep and associated events: rules, terminology and technical specifications version 2.0. Darien (IL): American Academy of Sleep Medicine; 2012.
6. Coote JH. Respiratory and circulatory control during sleep. J Exp Biol 1982;100: 223–44.
7. Kreider MB, Buskirk ER, Bass DE. Oxygen consumption and body temperatures during the night. J Appl Physiol 1958;12(3):361–6.
8. Ravussin E, Lillioja S, Anderson TE, et al. Determinants of 24-hour energy expenditure in man. Methods and results using a respiratory chamber. J Clin Invest 1986;78(6):1568–78.
9. Brebbia DR, Altshuler KZ. Oxygen consumption rate and electroencephalographic stage of sleep. Science 1965;150(3703):1621–3.
10. White DP, Weil JV, Zwillich CW. Metabolic rate and breathing during sleep. J Appl Physiol 1985;59(2):384–91.
11. Kong J, Shepel PN, Holden CP, et al. Brain glycogen decreases with increased periods of wakefulness: implications for homeostatic drive to sleep. J Neurosci 2002;22(13):5581–7.
12. Dworak M, McCarley RW, Kim T, et al. Sleep and brain energy levels: ATP changes during sleep. J Neurosci 2010;30(26):9007–16.
13. Nakanishi H, Sun Y, Nakamura RK, et al. Positive correlations between cerebral protein synthesis rates and deep sleep in *Macaca mulatta*. Eur J Neurosci 1997; 9(2):271–9.
14. Takahashi Y, Kipnis DM, Daughaday WH. Growth hormone secretion during sleep. J Clin Invest 1968;47(9):2079–90.
15. Van CE, Kerkhofs M, Caufriez A, et al. A quantitative estimation of growth hormone secretion in normal man: reproducibility and relation to sleep and time of day. J Clin Endocrinol Metab 1992;74(6):1441–50.
16. Van CE, Latta F, Nedeltcheva A, et al. Reciprocal interactions between the GH axis and sleep. Growth Horm IGF Res 2004;14(Suppl A):S10–7.
17. Moller N, Jorgensen JO. Effects of growth hormone on glucose, lipid, and protein metabolism in human subjects. Endocr Rev 2009;30(2):152–77.
18. Friess E, Wiedemann K, Steiger A, et al. The hypothalamic-pituitary-adrenocortical system and sleep in man. Adv Neuroimmunol 1995;5(2):111–25.
19. Sherwin RS. Role of the liver in glucose homeostasis. Diabetes Care 1980;3(2): 261–5.
20. Biggers DW, Myers SR, Neal D, et al. Role of brain in counterregulation of insulin-induced hypoglycemia in dogs. Diabetes 1989;38(1):7–16.

21. Peters A. The selfish brain: competition for energy resources. Am J Human Biol 2011;23(1):29–34.
22. Boyle PJ, Scott JC, Krentz AJ, et al. Diminished brain glucose metabolism is a significant determinant for falling rates of systemic glucose utilization during sleep in normal humans. J Clin Invest 1994;93(2):529–35.
23. Sawaya R, Ingvar DH. Cerebral blood flow and metabolism in sleep. Acta Neurol Scand 1989;80(6):481–91.
24. Zoccoli G, Cianci T, Lenzi P, et al. Shivering during sleep: relationship between muscle blood flow and fiber type composition. Experientia 1992;48(3):228–30.
25. Morris CJ, Aeschbach D, Scheer FA. Circadian system, sleep and endocrinology. Mol Cell Endocrinol 2012;349(1):91–104.
26. Clore JN, Nestler JE, Blackard WG. Sleep-associated fall in glucose disposal and hepatic glucose output in normal humans. Putative signaling mechanism linking peripheral and hepatic events. Diabetes 1989;38(3):285–90.
27. Frank SA, Roland DC, Sturis J, et al. Effects of aging on glucose regulation during wakefulness and sleep. Am J Physiol 1995;269(6 Pt 1):E1006–16.
28. Bolli GB, Gerich JE. The "dawn phenomenon"—a common occurrence in both non-insulin-dependent and insulin-dependent diabetes mellitus. N Engl J Med 1984;310(12):746–50.
29. Bolli GB, De FP, De CS, et al. Demonstration of a dawn phenomenon in normal human volunteers. Diabetes 1984;33(12):1150–3.
30. Schmidt MI, Lin QX, Gwynne JT, et al. Fasting early morning rise in peripheral insulin: evidence of the dawn phenomenon in nondiabetes. Diabetes Care 1984;7(1):32–5.
31. Rizza RA, Mandarino LJ, Gerich JE. Effects of growth hormone on insulin action in man. Mechanisms of insulin resistance, impaired suppression of glucose production, and impaired stimulation of glucose utilization. Diabetes 1982;31(8 Pt 1):663–9.
32. Carroll KF, Nestel PJ. Diurnal variation in glucose tolerance and in insulin secretion in man. Diabetes 1973;22(5):333–48.
33. Boyle PJ, Avogaro A, Smith L, et al. Absence of the dawn phenomenon and abnormal lipolysis in type 1 (insulin-dependent) diabetic patients with chronic growth hormone deficiency. Diabetologia 1992;35(4):372–9.
34. Boyle PJ, Avogaro A, Smith L, et al. Role of GH in regulating nocturnal rates of lipolysis and plasma mevalonate levels in normal and diabetic humans. Am J Physiol 1992;263(1 Pt 1):E168–72.
35. Cooper BG, White JE, Ashworth LA, et al. Hormonal and metabolic profiles in subjects with obstructive sleep apnea syndrome and the acute effects of nasal continuous positive airway pressure (CPAP) treatment. Sleep 1995;18(3):172–9.
36. Weitzman ED. Circadian rhythms and episodic hormone secretion in man. Annu Rev Med 1976;27:225–43.
37. Halberg F, Frank G, Harner R, et al. The adrenal cycle in men on different schedules of motor and mental activity. Experientia 1961;17:282–4.
38. Dzaja A, Dalal MA, Himmerich H, et al. Sleep enhances nocturnal plasma ghrelin levels in healthy subjects. Am J Physiol Endocrinol Metab 2004;286(6): E963–7.
39. Scheer FA, Hilton MF, Mantzoros CS, et al. Adverse metabolic and cardiovascular consequences of circadian misalignment. Proc Natl Acad Sci U S A 2009; 106(11):4453–8.
40. Bass J, Takahashi JS. Circadian integration of metabolism and energetics. Science 2010;330(6009):1349–54.

41. Kripke DF, Simons RN, Garfinkel L, et al. Short and long sleep and sleeping pills. Is increased mortality associated? Arch Gen Psychiatry 1979;36(1):103–16.
42. Schoenborn CA, Adams PE. Health behaviors of adults: United States, 2005-2007. Vital Health Stat 10 2010;(245):1–132.
43. Krueger PM, Friedman EM. Sleep duration in the United States: a cross-sectional population-based study. Am J Epidemiol 2009;169(9):1052–63.
44. Centers for Disease Control and Prevention. Short Sleep Duration Among Workers—United States, 2010. MMWR Morb Mortal Wkly Rep 2012;61(16):281–5.
45. National Sleep Foundation. NSF Bedroom Poll 2012. National Sleep Foundation 2012;1–56.
46. Centers for Disease Control and Prevention. Effect of short sleep duration on daily activities—United States, 2005-2008. MMWR Morb Mortal Wkly Rep 2011;60(8):239–42.
47. Shankar A, Koh WP, Yuan JM, et al. Sleep duration and coronary heart disease mortality among Chinese adults in Singapore: a population-based cohort study. Am J Epidemiol 2008;168(12):1367–73.
48. Tamakoshi A, Ohno Y. Self-reported sleep duration as a predictor of all-cause mortality: results from the JACC study, Japan. Sleep 2004;27(1):51–4.
49. Lauderdale DS, Knutson KL, Yan LL, et al. Objectively measured sleep characteristics among early-middle-aged adults: the CARDIA study. Am J Epidemiol 2006;164(1):5–16.
50. Redline S, Kirchner HL, Quan SF, et al. The effects of age, sex, ethnicity, and sleep-disordered breathing on sleep architecture. Arch Intern Med 2004;164(4):406–18.
51. Stickgold R, Walker MP. Sleep-dependent memory consolidation and reconsolidation. Sleep Med 2007;8(4):331–43.
52. Walker MP. The role of sleep in cognition and emotion. Ann N Y Acad Sci 2009;1156:168–97.
53. Cappuccio FP, D'Elia L, Strazzullo P, et al. Sleep duration and all-cause mortality: a systematic review and meta-analysis of prospective studies. Sleep 2010;33(5):585–92.
54. Chien KL, Chen PC, Hsu HC, et al. Habitual sleep duration and insomnia and the risk of cardiovascular events and all-cause death: report from a community-based cohort. Sleep 2010;33(2):177–84.
55. Punjabi NM, Caffo BS, Goodwin JL, et al. Sleep-disordered breathing and mortality: a prospective cohort study. PLoS Med 2009;6(8):e1000132.
56. Ikehara S, Iso H, Date C, et al. Association of sleep duration with mortality from cardiovascular disease and other causes for Japanese men and women: the JACC study. Sleep 2009;32(3):295–301.
57. Cappuccio FP, D'Elia L, Strazzullo P, et al. Quantity and quality of sleep and incidence of type 2 diabetes: a systematic review and meta-analysis. Diabetes Care 2010;33(2):414–20.
58. Buxton OM, Marcelli E. Short and long sleep are positively associated with obesity, diabetes, hypertension, and cardiovascular disease among adults in the United States. Soc Sci Med 2010;71(5):1027–36.
59. Gottlieb DJ, Punjabi NM, Newman AB, et al. Association of sleep time with diabetes mellitus and impaired glucose tolerance. Arch Intern Med 2005;165(8):863–7.
60. Tuomilehto H, Peltonen M, Partinen M, et al. Sleep duration is associated with an increased risk for the prevalence of type 2 diabetes in middle-aged women—the FIN-D2D survey. Sleep Med 2008;9(3):221–7.

61. Chaput JP, Despres JP, Bouchard C, et al. Association of sleep duration with type 2 diabetes and impaired glucose tolerance. Diabetologia 2007;50(11): 2298–304.
62. Najafian J, Mohamadifard N, Siadat ZD, et al. Association between sleep duration and diabetes mellitus: Isfahan Healthy Heart Program. Niger J Clin Pract 2013;16(1):59–62.
63. Altman NG, Izci-Balserak B, Schopfer E, et al. Sleep duration versus sleep insufficiency as predictors of cardiometabolic health outcomes. Sleep Med 2012; 13(10):1261–70.
64. Fiorentini A, Valente R, Perciaccante A, et al. Sleep's quality disorders in patients with hypertension and type 2 diabetes mellitus. Int J Cardiol 2007;114(2):E50–2.
65. Darukhanavala A, Booth JN III, Bromley L, et al. Changes in insulin secretion and action in adults with familial risk for type 2 diabetes who curtail their sleep. Diabetes Care 2011;34(10):2259–64.
66. Koren D, Levitt Katz LE, Brar PC, et al. Sleep architecture and glucose and insulin homeostasis in obese adolescents. Diabetes Care 2011;34(11):2442–7.
67. Qiu C, Enquobahrie D, Frederick IO, et al. Glucose intolerance and gestational diabetes risk in relation to sleep duration and snoring during pregnancy: a pilot study. BMC Womens Health 2010;10:17.
68. Facco FL, Grobman WA, Kramer J, et al. Self-reported short sleep duration and frequent snoring in pregnancy: impact on glucose metabolism. Am J Obstet Gynecol 2010;203(2):142–5.
69. Knutson KL, Van CE, Zee P, et al. Cross-sectional associations between measures of sleep and markers of glucose metabolism among subjects with and without diabetes: the Coronary Artery Risk Development in Young Adults (CARDIA) Sleep Study. Diabetes Care 2011;34(5):1171–6.
70. Jennings JR, Muldoon MF, Hall M, et al. Self-reported sleep quality is associated with the metabolic syndrome. Sleep 2007;30(2):219–23.
71. Flint J, Kothare SV, Zihlif M, et al. Association between inadequate sleep and insulin resistance in obese children. J Pediatr 2007;150(4):364–9.
72. Matthews KA, Dahl RE, Owens JF, et al. Sleep duration and insulin resistance in healthy black and white adolescents. Sleep 2012;35(10):1353–8.
73. Hung HC, Yang YC, Ou HY, et al. The association between self-reported sleep quality and metabolic syndrome. PLoS One 2013;8(1):e54304.
74. Hung HC, Yang YC, Ou HY, et al. The relationship between impaired fasting glucose and self-reported sleep quality in a Chinese population. Clin Endocrinol (Oxf) 2013;78(4):518–24.
75. Nakajima H, Kaneita Y, Yokoyama E, et al. Association between sleep duration and hemoglobin A1c level. Sleep Med 2008;9(7):745–52.
76. Hall MH, Muldoon MF, Jennings JR, et al. Self-reported sleep duration is associated with the metabolic syndrome in midlife adults. Sleep 2008;31(5):635–43.
77. Reutrakul S, Zaidi N, Wroblewski K, et al. Sleep disturbances and their relationship to glucose tolerance in pregnancy. Diabetes Care 2011;34(11):2454–7.
78. Knutson KL, Ryden AM, Mander BA, et al. Role of sleep duration and quality in the risk and severity of type 2 diabetes mellitus. Arch Intern Med 2006;166(16): 1768–74.
79. Ohkuma T, Fujii H, Iwase M, et al. Impact of sleep duration on obesity and the glycemic level in patients with type 2 diabetes mellitus: the Fukuoka Diabetes Registry. Diabetes Care 2013;36(3):611–7.
80. Song Y, Ye X, Ye L, et al. Disturbed subjective sleep in Chinese females with type 2 diabetes on insulin therapy. PLoS One 2013;8(1):e54951.

81. Pallayova M, Donic V, Gresova S, et al. Do differences in sleep architecture exist between persons with type 2 diabetes and nondiabetic controls? J Diabetes Sci Technol 2010;4(2):344–52.
82. Nakanishi-Minami T, Kishida K, Funahashi T, et al. Sleep-wake cycle irregularities in type 2 diabetics. Diabetol Metab Syndr 2012;4(1):18.
83. Ayas NT, White DP, Al-Delaimy WK, et al. A prospective study of self-reported sleep duration and incident diabetes in women. Diabetes Care 2003;26(2):380–4.
84. Nilsson PM, Roost M, Engstrom G, et al. Incidence of diabetes in middle-aged men is related to sleep disturbances. Diabetes Care 2004;27(10):2464–9.
85. Bjorkelund C, Bondyr-Carlsson D, Lapidus L, et al. Sleep disturbances in midlife unrelated to 32-year diabetes incidence: the prospective population study of women in Gothenburg. Diabetes Care 2005;28(11):2739–44.
86. Mallon L, Broman JE, Hetta J. High incidence of diabetes in men with sleep complaints or short sleep duration: a 12-year follow-up study of a middle-aged population. Diabetes Care 2005;28(11):2762–7.
87. Yaggi HK, Araujo AB, McKinlay JB. Sleep duration as a risk factor for the development of type 2 diabetes. Diabetes Care 2006;29(3):657–61.
88. Gangwisch JE, Heymsfield SB, Boden-Albala B, et al. Sleep duration as a risk factor for diabetes incidence in a large U.S. sample. Sleep 2007;30(12):1667–73.
89. Beihl DA, Liese AD, Haffner SM. Sleep duration as a risk factor for incident type 2 diabetes in a multiethnic cohort. Ann Epidemiol 2009;19(5):351–7.
90. Hayashino Y, Fukuhara S, Suzukamo Y, et al. Relation between sleep quality and quantity, quality of life, and risk of developing diabetes in healthy workers in Japan: the High-risk and Population Strategy for Occupational Health Promotion (HIPOP-OHP) Study. BMC Public Health 2007;7:129.
91. Kawakami N, Takatsuka N, Shimizu H. Sleep disturbance and onset of type 2 diabetes. Diabetes Care 2004;27(1):282–3.
92. Meisinger C, Heier M, Loewel H. Sleep disturbance as a predictor of type 2 diabetes mellitus in men and women from the general population. Diabetologia 2005;48(2):235–41.
93. von RA, Weikert C, Fietze I, et al. Association of sleep duration with chronic diseases in the European Prospective Investigation into Cancer and Nutrition (EPIC)-Potsdam study. PLoS One 2012;7(1):e30972.
94. Kita T, Yoshioka E, Satoh H, et al. Short sleep duration and poor sleep quality increase the risk of diabetes in Japanese workers with no family history of diabetes. Diabetes Care 2012;35(2):313–8.
95. Gonzalez-Ortiz M, Martinez-Abundis E, Balcazar-Munoz BR, et al. Effect of sleep deprivation on insulin sensitivity and cortisol concentration in healthy subjects. Diabetes Nutr Metab 2000;13(2):80–3.
96. VanHelder T, Symons JD, Radomski MW. Effects of sleep deprivation and exercise on glucose tolerance. Aviat Space Environ Med 1993;64(6):487–92.
97. Broussard JL, Ehrmann DA, Van CE, et al. Impaired insulin signaling in human adipocytes after experimental sleep restriction: a randomized, crossover study. Ann Intern Med 2012;157(8):549–57.
98. Benedict C, Hallschmid M, Lassen A, et al. Acute sleep deprivation reduces energy expenditure in healthy men. Am J Clin Nutr 2011;93(6):1229–36.
99. Kuhn E, Brodan V, Brodanova M, et al. Metabolic reflection of sleep deprivation. Act Nerv Super (Praha) 1969;11(3):165–74.
100. Vondra K, Brodan V, Bass A, et al. Effects of sleep deprivation on the activity of selected metabolic enzymes in skeletal muscle. Eur J Appl Physiol Occup Physiol 1981;47(1):41–6.

101. Wehrens SM, Hampton SM, Finn RE, et al. Effect of total sleep deprivation on postprandial metabolic and insulin responses in shift workers and non-shift workers. J Endocrinol 2010;206(2):205–15.
102. Reynolds AC, Dorrian J, Liu PY, et al. Impact of five nights of sleep restriction on glucose metabolism, leptin and testosterone in young adult men. PLoS One 2012;7(7):e41218.
103. Schmid SM, Hallschmid M, Jauch-Chara K, et al. Sleep loss alters basal metabolic hormone secretion and modulates the dynamic counterregulatory response to hypoglycemia. J Clin Endocrinol Metab 2007;92(8):3044–51.
104. Bosy-Westphal A, Hinrichs S, Jauch-Chara K, et al. Influence of partial sleep deprivation on energy balance and insulin sensitivity in healthy women. Obes Facts 2008;1(5):266–73.
105. Zielinski MR, Kline CE, Kripke DF, et al. No effect of 8-week time in bed restriction on glucose tolerance in older long sleepers. J Sleep Res 2008;17(4): 412–9.
106. Spiegel K, Leproult R, Van CE. Impact of sleep debt on metabolic and endocrine function. Lancet 1999;354(9188):1435–9.
107. Spiegel K, Leproult R, L'hermite-Baleriaux M, et al. Leptin levels are dependent on sleep duration: relationships with sympathovagal balance, carbohydrate regulation, cortisol, and thyrotropin. J Clin Endocrinol Metab 2004;89(11): 5762–71.
108. Buxton OM, Pavlova M, Reid EW, et al. Sleep restriction for 1 week reduces insulin sensitivity in healthy men. Diabetes 2010;59(9):2126–33.
109. Buxton OM, Cain SW, O'Connor SP, et al. Adverse metabolic consequences in humans of prolonged sleep restriction combined with circadian disruption. Sci Transl Med 2012;4(129):129ra43.
110. Schmid SM, Hallschmid M, Jauch-Chara K, et al. Disturbed glucoregulatory response to food intake after moderate sleep restriction. Sleep 2011;34(3): 371–7.
111. Nedeltcheva AV, Kessler L, Imperial J, et al. Exposure to recurrent sleep restriction in the setting of high caloric intake and physical inactivity results in increased insulin resistance and reduced glucose tolerance. J Clin Endocrinol Metab 2009;94(9):3242–50.
112. van Leeuwen WM, Hublin C, Sallinen M, et al. Prolonged sleep restriction affects glucose metabolism in healthy young men. Int J Endocrinol 2010;2010:108641.
113. Robertson MD, Russell-Jones D, Umpleby AM, et al. Effects of three weeks of mild sleep restriction implemented in the home environment on multiple metabolic and endocrine markers in healthy young men. Metabolism 2013;62(2): 204–11.
114. Donga E, van DM, van Dijk JG, et al. A single night of partial sleep deprivation induces insulin resistance in multiple metabolic pathways in healthy subjects. J Clin Endocrinol Metab 2010;95(6):2963–8.
115. Leproult R, Copinschi G, Buxton O, et al. Sleep loss results in an elevation of cortisol levels the next evening. Sleep 1997;20(10):865–70.
116. Kumari M, Badrick E, Ferrie J, et al. Self-reported sleep duration and sleep disturbance are independently associated with cortisol secretion in the Whitehall II study. J Clin Endocrinol Metab 2009;94(12):4801–9.
117. Omisade A, Buxton OM, Rusak B. Impact of acute sleep restriction on cortisol and leptin levels in young women. Physiol Behav 2010;99(5):651–6.
118. Leproult R, Van CE. Effect of 1 week of sleep restriction on testosterone levels in young healthy men. JAMA 2011;305(21):2173–4.

119. Spiegel K, Leproult R, Colecchia EF, et al. Adaptation of the 24-h growth hormone profile to a state of sleep debt. Am J Physiol Regul Integr Comp Physiol 2000;279(3):R874–83.
120. Patel SR, Zhu X, Storfer-Isser A, et al. Sleep duration and biomarkers of inflammation. Sleep 2009;32(2):200–4.
121. Hayes AL, Xu F, Babineau D, et al. Sleep duration and circulating adipokine levels. Sleep 2011;34(2):147–52.
122. Al-Disi D, Al-Daghri N, Khanam L, et al. Subjective sleep duration and quality influence diet composition and circulating adipocytokines and ghrelin levels in teen-age girls. Endocrinol Jpn 2010;57(10):915–23.
123. Brondel L, Romer MA, Nougues PM, et al. Acute partial sleep deprivation increases food intake in healthy men. Am J Clin Nutr 2010;91(6):1550–9.
124. St-Onge MP, Roberts AL, Chen J, et al. Short sleep duration increases energy intakes but does not change energy expenditure in normal-weight individuals. Am J Clin Nutr 2011;94(2):410–6.
125. Nedeltcheva AV, Kilkus JM, Imperial J, et al. Sleep curtailment is accompanied by increased intake of calories from snacks. Am J Clin Nutr 2009;89(1):126–33.
126. Calvin AD, Carter RE, Adachi T, et al. Effects of experimental sleep restriction on caloric intake and activity energy expenditure. Chest 2013. [Epub ahead of print].
127. Spiegel K, Tasali E, Penev P, et al. Brief communication: sleep curtailment in healthy young men is associated with decreased leptin levels, elevated ghrelin levels, and increased hunger and appetite. Ann Intern Med 2004;141(11): 846–50.
128. Santana AA, Pimentel GD, Romualdo M, et al. Sleep duration in elderly obese patients correlated negatively with intake fatty. Lipids Health Dis 2012;11:99.
129. Weiss A, Xu F, Storfer-Isser A, et al. The association of sleep duration with adolescents' fat and carbohydrate consumption. Sleep 2010;33(9):1201–9.
130. Grandner MA, Kripke DF, Naidoo N, et al. Relationships among dietary nutrients and subjective sleep, objective sleep, and napping in women. Sleep Med 2010; 11(2):180–4.
131. Chapman CD, Benedict C, Brooks SJ, et al. Lifestyle determinants of the drive to eat: a meta-analysis. Am J Clin Nutr 2012;96(3):492–7.
132. Suzuki K, Jayasena CN, Bloom SR. Obesity and appetite control. Exp Diabetes Res 2012;2012:824305.
133. Guilleminault C, Powell NB, Martinez S, et al. Preliminary observations on the effects of sleep time in a sleep restriction paradigm. Sleep Med 2003;4(3):177–84.
134. St-Onge MP, O'Keeffe M, Roberts AL, et al. Short sleep duration, glucose dysregulation and hormonal regulation of appetite in men and women. Sleep 2012; 35(11):1503–10.
135. Nedeltcheva AV, Kilkus JM, Imperial J, et al. Insufficient sleep undermines dietary efforts to reduce adiposity. Ann Intern Med 2010;153(7):435–41.
136. Schmid SM, Hallschmid M, Jauch-Chara K, et al. A single night of sleep deprivation increases ghrelin levels and feelings of hunger in normal-weight healthy men. J Sleep Res 2008;17(3):331–4.
137. Taheri S, Lin L, Austin D, et al. Short sleep duration is associated with reduced leptin, elevated ghrelin, and increased body mass index. PLoS Med 2004;1(3):e62.
138. Chaput JP, Despres JP, Bouchard C, et al. Short sleep duration is associated with reduced leptin levels and increased adiposity: results from the Quebec family study. Obesity (Silver Spring) 2007;15(1):253–61.

139. Schmid SM, Hallschmid M, Jauch-Chara K, et al. Short-term sleep loss decreases physical activity under free-living conditions but does not increase food intake under time-deprived laboratory conditions in healthy men. Am J Clin Nutr 2009;90(6):1476–82.

140. Simpson NS, Banks S, Dinges DF. Sleep restriction is associated with increased morning plasma leptin concentrations, especially in women. Biol Res Nurs 2010; 12(1):47–53.

141. Magee CA, Huang XF, Iverson DC, et al. Acute sleep restriction alters neuroendocrine hormones and appetite in healthy male adults. Sleep Biol Rhythm 2009; 7(2):125–7.

142. Morselli LL, Guyon A, Spiegel K. Sleep and metabolic function. Pflugers Arch 2012;463(1):139–60.

143. Knutson KL. Sleep duration and cardiometabolic risk: a review of the epidemiologic evidence. Best Pract Res Clin Endocrinol Metab 2010;24(5):731–43.

144. Jun JC, Polotsky VY. Sleep and sleep loss: an energy paradox? Sleep 2012; 35(11):1447–8.

145. Luyster FS, Strollo PJ Jr, Zee PC, et al. Sleep: a health imperative. Sleep 2012; 35(6):727–34.

146. U.S. Department of Labor. Workers on flexible and shift schedules in 2004. Washington, DC: Bureau of Labor Statistics; 2005.

147. Folkard S. Do permanent night workers show circadian adjustment? A review based on the endogenous melatonin rhythm. Chronobiol Int 2008;25(2): 215–24.

148. Sack RL, Blood ML, Lewy AJ. Melatonin rhythms in night shift workers. Sleep 1992;15(5):434–41.

149. Jennum P, Riha RL. Epidemiology of sleep apnoea/hypopnoea syndrome and sleep-disordered breathing. Eur Respir J 2009;33(4):907–14.

150. Meslier N, Lebrun T, Grlllier-Lanoir V, et al. A French survey of 3,225 patients treated with CPAP for obstructive sleep apnoea: benefits, tolerance, compliance and quality of life. Eur Respir J 1998;12(1):185–92.

151. Kawahara S, Akashiba T, Akahoshi T, et al. Nasal CPAP improves the quality of life and lessens the depressive symptoms in patients with obstructive sleep apnea syndrome. Intern Med 2005;44(5):422–7.

152. Lopez-Jimenez F, Sert Kuniyoshi FH, Gami A, et al. Obstructive sleep apnea: implications for cardiac and vascular disease. Chest 2008;133(3):793–804.

153. Caples SM, Garcia-Touchard A, Somers VK. Sleep-disordered breathing and cardiovascular risk. Sleep 2007;30(3):291–303.

154. Stamatakis KA, Punjabi NM. Effects of sleep fragmentation on glucose metabolism in normal subjects. Chest 2010;137(1):95–101.

155. Tasali E, Leproult R, Ehrmann DA, et al. Slow-wave sleep and the risk of type 2 diabetes in humans. Proc Natl Acad Sci U S A 2008;105(3):1044–9.

156. Larsen JJ, Hansen JM, Olsen NV, et al. The effect of altitude hypoxia on glucose homeostasis in men. J Physiol 1997;504(Pt 1):241–9.

157. Barnholt KE, Hoffman AR, Rock PB, et al. Endocrine responses to acute and chronic high-altitude exposure (4,300 meters): modulating effects of caloric restriction. Am J Physiol Endocrinol Metab 2006;290(6):E1078–88.

158. Braun B, Rock PB, Zamudio S, et al. Women at altitude: short-term exposure to hypoxia and/or alpha(1)-adrenergic blockade reduces insulin sensitivity. J Appl Physiol 2001;91(2):623–31.

159. Oltmanns KM, Gehring H, Rudolf S, et al. Hypoxia causes glucose intolerance in humans. Am J Respir Crit Care Med 2004;169(11):1231–7.

160. Louis M, Punjabi NM. Effects of acute intermittent hypoxia on glucose metabolism in awake healthy volunteers. J Appl Physiol 2009;106(5):1538–44.
161. Peng YJ, Yuan G, Ramakrishnan D, et al. Heterozygous HIF-1alpha deficiency impairs carotid body-mediated systemic responses and reactive oxygen species generation in mice exposed to intermittent hypoxia. J Physiol 2006;577(Pt 2):705–16.
162. Fletcher EC. Sympathetic over activity in the etiology of hypertension of obstructive sleep apnea. Sleep 2003;26(1):15–9.
163. Ryan S, Taylor CT, McNicholas WT. Selective activation of inflammatory pathways by intermittent hypoxia in obstructive sleep apnea syndrome. Circulation 2005;112(17):2660–7.
164. Yokoe T, Alonso LC, Romano LC, et al. Intermittent hypoxia reverses the diurnal glucose rhythm and causes pancreatic beta-cell replication in mice. J Physiol 2008;586(3):899–911.
165. Xu J, Long YS, Gozal D, et al. Beta-cell death and proliferation after intermittent hypoxia: role of oxidative stress. Free Radic Biol Med 2009;46(6):783–90.
166. Polotsky VY, Rubin AE, Balbir A, et al. Intermittent hypoxia causes REM sleep deficits and decreases EEG delta power in NREM sleep in the C57BL/6J mouse. Sleep Med 2006;7(1):7–16.
167. Pamidi S, Tasali E. Obstructive sleep apnea and type 2 diabetes: is there a link? Front Neurol 2012;3:126.
168. Foster GD, Sanders MH, Millman R, et al. Obstructive sleep apnea among obese patients with type 2 diabetes. Diabetes Care 2009;32(6):1017–9.
169. Levinson PD, McGarvey ST, Carlisle CC, et al. Adiposity and cardiovascular risk factors in men with obstructive sleep apnea. Chest 1993;103(5):1336–42.
170. Ip MS, Lam B, Ng MM, et al. Obstructive sleep apnea is independently associated with insulin resistance. Am J Respir Crit Care Med 2002;165(5):670–6.
171. Punjabi NM, Sorkin JD, Katzel LI, et al. Sleep-disordered breathing and insulin resistance in middle-aged and overweight men. Am J Respir Crit Care Med 2002;165(5):677–82.
172. McArdle N, Hillman D, Beilin L, et al. Metabolic risk factors for vascular disease in obstructive sleep apnea: a matched controlled study. Am J Respir Crit Care Med 2007;175(2):190–5.
173. Punjabi NM. Do sleep disorders and associated treatments impact glucose metabolism? Drugs 2009;69(Suppl 2):13–27.
174. Reichmuth KJ, Austin D, Skatrud JB, et al. Association of sleep apnea and type II diabetes: a population-based study. Am J Respir Crit Care Med 2005;172(12):1590–5.
175. Celen YT, Hedner J, Carlson J, et al. Impact of gender on incident diabetes mellitus in obstructive sleep apnea: a 16-year follow-up. J Clin Sleep Med 2010;6(3):244–50.
176. Marshall NS, Wong KK, Phillips CL, et al. Is sleep apnea an independent risk factor for prevalent and incident diabetes in the Busselton Health Study? J Clin Sleep Med 2009;5(1):15–20.
177. Botros N, Concato J, Mohsenin V, et al. Obstructive sleep apnea as a risk factor for type 2 diabetes. Am J Med 2009;122(12):1122–7.
178. Lindberg E, Theorell-Haglow J, Svensson M, et al. Sleep apnea and glucose metabolism: a long-term follow-up in a community-based sample. Chest 2012;142(4):935–42.
179. Sharma SK, Agrawal S, Damodaran D, et al. CPAP for the metabolic syndrome in patients with obstructive sleep apnea. N Engl J Med 2011;365(24):2277–86.

180. Weinstock TG, Wang X, Rueschman M, et al. A controlled trial of CPAP therapy on metabolic control in individuals with impaired glucose tolerance and sleep apnea. Sleep 2012;35(5):617–625B.
181. Lam JC, Lam B, Yao TJ, et al. A randomised controlled trial of nasal continuous positive airway pressure on insulin sensitivity in obstructive sleep apnoea. Eur Respir J 2010;35(1):138–45.
182. Malhotra A, White DP. Obstructive sleep apnoea. Lancet 2002;360(9328): 237–45.
183. Valencia-Flores M, Orea A, Castano VA, et al. Prevalence of sleep apnea and electrocardiographic disturbances in morbidly obese patients. Obes Res 2000;8(3):262–9.
184. Young T, Palta M, Dempsey J, et al. The occurrence of sleep-disordered breathing among middle-aged adults. N Engl J Med 1993;328(17):1230–5.
185. Smith PL, Gold AR, Meyers DA, et al. Weight loss in mildly to moderately obese patients with obstructive sleep apnea. Ann Intern Med 1985;103(6 (Pt 1)):850–5.
186. Schwartz AR, Gold AR, Schubert N, et al. Effect of weight loss on upper airway collapsibility in obstructive sleep apnea. Am Rev Respir Dis 1991;144(3 Pt 1): 494–8.
187. Sampol G, Munoz X, Sagales MT, et al. Long-term efficacy of dietary weight loss in sleep apnoea/hypopnoea syndrome. Eur Respir J 1998;12(5):1156–9.
188. Loube DI, Loube AA, Erman MK. Continuous positive airway pressure treatment results in weight less in obese and overweight patients with obstructive sleep apnea. J Am Diet Assoc 1997;97(8):896–7.
189. Redenius R, Murphy C, O'Neill E, et al. Does CPAP lead to change in BMI? J Clin Sleep Med 2008;4(3):205–9.
190. Chin K, Shimizu K, Nakamura T, et al. Changes in intra-abdominal visceral fat and serum leptin levels in patients with obstructive sleep apnea syndrome following nasal continuous positive airway pressure therapy. Circulation 1999; 100(7):706–12.

Asthma and Obesity
The Dose Effect

Amy Manion, PhD, RN, PNP[a,b],*

KEYWORDS

- Asthma • Obesity • Dose effect

KEY POINTS

- Asthma is one of the most common chronic illnesses in the world, affecting an estimated 300 million people.
- Globally, the prevalence of asthma has continued to spread as economic improvements in developing countries create a population trend toward urbanization and adoption of a western lifestyle.
- Research supports an association between obesity and asthma.

As the populations of the world have evolved from a mainly rural, mainly agrarian society, to a more urban and industrial society, the challenges facing modern medicine have also evolved. What were once the mainstays of concern, infectious diseases, such as polio, tuberculosis, and typhoid, have now been replaced with an equally fatal, if not more insidious problem. As the new millennium begins, the high rate of mortality from infectious diseases has been replaced with chronic illnesses, such as heart disease, diabetes, and asthma.

ASTHMA

Asthma is one of the most common chronic illnesses in the world, affecting an estimated 300 million people.[1] Over the period 1980 through 1996, there was a dramatic increase in the prevalence of asthma among all ages, genders, and racial groups, especially in more urbanized nations such as the United States.[2] Currently, 24.6 million people living in the United States have been diagnosed with asthma.[3] Globally, the prevalence of asthma has continued to spread as economic improvements in

This article originally appeared in Nursing Clinics of North America, Volume 48, Issue 1, March 2013.
Funding Sources: Nil.
Conflict of Interest: Nil.
[a] Northwestern Children's Practice, Chicago, IL, USA; [b] College of Nursing, Rush University, 600 South Paulina Street, Chicago, IL 60612, USA
* Armour Academic Center, College of Nursing, Rush University, 600 South Paulina Street, 1080, Chicago, IL 60612.
E-mail address: Amy_manion@rush.edu

Clinics Collections 3 (2014) 139–146
http://dx.doi.org/10.1016/j.ccol.2014.09.036
2352-7986/14/$ – see front matter © 2014 Elsevier Inc. All rights reserved.

developing countries create a population trend toward urbanization and adoption of a western lifestyle.[4,5] Based on this urbanization trend, it has been predicted that by 2025 an additional 100 million people will be diagnosed with asthma, increasing the global impact to 400 million.[1]

There is no cure for asthma. However, it can be controlled and managed with proper treatment. The general goals of asthma therapy consist of preventing chronic asthma symptoms and exacerbations, maintaining normal levels of activity, having normal or near-normal lung function, and having minimal side effects, while receiving optimal medication management.[6] Standard treatment of asthma consists of bronchodilators to relieve airway constriction, inhaled or oral corticosteroids to control inflammation, and avoidance of asthma triggers, such as smoke and other environmental irritants.[6]

Recently, combination therapy, consisting of an inhaled long-acting β_2-agonist along with an inhaled corticosteroid, has become the center of therapy for patients with moderate or severe persistent asthma.[7] In addition, leukotriene modifiers, which can prevent bronchoconstriction at a cellular level, are being used as add-on therapy.[7]

Despite the advances in therapeutic options, the economic burden of treating asthma in the United States has been expanding at an alarming rate because of the ever-increasing number of individuals diagnosed with the disease. In 1990, total costs due to asthma were estimated to be $6.2 billion.[8] By 1998, the cost of asthma had almost doubled to $11.3 billion, with direct costs accounting for $7.5 billion and indirect costs amounting to $3.8 billion.[9] Currently, the economic burden of asthma in the United States is staggering, with direct health care costs estimated at over $50 billion and indirect costs at $5.9 billion annually.[10]

Although asthma affects people of all ages, it disproportionately affects more children than adults, especially minority and poor children.[11,12] Currently, in the United States, over 10 million children and adolescents have been diagnosed with asthma, making it the leading chronic childhood illness.[13] Since 1999, children 5 to 17 years of age have demonstrated the highest prevalence rates with 109.3 per 1000 diagnosed with asthma, compared with 76.8 per 1000 in those over 18 years of age.[10] In 2009, the Centers for Disease Control and Prevention in the United States reported asthma prevalence ratios to be higher in children with approximately 1 in 12 for adults having asthma compared with 1 in 10 children.[14] The higher prevalence of asthma among children is not restricted to the United States; it is evident worldwide, especially in other industrial countries, such as the United Kingdom, where 1 in 7 children have been diagnosed with asthma compared with 1 in 25 adults.[15]

Furthermore, besides economic and age-related disparities, significant racial inequalities exist as well, especially in the more industrialized countries with the highest numbers of asthma prevalence. For example, in the United States, the asthma rate of prevalence is 43% higher for non-Hispanic blacks compared with non-Hispanic whites.[10] Even among children, these differences are evident. An analysis using results from the National Health Interview Survey 1997 to 2003 found that rate of asthma prevalence was consistently greater among non-Hispanic black children (15.7%) compared with non-Hispanic white children (11.5%) across all levels of income.[12] In addition, non-Hispanic black children are 3.6 times more likely to use the emergency department for asthma-related issues than non-Hispanic white children.[16] Multiple asthma-related emergency department visits are considered risk factors for fatal asthma, which is reflected in the rates of asthma mortality seen among minority groups, especially African Americans.[17] In 2006, non-Hispanic blacks had a rate of asthma mortality over 200% higher than non-Hispanic whites.[18] Furthermore, from 2003 to 2005, the Centers for Disease Control and Prevention reported that African American children had a rate of asthma mortality 7 times higher than non-Hispanic white children.[19] The World Health Organization has estimated the global rate of mortality from asthma to be 250,000 people annually.[20]

OBESITY

The high global prevalence of asthma and its continued drain on medical resources make it a major cause for concern. Nevertheless, another disturbing trend in health care use has revealed itself in the past decade as millions of American waistlines have grown to uncomfortable and unhealthy sizes. The prevalence of obesity in the United States is increasing at an alarming rate. Body mass index (BMI), defined as the weight in kilograms divided by the square of the height in meters, is commonly used to classify overweight and obesity among adults.[21] In adults, a BMI between 25 and 29.9 is defined as overweight, and a BMI of 30 or higher is considered obese. For children, overweight is defined as a BMI between the 85th and 94th percentile for age and gender, and obese is defined at a BMI at or above the 95th percentile for age and gender.[21]

According to data from the 2005 to 2006 National Health and Nutrition Examination Survey (NHANES), more than one-third of adults, or over 72 million people, are obese.[22] The incidence of obesity is increasing not only in the United States but also globally. Worldwide there are more than 1.5 billion overweight adults, with at least 500 million clinically obese adults.[23] The World Health Organization has predicted that by 2015, approximately 2.3 billion adults will be overweight and over 700 million will be obese.[24]

The worldwide increase in the prevalence of obesity is especially concerning because of the multitude of health problems associated with obesity. Obese and overweight adults are at greater risk of cardiovascular disease, hypertension, stroke, type 2 diabetes, and certain forms of cancer, such as breast, pancreas, kidney, thyroid, and esophagus.[25] Approximately 85% of people with diabetes are type 2, and of these, 90% are overweight or obese.[23]

The true economic impact associated with the rise in obesity prevalence is difficult to determine due to the number of obesity-related conditions. The direct obesity-related medical costs in the United States have been estimated at $51.6 billion, whereas the indirect costs have been estimated at $47.6 billion.[26]

The increase in the prevalence of obesity in adults has been accompanied by a similar increase in the prevalence of obesity in children.[27] Furthermore, there is a strong cyclical relationship between adult and childhood obesity. For example, parental obesity more than doubles the risk of adult obesity in both obese and nonobese children.[28,29] If both parents are lean, a healthy child has a 14% chance of becoming overweight; however, if both parents are obese, the risk jumps to 80%.[30]

In the United States, the number of overweight children has doubled and the number of overweight adolescents has tripled over the last 2 decades.[31] The results from the 2003 to 2006 NHANES study showed an estimated 17% of children ages 6 to 11 years are overweight, which represents more than a 60% increase from the overweight estimates of 11% obtained from the 1988 to 1994 NHANES.[21]

The increasing prevalence of childhood overweight is not restricted to the United States alone. An estimated 22 million children under the age of 5 are considered overweight worldwide.[24] Childhood overweight is becoming prevalent even in the developing world; for example, in Thailand, the prevalence of overweight in children 5 to 12 years of age increased from 12.2% to 15.6% in just 2 years.[23]

Similar to asthma, racial and ethnic disparities exist with obesity prevalence as well. In the United States, non-Hispanic blacks have a 51% higher rate of obesity, and

Hispanics have a 21% higher rate of obesity compared with non-Hispanic whites.[32] Similar to adults, NHANES data have shown the prevalence of obesity and overweight combined to be higher in non-Hispanic black children (35.4%) compared with non-Hispanic white children (28.2%).[33] The NHANES data found Mexican American boys ages 6 to 11 to have the highest combined obesity and overweight prevalence (43.9%).[33]

ASTHMA AND OBESITY

The increase in prevalence of both asthma and obesity has led to several studies examining the possible relationship between these 2 variables. Much of the research in this area has focused on the adult population. A study examining the trends in obesity among adults, using data from the NHANES I (1971–1975), II (1976–1980), and III (1988–1994), found that BMI increased universally among adults with asthma and those without; however, the prevalence of obesity rose more in the asthma group (21.3-32.8%) compared with the nonasthma group (14.6-22.8%).[34] A retrospective study of 143 individuals ages 18 to 88 found that the prevalence of obesity increased along with increasing asthma severity.[35]

The relationship between asthma and obesity demonstrated in studies conducted with adults has also been replicated in the pediatric population. A cross-sectional study using data from the Third National Health and Nutrition Examination Survey 1988 to 1994 showed that 2 of the highest risk groups for developing asthma were children over the age of 10 with a BMI greater than or equal to the 85th percentile (overweight and obese category) and children with a parental history of asthma who were 10 years or younger and of African American ethnicity.[36] A study conducted in the United Kingdom found that obesity among children 4 to 11 years of age was associated with asthma regardless of ethnicity, especially among girls.[37] Findings from the National Longitudinal Survey of Youth, which followed more than 4000 asthma-free children for 14 years, discovered a BMI at or greater than the 85th percentile at age 2 to 3 years was a risk factor for subsequent asthma development in boys.[38]

DOSE EFFECT

Research seems to support a relationship between obesity and asthma. Obesity has proven to be a risk factor for asthma in both adults and children.[39,40] There is a growing body of evidence to support a dose effect for asthma severity with obesity; however, a causal relationship has not been proven.

The evidence of a dose effect between obesity and asthma symptoms and severity is most strongly supported by the results from research conducted with patients who have experienced weight loss. In a study of 500 morbidly obese patients who underwent laparoscopic adjustable gastric banding surgery, greater than 80% of the patients who had asthma symptoms before surgery reported resolution or improvement in their symptoms.[41] A systematic review of studies examining asthma and weight loss found there was reversibility of at least 1 asthma outcome irrespective of whether weight loss was a result of surgical or medical intervention.[42] A meta-analysis of prospective studies involving obesity and asthma risk found asthma incidence increased by 50% in overweight and obese individuals regardless of gender, demonstrating a dose-dependent relationship between obesity and asthma.[43]

The dose effect relationship between obesity and asthma has also been researched in children. A study examining non-Hispanic black and Hispanic children age 2 to 18 years with asthma found the prevalence of overweight to be higher in children with moderate to severe asthma symptoms compared with the control group.[44] A more recent study found obese children with asthma used more asthma medications, wheezed more, and had a higher number of unscheduled emergency department visits than the nonobese children with asthma.[45] A large cross-sectional study of more than 400,000 adolescents found a significantly higher likelihood of asthma diagnosis occurring at higher BMI percentiles regardless of gender and race/ethnicity, indicating a positive dose response relationship between increasing BMI and asthma risk.[46]

Internationally, the dose effect relationship between obesity and asthma has also been documented. A large Norwegian study of more than 135,000 men and women found a 10% increase in asthma prevalence per unit of increase in BMI in men and a 7% increase in prevalence per unit increase in BMI in women.[47] A study in Taiwan of greater than 15,000 school-aged children found the prevalence of asthma increased as BMI elevated and high BMI coincided with low FEV_1/FCV scores on lung function testing, which is associated with lung impairment.[48] A similar result was found in a study conducted in Nova Scotia, Canada, that examined over 3000 students 10 to 11 years of age and found a linear association between BMI and asthma with a 6% increase in prevalence per unit increase of BMI.[49]

The exact mechanism creating the dose effect seen between obesity and asthma still needs further investigation. One theory proposed, which supports the less common view that asthma causes obesity, is that individuals with asthma restrict their levels of activity for fear of inducing an asthma exacerbation, which then leads to a more sedentary lifestyle and an increased risk of obesity.[37] Although many individuals with asthma might avoid vigorous physical activity and thus put on weight, this would seem, at best, an incomplete explanation for asthma causing obesity.[50]

The reverse association, that obesity causes asthma, and is the driving force behind the dose effect seen between these diseases has the most support. Proposed theories include mechanical, dietary, genetic, and hormonal.[46,51] One main theory that has generated the most discussion is the role pro-inflammatory cytokines such as leptin play in the process because adipose tissue is known as a primary source of these systemic immunomodulating agents and could be contributing to the chronic inflammation seen in asthma, creating more symptoms of the disease.[46,52] Cytokines are already believed to play a role in exercise-induced asthma, which could lead to proposals to add similar obesity-induced asthma nomenclature to the list of asthma categories.[53]

IMPLICATIONS

Whether the relationship between obesity and asthma is direct or indirect has yet to be determined. Nevertheless, the affects of obesity on asthma are evident and need to be incorporated into the management of the disease. Because prevention is the key to combating the steady rise in obesity, weight management should be addressed at each health care visit regardless of the individual's weight. For those individuals who are overweight or obese, nutritional counseling should be provided and a follow-up plan for weight loss should be developed. The positive effects of weight loss on asthma symptoms should be shared with patients to provide motivation and encouragement. Only by making weight management a priority in the treatment of asthma can the rising prevalence of both diseases be hindered and global health improved.

REFERENCES

1. Global Initiative for Asthma (GINA). The Global Strategy for Asthma Management and Prevention. 2011. Available at: http://www.Ginasthma.org/. Accessed June 15, 2012.

2. Akinbami LJ, Moorman JE, Garbe PL, et al. Status of childhood asthma in the United States, 1980–2007. Pediatrics 2009;123(Suppl 3):S131–45.
3. Centers for Disease Control and Prevention (CDC). Vital signs: asthma prevalence, disease characteristics, and self-management education: United States, 2001-2009. MMWR Morb Mortal Wkly Rep 2011;60(17):547–52 [0149-2195].
4. Bai J, Zhao J, Shen K, et al. Current trends of the prevalence of childhood asthma in three Chinese cities: a multicenter epidemiological survey. Biomed Environ Sci 2010;23:453–7.
5. Ait-Khaled N, Enarson DA, Bissell K, et al. Access to inhaled corticosteroids is key to improving quality of care for asthma in developing countries. Allergy 2007;62:230–6.
6. National Asthma Education and Prevention Program. Expert panel report 3: Guidelines for the diagnosis and management of asthma (No. NIH publication no. 07-4051). Bethesda (MD): National Heart Lung and Blood Institute; 2007.
7. Arellano FM, Arana A, Wentworth CE, et al. Prescription patterns for asthma medications in children and adolescents with health care insurance in the United States. Pediatr Allergy Immunol 2011;22:469–76.
8. Weiss KB, Sullivan SD. The health economics of asthma and rhinitis. Assessing the economic impact. J Allergy Clin Immunol 2001;107:3–8.
9. National Heart Lung and Blood Institute. Data fact sheet: asthma statistics. 1999. Available at: http://www.nhlbi.nih.gov/health/prof/lung/asthma/asthstat.pdf. Accessed March 3, 2006.
10. American Lung Association. Trends in morbidity and mortality. 2011. Available at: www.lung.org/finding-cures/our-research/trend-reports/asthma-trend-report.pdf. Accessed August 5, 2012.
11. Flores G, The Committee on Pediatric Research. Technical report- Racial and ethnic disparities in the health and health care of children. Pediatrics 2010;125(4):e979–1021.
12. McDaniel M, Paxson C, Waldfogel J. Racial disparities in childhood asthma in the United States: Evidence from the National Health Interview Survey, 1997 to 2003. Pediatrics 2006;117(5):868–77.
13. Bloom B, Cohen RA, Freeman G. Summary health statistics for U.S. children: National health interview survey, 2010. Vital Health Stat 10 2010;(250):1–89.
14. CDC. 2011 Asthma in the U.S., Vital Signs. 2011. Available at: http://www.cdc.gov/VitalSigns/Asthma/. Accessed August 5, 2012.
15. Braman SS. The global burden of asthma. Chest 2006;130(1):4S–12S.
16. U.S. Department of Health and Human Services, Agency for Healthcare Research and Quality, National Healthcare Quality and Disparities Reports. 2011. Available at: www.ahrq.gov/qual/qrdr11/6_maternalchildhealth/T6_4_14_1_1.htm. Accessed June 19, 2012.
17. Carroll CL, Uygungil B, Zucker AR, et al. Identifying an at-risk population of children with recurrent near-fatal asthma exacerbations. J Asthma 2010;47:460–4.
18. CDC. Asthma prevalence, health care use and mortality: United States, 2003-2005. 2006. Available at: http://www.cdc.gov/nchs. Accessed August 15, 2009.
19. Akinbami LJ. The state of childhood asthma, United States, 1980-2005, Advance data from vital health statistics; no. 381. Hyattsville (MD): National Center for Health Statistics; 2006.
20. World Health Organization. Global surveillance, prevention and control of chronic respiratory diseases: a comprehensive approach. Geneva, Switzerland: World Health Organization; 2007.

21. CDC. Overweight and obesity. 2012. Available at: http://www.cdc.gov/obesity/adult/defining.html. Accessed June 19, 2012.
22. Ogden CL, Carroll MD, McDowell MA, et al. Obesity among adults in the United States- no change since 2003-2004. Hyattsville (MD): National Center for Health Statistics; 2007.
23. World Health Organization. Obesity and overweight. 2011. Available at: http://www.who.int/mediacentre/factsheets/fs311/en/index.html. Accessed July 6, 2012.
24. World Health Organization. WHO: global database on body mass index. 2012. Available at: http://www.who.int/bmi/index.jsp. Accessed July 6, 2012.
25. Kopelman P. Health risks associated with overweight and obesity. Obes Rev 2007;8(Suppl 1):13–7.
26. Li Z, Bowerman S, Heber D. Health ramifications of the obesity epidemic. Surg Clin North Am 2005;85(4):681–701.
27. Maffeis C, Tato L. Long-term effects of childhood obesity on morbidity and morality. Horm Res 2001;55(Suppl 1):42–5.
28. Krebs NF, Jacobson MS, American Academy of Pediatrics Committee on Nutrition. Prevention of pediatric overweight and obesity. Pediatrics 2003;112(2):424–30.
29. Whitaker RC, Wright JA, Pepe MS, et al. Predicting obesity in young adulthood from childhood and parental obesity. N Engl J Med 1997;337(13):869–73.
30. Hagarty MA, Schmidt C, Bernaix L, et al. Adolescent obesity: Current trends in identification and management. J Am Acad Nurse Pract 2004;16(11):481–9.
31. U.S. Preventative Services Task Force. Screening and interventions for overweight in children and adolescents: recommendation statement. Pediatrics 2005;116(1):205–9.
32. CDC. Differences in prevalence of obesity among black, white, and hispanic adults–United States, 2006-2008. MMWR Morb Mortal Wkly Rep 2009;58(27):740–4.
33. Wang Y, Beydoun MA. The obesity epidemic in the United States—Gender, age socioeconomic, racial/ethnic, and geographic characteristics: A systemic review and meta-regression analysis. Epidemiol Rev 2007;29:6–28.
34. Ford ES, Mannino DM. Time trends in obesity among adults with asthma in the United States: findings from three national surveys. J Asthma 2005;42(2):91–5.
35. Akerman MJ, Calacanis CM, Madsen MK. Relationship between asthma severity and obesity. J Asthma 2004;41(5):521–6.
36. Rodriguez MA, Winkleby MA, Ahn D, et al. Identification of population subgroups of children and adolescents with high asthma prevalence: findings from the Third National Health and Nutrition Examination Survey. Arch Pediatr Adolesc Med 2002;156(3):269–75.
37. Figueroa-Munoz JI, Chinn S, Rona RJ. Association between obesity and asthma in 4-11 year old children in the U.K. Thorax 2001;56:133–7.
38. Mannino DM, Mott J, Ferdinands JM, et al. Boys with high body masses have an increased risk of developing asthma: findings from the National Longitudinal Survey of Youth (NLSY). Int J Obes 2006;30(1):6–13.
39. Guerra S, Sherrill DL, Bobadilla A, et al. The relation of body mass index to asthma, chronic bronchitis, and emphysema. Chest 2002;122:1256–63.
40. Hjellvik V, Tverdal A, Furu K. Body mass index as predictor for asthma: a cohort study of 118, 723 males and females. Eur Respir J 2010;35(6):1235–42.
41. Spivak H, Hewitt MF, Onn A, et al. Weight loss and improvement of obesity-related illness in 500 U.S. patients following laparoscopic adjustable gastric banding procedure. Am J Surg 2005;189(1):27–32.

42. Eneli IU, Skybo T, Camargo CA Jr. Weight loss and asthma: a systematic review. Thorax 2008;63:671–6.
43. Beuther DA, Sutherland ER. Overweight, obesity, and incident of asthma. Am J Respir Crit Care Med 2007;175:661–6.
44. Luder E, Melnik TA, DiMaio M. Association of being overweight with greater asthma symptoms in inner city black and Hispanic children. J Pediatr 1998; 132(4):699–703.
45. Belamarich PF, Luder E, Kattan M, et al. Do obese inner-city children with asthma have more symptoms than nonobese children with asthma? Pediatrics 2000; 106(6):1436–41.
46. Davis A, Lipsett M, Milet M, et al. An association between asthma and BMI in adolescents: results from the California Healthy Kids survey. J Asthma 2007;44: 873–9.
47. Nystad W, Meyer HE, Nafstad P, et al. Body mass index in relation to adult asthma among 135,000 Norwegian men and women. Am J Epidemiol 2004;160:969–76.
48. Chiu YT, Chen WY, Wang TN, et al. Extreme BMI predicts higher asthma prevalence and is associated with lung function impairment in school-aged children. Pediatr Pulmonol 2009;44:472–9.
49. Sithole F, Douwes J, Burstyn I, et al. Body mass index and childhood asthma: a linear association? J Asthma 2008;45:473–7.
50. Shaneen SO. Obesity and asthma: cause for concern? Clin Exp Allergy 1999; 29(3):291–3.
51. Chin S. Obesity and asthma: evidence for and against a causal relation. J Asthma 2003;40(1):1–16.
52. Silva P, Mello M, Cheik N, et al. The role of pro-inflammatory and anti-inflammatory adipokines on exercise-induced bronchospasm in obese adolescents undergoing treatment. Respir Care 2012;57(4):572–82.
53. Hallstrand TS, Moody MW, Aitken ML, et al. Airway immunopathology of asthma with exercise-induced bronchoconstriction. J Allergy Clin Immunol 2005;116(3): 586–93.

Obesity Hypoventilation Syndrome and Anesthesia

Edmond H.L. Chau, MD[a], Babak Mokhlesi, MD, MSc[b],
Frances Chung, MBBS, FRCPC[a],*

KEYWORDS

- Obesity hypoventilation syndrome • Perioperative management
- Positive airway pressure

KEY POINTS

- Obesity hypoventilation syndrome (OHS) is an important disease entity that requires the anesthesiologist's thorough understanding.
- Patients with OHS present with severe upper airway obstruction, restrictive pulmonary physiology, blunted central respiratory drive, and pulmonary hypertension. The primary therapy for OHS is positive airway pressure (PAP) therapy.
- Screening questionnaires such as the validated STOP-Bang questionnaire can identify patients at high risk of obstructive sleep apnea.
- Before major elective surgery, these patients should be referred to sleep medicine for polysomnography and PAP titration.
- Future research should focus on the perioperative strategies of screening, monitoring, and treatment of OHS and associated complications.

INTRODUCTION

Obesity is a global health concern. One of the complications associated with morbid obesity is obesity hypoventilation syndrome (OHS). OHS is defined by the triad of obesity (body mass index [BMI] $\geq$30 kg/m^2), daytime hypoventilation with hypercapnia (partial pressure of arterial carbon dioxide [$Paco_2$] $\geq$45 mm Hg at sea level), and hypoxemia (partial pressure of arterial oxygen [Pao_2] less than 70 mm Hg at sea level), and sleep-disordered breathing.[1] OHS is diagnosed after excluding other known causes of hypoventilation, such as severe obstructive or restrictive parenchymal lung disease,

This article originally appeared in Sleep Medicine Clinics, Volume 8, Issue 1, March 2013.
[a] Department of Anesthesiology, Toronto Western Hospital, University Health Network, University of Toronto, Bathurst Street, Toronto, Ontario M5T2S8, Canada; [b] Section of Pulmonary and Critical Care Medicine, Department of Medicine, Sleep Disorders Center, University of Chicago Pritzker School of Medicine, Maryland Avenues, Chicago, IL 60637, USA
* Corresponding author. Department of Anesthesia, Room 405, 2McL, 399 Bathurst Street, Toronto, Ontario, Canada M5T 2S8.
E-mail address: frances.chung@uhn.on.ca

Clinics Collections 3 (2014) 147–164
http://dx.doi.org/10.1016/j.ccol.2014.09.037
2352-7986/14/$ – see front matter © 2014 Elsevier Inc. All rights reserved.

kyphoscoliosis, severe hypothyroidism, neuromuscular disease, and congenital central hypoventilation syndrome. In 90% of cases of OHS, the sleep-disordered breathing present is obstructive sleep apnea (OSA).[2] The prevalence of OHS in the general adult population is estimated to be 0.15% to 0.3%.[2] In patients undergoing bariatric surgery, approximately 8% present with OHS.[3]

Patients with OHS have a higher burden of comorbidities and increased risk for perioperative morbidity and mortality.[4–6] Therefore, a thorough plan of evaluation and management is essential for patients with OHS who undergo surgery. Currently, information on the perioperative management of OHS is extremely limited in the literature. As the prevalence of OHS is likely to increase as a result of the current global obesity epidemic, it is crucial for physicians to recognize and manage patients with this syndrome. This review examines the current data on OHS and discusses its optimal perioperative management.

PATHOPHYSIOLOGY

Daytime hypercapnia is a distinguishing feature in OHS and is entirely due to hypoventilation; a short course of noninvasive positive airway pressure (PAP) therapy (<2 weeks) improves hypercapnia without any significant changes in body weight, carbon dioxide (CO_2) production, or dead space volume.[7] There are currently 3 main hypotheses regarding the development of OHS: obesity-induced impairment in respiratory mechanics, leptin resistance, and impaired compensation for acute hypercapnia in OSA.[2,8]

Obesity-Induced Impairment in Respiratory Mechanics

Obesity induces hypoventilation by increasing the mechanical load on the respiratory system, resulting in fatigue and weakness of the respiratory muscles.[9–11] In several studies, patients with OHS were shown to have higher BMI than eucapnic obese individuals.[12–15] However, because less than one third of morbidly obese individuals develop hypercapnia, other mechanisms may contribute to hypoventilation.[14–16]

Leptin Resistance

Leptin is a protein secreted specifically by adipocytes to regulate appetite and energy expenditure.[17–19] Leptin crosses the blood-brain barrier and exerts its effect by binding to leptin receptors in various areas of the brain.[18] In obese individuals, a higher level of leptin is found to be associated with an increase in ventilation to compensate for the increased CO_2 production by excess body mass.[17,20,21] Patients with OHS have an even higher serum leptin level than eucapnic individuals matched for BMI.[22,23] Although the precise relationship between leptin and OHS remains to be determined, it is speculated that leptin resistance may lead to central hypoventilation in OHS.

Impaired Compensation of Acute Hypercapnia in OSA

Hypoventilation during sleep secondary to obstructive apneas and hypopneas results in transient episodes of acute hypercapnia and serum bicarbonate (HCO_3^-) retention. Eucapnic patients with OSA present several compensatory mechanisms to maintain acid-base homeostasis. During sleep, they hyperventilate between periods of apnea.[24] In addition, during wakefulness in daytime, acute hypercapnia is corrected and the excess HCO_3^- is excreted. On the other hand, patients with OHS have a reduced duration of ventilation between periods of apnea while sleeping.[25] The resulting acute hypercapnia persists during wakefulness and HCO_3^- retention occurs, causing gradual adaptation by chemoreceptors and further blunting of ventilatory CO_2 responsiveness. In a computer model, when both CO_2 response and the rate of renal HCO_3^- excretion was abnormally low, an increase in awake $Paco_2$ and HCO_3^- developed over multiple days.[26]

DISTINGUISHING CLINICAL FEATURES

Compared with eucapnic obese individuals with and without OSA, patients with OHS demonstrate more severe upper airway obstruction, restrictive pulmonary physiology, blunted central respiratory drive, and increased incidence of pulmonary hypertension. Patients with OHS display increased upper airway resistance in both the sitting and supine position in comparison with obese individuals with eucapnia.[27] In perioperative settings, patients with OHS are at increased risk of life-threatening apneic events because sedatives and narcotics increase the collapsibility of the upper airway and attenuate respiratory drive.[28,29]

Spirometric values from morbidly obese patients typically reveal a restrictive pattern with a reduction in forced expiratory volume in the first second (FEV_1) and forced vital capacity (FVC) but normal FEV_1/FVC ratio. This restrictive pulmonary physiology is further impaired in OHS.[3] Chest wall compliance is reduced and respiratory resistance is increased, likely secondary to the reduction in functional residual capacity and expiratory reserve volume. As a result, the work of breathing in OHS patients is twice that of obese eucapnic individuals[30,31] and increases further when these patients are positioned supine from sitting as a result of the cephaled shift of abdominal contents.[30,32]

In contrast to obese eucapnic individuals who possess a substantially increased central respiratory drive,[32] patients with OHS have a blunted central respiratory drive to both hypercapnia and hypoxia. They do not hyperventilate to the same extent as obese eucapnic individuals when forced to rebreathe CO_2[33–35] or breathe a hypoxic gas mixture.[35]

The prevalence of pulmonary hypertension in patients with OHS is high, ranging from 30% to 88%.[4,36–38] Seventy-seven percent of patients with OHS with respiratory failure in the intensive care unit have moderate to severe pulmonary hypertension (pulmonary systolic pressure >45 mm Hg).[37] The cause of pulmonary hypertension is likely secondary to chronic alveolar hypoxia and hypercapnia. In morbidly obese patients, left-heart failure is not uncommon and may increase pulmonary arterial pressure.[39]

MORBIDITY AND MORTALITY

Obesity and OSA are associated with a spectrum of comorbidities such as coronary artery disease, heart failure, stroke, and metabolic syndrome, which result in increased morbidity and mortality.[40–44] Furthermore, patients with OSA are at increased risk of developing postoperative complications including arrhythmias and hypoxemia.[45–47] An increased risk of transfer to the intensive care unit and increased length of hospital stay were also observed among patients with OSA who underwent noncardiac surgery.[46]

Several studies have shown that patients with OHS may experience higher morbidity and mortality than patients who are similarly obese and have OSA. Compared with obese individuals with eucapnia, patients with OHS were more likely to develop heart failure (odds ratio [OR] 9, 95% confidence interval [CI] 2.3–35), angina pectoris (OR 9, 95% CI 1.4–57.1), and cor pulmonale (OR 9, 95% CI 1.4–57.1).[4] They also received higher rates of long-term care at discharge (19% vs 2%, $P = .01$), and invasive mechanical ventilation (6% vs 0%, $P = .01$).[48]

Hospitalized patients with untreated OHS had a high mortality rate of 46% during a 50-month follow-up period after discharge.[49] In addition, their mortality rate is higher compared with obese eucapnic patients after hospital discharge at 18 months (23% vs 9%).[48] In patients undergoing open bariatric surgery, those with either OHS or OSA suffered a surgical mortality rate of 4%, significantly higher than those without the disease (0.2%, $P<.01$).[50] In patients with OHS with additional risk factors (previous history of venous thromboembolism, BMI ≥ 50 kg/m^2, male sex, hypertension and age ≥ 45 years) undergoing bariatric surgery, mortality ranges between 2% and 8%.[5,6,51]

In summary, patients with OHS experience higher morbidity and mortality than those with eucapnia who are obese. Previous history of venous thromboembolism, morbid obesity, male sex, hypertension, increasing age, and noncompliance with PAP treatment may further increase mortality risk. The surgical mortality rate in high-risk patients with OHS undergoing bariatric surgery is between 2% and 8%.

TREATMENT

Therapeutic interventions for OHS include 4 main components: PAP therapy, supplemental oxygen, bariatric surgery, and pharmacologic respiratory stimulants.

PAP Therapy

The 2 main forms of PAP therapy currently being used are continuous positive airway pressure (CPAP) and bilevel PAP. The overall short-term and long-term benefits were summarized in a recent systematic review.[3]

Short-term benefits of PAP include an improvement in gas exchange and sleep-disordered breathing. A short course (≤ 3 weeks) of PAP results in a significant decrease in $Paco_2$ and an increase in Pao_2.[49,52–54] Furthermore, sleep study parameters, including the apnea-hypopnea index (AHI) and oxygen saturation during sleep, were reported to be significantly improved.[53–56]

Long-term benefits of PAP include an improvement in pulmonary function and central respiratory drive to CO_2. A course of PAP therapy for 24 to 48 weeks significantly increased FEV_1 and FVC.[57–59] The effect of PAP on central respiratory drive, measured as the change in minute ventilation per unit change in end-tidal CO_2, was reported in several studies to be favorable.[52,58,60]

PAP may also reduce mortality in OHS. Two retrospective studies have reported a mortality rate of 13% to 19% in patients with OHS on PAP throughout a mean period of 4 years.[57,61] Through indirect comparison, this mortality rate is lower than the 23% mortality rate reported in patients with untreated OHS at 18 months of follow-up.[48]

CPAP failure, defined by a residual AHI of 5 or more or a mean nocturnal pulse oximeter oxygen saturation (Spo_2) less than 90%, has been reported.[62] A recent prospective randomized study compared the long-term efficacy of bilevel PAP versus CPAP.[63] Two groups of 18 patients with OHS who underwent successful CPAP titration were randomized to either bilevel PAP or CPAP for 3 months. Both groups experienced a similar degree of improvement in $Paco_2$ and daytime sleepiness. Overall, bilevel PAP was not considerably superior to CPAP if CPAP titration was successful. However, if CPAP titration is unsuccessful, bilevel PAP should be strongly considered and treatment should be individualized to each patient.[2] Bilevel PAP should be instituted if the patient is intolerant of higher CPAP pressure (>15 cm H_2O) or if hypoxemia persists despite adequate resolution of obstructive respiratory events.[64] A therapeutic algorithm for CPAP titration in OHS patients is shown in **Fig. 1**.

A new treatment modality in patients with OHS is average volume-assured pressure-support (AVAPS) ventilation. This mode of PAP therapy ensures the delivery of

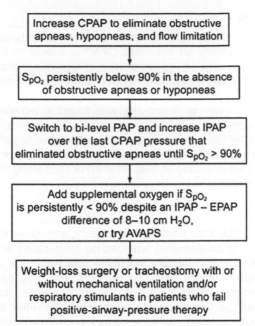

Fig. 1. Algorithm for continuous PAP titration in patients with OHS. AVAPS, average volume-assured pressure-support ventilation; CPAP, continuous positive airway pressure; EPAP, expiratory positive airway pressure; IPAP, inspiratory positive airway pressure.

a preset tidal volume during bilevel PAP mode. The expiratory tidal volume and leak are estimated based on pneumotacographic inspiratory and expiratory flows. Target tidal volume is typically set at 8 to 10 mL/kg of ideal body weight. The expiratory PAP is set to resolve upper airway obstruction and the inspiratory PAP is automatically adjusted to achieve the targeted tidal volume. This mode of PAP also provides a backup rate to alleviate central apneas that may emerge during PAP therapy.[65] In 1 clinical trial, AVAPS was more effective in improving nocturnal hypoventilation compared with CPAP and bilevel PAP in ST mode (activated backup rate). However, the degree of improvement in daytime $Paco_2$ did not reach statistical significance.[66] In a recent randomized controlled trial of patients with OHS, there was no significant difference between AVAPS and bilevel PAP ST mode in the degree of improvement in daytime and nocturnal gas exchange.[67] However, in this study, those randomized to bilevel PAP ST mode underwent aggressive bilevel PAP titration focusing on achieving adequate tidal volumes (mean inspiratory PAP of 23 cm H_2O and mean expiratory PAP of 10 cm H_2O), as recommended by the American Academy of Sleep Medicine guidelines on noninvasive ventilation.[68]

In summary, PAP therapy improves gas exchange, sleep-disordered breathing, lung function, and central respiratory drive to CO_2. Long-term PAP therapy also lowers the mortality rate in patients with OHS. Because of its noninvasiveness and effectiveness, PAP is the first-line therapy for OHS. CPAP is usually the initials modality of choice because of its relative simplicity and low cost. However, if CPAP titration fails, bilevel PAP or AVAPS should be applied. A need for a backup rate should be strongly considered because central apneas occur commonly in patients with OHS undergoing PAP therapy.

Supplemental Oxygen

Approximately 20% to 30% of patients with OHS continue to desaturate to Spo_2 less than 90% during sleep while on adequate CPAP or bilevel PAP settings, thereby requiring supplemental oxygen.[55] Administration of high-concentration supplemental oxygen without PAP therapy may induce hypoventilation and worsen hyercapnia.[69,70] In a recent study, a significant decrease in minute ventilation, resulting in an increase in transcutaneous CO_2 tension by 5 mm Hg, was found in patients with OHS while breathing 100% oxygen compared with those breathing room air.[71] Therefore, clinicians should administer the lowest concentration of oxygen to patients with OHS to avoid worsening of hypercapnia while maintaining optimized oxygenation, particularly in patients with OHS experiencing an exacerbation or recovering from sedatives/narcotics or general anesthesia.[72]

Bariatric Surgery

Bariatric surgery is a mainstay treatment of obesity, especially for morbidly obese patients in whom more conservative approaches have failed or who have developed comorbidities. Bariatric surgery improves gas exchange and lung function in OHS. At 1 year after surgery, Pao_2, $Paco_2$, FEV_1, and FVC all improved significantly.[50,73] To better understand the effect of surgical weight loss on OSA, Greenburg and colleagues[74] performed a meta-analysis of 12 studies including a total of 342 patients in whom polysomnography before and after maximum weight loss were available. They found that bariatric surgery led to significant weight loss with a mean reduction in BMI from 55.3 kg/m^2 to 37.7 kg/m^2. This robust weight loss was accompanied by a reduction in the AHI from baseline values of 55 events/h (95% CI 49–60) to 16 events/h (95% CI 13–19). However, many of these patients (62%) had persistent OSA of moderate severity (AHI $\geq$15 events/h). Thus, although improvements should be anticipated, OSA does not resolve in all patients after surgically achieved weight loss. CPAP therapy could still benefit patients with residual OSA after maximum weight loss. Similarly, 14% of patients with OHS still require PAP therapy after weight loss.[73] Therefore, patients with OHS should undergo reevaluation after bariatric surgery before discontinuing PAP therapy. As patients age and/or regain some weight over the years, the severity of OSA can increase.

Bariatric surgery is associated with significant risk. The overall perioperative mortality ranges between 0.5% and 1.5%.[75,76] The presence of OSA and extreme preoperative weight are independent risk factors associated with perioperative death and adverse events including venous thromboembolism, surgical reintervention, and prolonged hospital stay.[76,77] Ideally, PAP should be initiated in all patients with OHS and bariatric surgery should be considered as a second-line intervention.

Pharmacotherapy

Medications that increase respiratory drive have been investigated for the treatment of OHS. Limited evidence is available for 2 respiratory stimulants: medroxyprogesterone acetate and acetazolamide.

Medroxyprogesterone acetate stimulates respiration at the hypothalamic level.[78] Its role in OHS is uncertain. An early study reported an increase in Pao_2 and a decrease in $Paco_2$ in patients with OHS treated with medroxyprogesterone acetate.[79] However, a later study did not demonstrate the same benefits.[7] Because medroxyprogesterone acetate increases the risk of venous thromboembolism,[80] administration to patients with OHS whose mobility is limited may be unsafe.

Acetazolamide is a carbonic anhydrase inhibitor that increases minute ventilation by inducing metabolic acidosis through increased excretion of bicarbonate by the kidneys. Acetazolamide has been shown to improve AHI, increase Pa_{O_2}, and reduce Pa_{CO_2} in patients with OSA.[81,82] More recently, in mechanically ventilated patients with OHS, acetazolamide reduced plasma HCO_3^- and increased hypercapnic drive response.[83] Given the limited data on pharmacotherapy and because it is not widely used, the authors do not recommend it as a mainstay therapy but rather an adjunctive therapy in patients with OHS who remain hypercapnic despite adequate adherence to optimally titrated PAP therapy. Specifically, OHS patients requiring high doses of loop diuretics, which can lead to further HCO_3^- retention, may be ideal candidates for acetazolamide. Caution should be exercised in prescribing a respiratory stimulant in patients with ventilatory limitation because it can lead to exacerbation of acidosis and worsening of dyspnea. Acetazolamide should not be prescribed as a respiratory stimulant if a patient cannot normalize or near normalize their Pa_{CO_2} (or end-tidal CO_2) levels with 1 to 2 minutes of voluntary hyperventilation.

PREOPERATIVE ASSESSMENT OF PATIENTS WITH OHS

The 3 main challenges in OHS are OSA, obesity, and hypoventilation (hypercapnia and hypoxemia). For a patient with suspected OHS presenting for elective surgery, the preoperative assessment should begin with the history and physical examination directed to identify comorbidities in OHS, including coronary artery disease, congestive heart failure, pulmonary hypertension, and diabetes mellitus. A detailed examination of the airway and sites for venous access should also be performed. Further laboratory and imaging investigations should be focused on screening for sleep-disordered breathing and stratification of surgical risk. An algorithm for the perioperative evaluation and management of OHS is given in **Fig. 2**.

Preoperative Screening for OHS

OHS is often undiagnosed and may increase perioperative risk. Appropriate screening facilitates the identification of patients at risk for OHS, referral to sleep medicine for PAP therapy, and modifications in the surgical approach, anesthetic technique, and postoperative monitoring.

The definitive test for alveolar hypoventilation is an arterial blood gas performed on room air during wakefulness. As this is a relatively invasive procedure, several screening tools have been proposed. Mokhlesi and colleagues[15] suggested 3 clinical predictors of OHS: serum HCO_3^-, AHI, and lowest oxygen saturation during sleep. Increased serum HCO_3^- level caused by metabolic compensation of chronic respiratory acidosis is common in patients with OHS. In a cohort of obese patients with OSA referred to the sleep laboratory for suspicion of OSA, a serum HCO_3^- threshold of 27 mEq/L demonstrated a 92% sensitivity in predicting hypercapnia on arterial blood gas.[15] To complement the highly sensitive serum HCO_3^-, a highly specific (95%) AHI threshold of 100 was identified. A 2-step screening process was proposed, with serum HCO_3^- as the initial test to exclude patients without OHS and then AHI as the second test to improve specificity. In addition, hypoxemia (Sp_{O_2} <90%, corresponding to Pa_{O_2} <60 mm Hg)[84] during wakefulness should lead clinicians to suspect OHS in patients with OSA. In a recent meta-analysis, patients with OSA and higher BMI, higher AHI, and more restrictive chest wall mechanics were more likely to develop OHS.[85] In these patients with OHS, the mean BMI, AHI, percent predicted FEV_1, and percent predicted FVC were 39 kg/m^2, 64 events/h, 71%, and 85%, respectively.

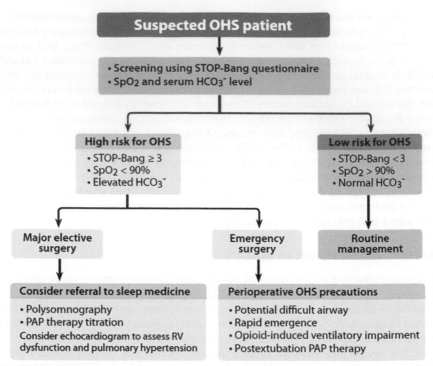

Fig. 2. Perioperative management of the patient suspected to have OHS. HCO_3^-, serum bicarbonate; RV, right ventricular. (*Adapted from* Mokhlesi B. Obesity hypoventilation syndrome: a state-of-the-art review. Respir Care 2010;55:1347–62; with permission.)

In summary, patients presenting with a high BMI and AHI should alert the physician to screen for OHS. The serum HCO_3^- is an easy initial screening test. If it is increased or hypoxemia by room air Spo_2 during wakefulness is present, a measurement of arterial blood gases, or end-tidal CO_2, is recommended. Once hypercapnia is confirmed, referral to sleep medicine and further testing, such as pulmonary function testing, chest imaging, measurement of thyroid-stimulating hormone level, and clinical assessment of neuromuscular strength, should be considered to rule out other important causes of hypoventilation.

Preoperative Screening for OSA

OSA screening in patients suspected to have OHS provides valuable information that may modify perioperative management. Approximately 90% of patients with OHS present with OSA, therefore a positive screen increases the index of suspicion for OHS. Multiple screening tools have been developed to evaluate patients at risk for OSA. The STOP-Bang questionnaire was used in preoperative patients.[86,87] It is a scoring model combining the STOP (snoring, tiredness, observed apneas, and increased blood pressure) questionnaire and Bang (BMI $\geq$35 kg/m², age >50 years, neck circumference >40 cm, and male gender). A systematic review has suggested using the STOP-Bang questionnaire in the surgical population due to its high methodological quality and easy-to-use features.[88] A positive screen ($\geq$3 questions answered yes) is highly sensitive for moderate to severe OSA and is useful to exclude patients with the disease. On the other hand, patients with an STOP-Bang score of 5 to 8 have been shown to be at higher risk for moderate to severe OSA.[89] If these patients present with concurrent morbid obesity, they are at high risk for OHS and should be referred to sleep medicine for further evaluation.

In summary, the STOP-Bang questionnaire is a validated and easy tool to screen for OSA as part of the preoperative evaluation for patients with suspected OHS. A high STOP-Bang score with coexisting morbid obesity indicates an increased risk for OHS.

Preoperative Risk Stratification and Cardiopulmonary Testing

The Lee revised cardiac risk index represents a valuable tool to predict cardiac risk for elective major noncardiac surgery in the general population.[90] However, other risk factors specifically related to OHS, such as pulmonary hypertension and a history of venous thromboembolism, should be considered when evaluating perioperative risk. The Obesity Surgery Mortality Risk Score was developed for patients undergoing gastric bypass, and includes 5 risk factors: hypertension, BMI of 50 kg/m^2 or greater, male sex, age 45 years or more, and known risk factors for pulmonary embolism (OHS, previous thromboembolism, preoperative vena cava filter, pulmonary hypertension).[5,6,51] This risk score stratifies mortality risk into low (0 or 1 comorbidity), intermediate (2 to 3 comorbidities) and high (4 to 5 comorbidities). Mortality rates were 0.2%, 1.2%, and 2.4% for low-risk, intermediate-risk, and high-risk classes, respectively.[6] The most common causes of death were pulmonary embolism (30%), cardiac causes (27%), and gastrointestinal leak (21%).

A 12-lead electrocardiogram and chest radiograph should be obtained in patients suspected to have OHS to evaluate for coronary artery disease, congestive heart failure, and pulmonary hypertension. Indications for further cardiovascular testing should be based on the patient's cardiovascular risk factors and the invasiveness of surgery according to current American Heart Association guidelines.[90,91] The assessment of functional capacity is of particular importance in obese individuals because cardiorespiratory fitness levels and the postoperative complication rate are inversely related to BMI.[92,93] If these patients are undergoing major surgery and present with multiple cardiac risk factors, stress testing and transthoracic echocardiogram may be considered if management may be changed.[91]

Studies evaluating postoperative pulmonary complications have generally found no increased risk attributable to obesity.[94] However, patients with OSA were found to have a higher risk of pulmonary complications than patients without OSA in a recent retrospective study.[95] Routine pulmonary function tests may not translate into an effective risk prediction for postoperative pulmonary complications in noncardiothoracic surgery.[96] However, if coexisting chronic obstructive pulmonary disease is suspected in the patient with OHS, spirometry may be considered for diagnosis and subsequent optimization.

INTRAOPERATIVE MANAGEMENT OF OHS

Key considerations specific to the intraoperative management of OHS include airway management and emergence from anesthesia.

Airway Management

OSA is a risk factor for both difficult mask ventilation and tracheal intubation.[97] In addition, patients with severe OSA (AHI ≥40 events/h) showed a significantly higher prevalence of difficult intubation than patients with lower AHI.[98]

Obesity results in a threefold increase in difficulty with mask ventilation.[99] Whether obesity increases the difficulty of tracheal intubation is more controversial. A retrospective study of 18,500 surgical patients reported that obesity is a risk factor for difficult intubation.[100] However, other studies have not found an association between BMI and intubation difficulties.[101,102] More recently, Kheterpal and colleagues[103] identified 5 risk factors (limited mandibular protrusion, thick/obese neck anatomy, OSA, snoring, and BMI more than 30 kg/m^2) as independent predictors of difficult mask ventilation and intubation during anesthesia induction, which suggests that patients with OHS with limited mandibular protrusion are in the highest risk group for airway complications.

During induction of anesthesia, patients with OHS should be placed in the ramp position with tilting of the torso and head by 25°. This position has been shown to improve the glottic view during intubation and reduce atelectasis.[104] Preoxygenation for more than 3 minutes with a tightly fitted mask can increase apnea tolerance time. A variety of airway adjuncts and skilled anesthesiology assistance should be made available in advance. Awake fiber optic intubation should be considered in patients with OHS with markers for difficult mask ventilation and intubation. In situations during which a patient with OHS is hypoxemic, concomitant use of PAP during fiber optic intubation prevents further deterioration of oxygen saturation.[105,106] In addition, PAP splints the airway open and thus facilitates the visualization of anatomic landmarks.[107]

Emergence from Anesthesia

Patients with OHS are sensitive to the respiratory depressant effects of anesthetic agents due to the propensity for airway collapse, sleep deprivation, and blunting of physiologic response to hypercapnia and hypoxemia. A semi-upright or lateral position is recommended at the end of surgery for better oxygenation and airway maintenance.[108] Rapid emergence from anesthesia is preferred because tracheal extubation should be performed only after the patient is fully conscious. A systematic analysis of the literature comparing postoperative recovery after propofol, isoflurane, desflurane, and sevoflurane-based anesthesia in adults demonstrated that early recovery was faster in the desflurane and sevoflurane groups.[109] Another strategy to accelerate emergence is to decrease volatile anesthetic requirement and minimize washout time from fat/muscle by using other short-acting anesthetic adjuvants, such as remifentanil, or a combined general regional anesthetic.[29]

POSTOPERATIVE MANAGEMENT OF OHS

Key considerations specific to the postoperative management of OHS include monitoring for opioid-induced ventilatory impairment (OIVI) and prompt use of PAP therapy. The dual roles of postoperative PAP therapy are to prevent and treat respiratory failure secondary to sleep-disordered breathing.

OIVI

OIVI induces central respiratory depression, decreased level of consciousness, and upper airway obstruction, ultimately resulting in alveolar ventilation. The incidence of OIVI after major surgery varies with the different routes of opioid administration. The incidence of decreased respiratory rate was 0.8%, 1.2%, and 1.1% for intramuscular, intravenous patient-controlled analgesia, and epidural analgesia, respectively.[110] The incidence of oxygen desaturation was 37%, 11.5%, and 15.1% for intramuscular, intravenous patient-controlled analgesia, and epidural analgesia, respectively.[110] Patients with OHS could be at significant risk for OIVI because of their susceptibility to upper airway obstruction, depressed central respiratory drive, and impaired pulmonary mechanics. An opioid-sparing analgesic regimen, including local anesthetic–infused nerve block catheters and nonopioid adjuncts (acetaminophen, nonsteroidal antiinflammatory drugs), should be considered in these patients.

Improved postoperative monitoring is key in reducing the risk of OIVI. Patient-specific, anesthetic, and surgical factors determine the requirements for postoperative monitoring. Patients with OHS undergoing major surgery who require high doses of postoperative opioid should be monitored with continuous oximetry. Recurrent respiratory events in the postanesthesia care unit, including apnea for 10 seconds or more, bradypnea of less than 8 breaths/min, pain-sedation mismatch, or desaturations to less than 90%, can be used to identify patients at high risk of postoperative respiratory complications.[111] Recently, Macintyre and colleagues[112] proposed that sedation level is a more reliable sign of OIVI than respiratory rate because multiple reports suggest that OIVI is not always accompanied by a decrease in respiratory rate.[112–114] Thus, sedation scoring systems should be used postoperatively to recognize OIVI so that appropriate interventions are triggered. In patients with OHS requiring high doses of postoperative opioids, sedation monitoring should be considered every 1 to 2 hours for the first 24 hours.[115]

Postoperative PAP Therapy: Prevention of Respiratory Failure

There is limited evidence demonstrating a reduction in postoperative complications with PAP in patients with OHS. However, a case series of 14 patients with OSA suggested that the use of CPAP continuously for 24 to 48 hours after extubation may reduce the risk of postoperative complications.[116] In addition, PAP was found to decrease respiratory failure after extubation in severely obese patients admitted to the intensive care unit (absolute risk reduction of 16%).[117] Subgroup analysis of patients with hypercapnia showed reduced hospital mortality in the PAP group compared with the control group. Other potential benefits of postoperative PAP include reduced hemodynamic fluctuations and arrhythmia related to hypoxemia.

In summary, patients with OHS who were previously on PAP should resume therapy as soon as possible postoperatively. In patients suspected to have OHS experiencing postoperative ventilatory impairment, PAP should be considered. Based on the available literature, patients with OHS typically require an inspiratory PAP and the expiratory PAP of 16 to 22 cm H_2O and 9 to 10 cm H_2O, respectively, to achieve adequate resolution of upper airway obstruction and to improve ventilation. Bilevel PAP can be empirically set at these pressures in patients suspected of having OHS.

Postoperative PAP Therapy: Treatment of Respiratory Failure

Although the incidence of postoperative respiratory failure in patients with OHS is unknown, these patients are particularly susceptible to cardiopulmonary complications secondary to increased respiratory load, blunted central drive, pulmonary hypertension, and impaired ventricular function. In the postoperative period, these patients may decompensate acutely due to multiple factors, including sedation, sleep deprivation, and deconditioning.[118] Of concern, misdiagnosis is common if the physician is not aware of the potential for sleep-disordered breathing causing acute cardiopulmonary failure.[37,118] It was reported that 77% of patients with OHS admitted to the intensive care unit for hypercapnic respiratory failure were erroneously diagnosed and treated for chronic obstructive pulmonary disease/asthma.[37]

Four presentations of acute cardiopulmonary failure may be encountered postoperatively: hypercapnic respiratory failure, acute congestive heart failure, acute cor pulmonale, and sudden death, an extreme manifestation. The mechanisms leading to the development of such complications were described by Carr and colleagues[118] in detail. A high index of suspicion and early initiation of PAP therapy are key in managing patients with suspected OHS who develop respiratory failure postoperatively. Adjunctive interventions include judicious sedation/analgesia, minimal sleep disruption at night, and close follow-up with a sleep specialist.

SUMMARY

OHS is an important disease entity that requires the anesthesiologist's thorough understanding. The prevalence of OHS is estimated to be 0.15% to 0.3% in the general population and 8% in patients undergoing bariatric surgery.[2,3] Patients with OHS present with severe upper airway obstruction, restrictive pulmonary physiology, blunted central respiratory drive, and pulmonary hypertension. The primary therapy for OHS is PAP.

Perioperative management begins with a high index of suspicion for OHS in the morbidly obese patient. Screening questionnaires such as the validated STOP-Bang questionnaire can identify patients at high risk of OSA. This screening tool can be further complemented by the presence of low Spo_2, increased end-tidal CO_2 or $Paco_2$, and serum HCO_3^- level to identify patients at high risk of OHS. Before major elective surgery, these patients should be referred to sleep medicine for polysomnography and PAP titration. An echocardiogram should be considered to assess right ventricular function and pulmonary hypertension. Perioperative precautions for OHS include prudent airway management, rapid emergence, monitoring for ventilatory impairment, and early resumption of PAP therapy. Future research should focus on the perioperative strategies of screening, monitoring, and treatment of OHS and associated complications.

REFERENCES

1. Olson A, Zwillich C. The obesity hypoventilation syndrome. Am J Med 2005;118: 948–56.
2. Mokhlesi B. Obesity hypoventilation syndrome: a state-of-the-art review. Respir Care 2010;55:1347–62.
3. Chau E, Lam D, Wong J, et al. Obesity hypoventilation syndrome: a review of epidemiology, pathophysiology, and perioperative considerations. Anesthesiology 2012;117:188–205.
4. Berg G, Delaive K, Manfreda J, et al. The use of health-care resources in obesity-hypoventilation syndrome. Chest 2001;120:377–83.
5. DeMaria E, Portenier D, Wolfe L. Obesity surgery mortality risk score: proposal for a clinically useful score to predict mortality risk in patients undergoing gastric bypass. Surg Obes Relat Dis 2007;3:134–40.
6. DeMaria E, Murr M, Byrne TK, et al. Validation of the obesity surgery mortality risk score in a multicenter study proves it stratifies mortality risk in patients undergoing gastric bypass for morbid obesity. Ann Surg 2007;246:578–82.
7. Rapoport DM, Garay SM, Epstein H, et al. Hypercapnia in the obstructive sleep apnea syndrome. A reevaluation of the "Pickwickian syndrome". Chest 1986;89: 627–35.
8. Piper AJ, Grunstein RR. Obesity hypoventilation syndrome: mechanisms and management. Am J Respir Crit Care Med 2011;183:292–8.
9. Aldrich T, Arora NS, Rochester DF. The influence of airway obstruction and respiratory muscle strength on maximal voluntary ventilation. Am Rev Respir Dis 1982;126:195–9.
10. Ladosky W, Botelho MA, Albuquerque JP Jr. Chest mechanics in morbidly obese non-hypoventilated patients. Respir Med 2001;95:281–6.

11. Lavietes M, Clifford E, Silverstein D, et al. Relationship of static respiratory muscle pressure and maximum ventilatory ventilation. Respiration 1979;38:121–6.
12. Akashiba T, Akahoshi T, Kawahara S, et al. Clinical characteristics of obesity-hypoventilation syndrome in Japan: a multi-center study. Intern Med 2006;45: 1121–5.
13. Kawata N, Tatsumi K, Terada J, et al. Daytime hypercapnia in obstructive sleep apnea syndrome. Chest 2007;132:1832–8.
14. Laaban J, Chailleux E. Daytime hypercapnia in adult patients with obstructive sleep apnea syndrome in France, before initiating nocturnal nasal continuous positive airway pressure therapy. Chest 2005;127:710–5.
15. Mokhlesi B, Tulaimat A, Faibussowitsch I, et al. Obesity hypoventilation syndrome: prevalence and predictors in patients with obstructive sleep apnea. Sleep Breath 2007;11:117–24.
16. Javaheri S, Colangelo G, Lacey W, et al. Chronic hypercapnia in obstructive sleep apnea-hypopnea syndrome. Sleep 1994;17:416–23.
17. Considine R, Sinha MK, Heiman ML, et al. Serum immunoreactive-leptin concentrations in normal-weight and obese humans. N Engl J Med 1996;334:292–5.
18. Kalra S. Central leptin insufficiency syndrome: an interactive etiology for obesity, metabolic and neural diseases and for designing new therapeutic interventions. Peptides 2008;29:127–38.
19. Tankersley C, O'Donnell C, Daood MJ, et al. Leptin attenuates respiratory complications associated with the obese phenotype. J Appl Physiol 1998;85: 2261–9.
20. Gilbert R, Sipple JH, Auchincloss JH Jr. Respiratory control and work of breathing in obese subjects. J Appl Physiol 1961;16:21–6.
21. Kress J, Pohlman AS, Alverdy J, et al. The impact of morbid obesity on oxygen cost of breathing (VO2(RESP)) at rest. Am J Respir Crit Care Med 1999;160: 883–6.
22. Phipps P, Starritt E, Caterson I, et al. Association of serum leptin with hypoventilation in human obesity. Thorax 2002;57:75–6.
23. Shimura R, Tatsumi K, Nakamura A, et al. Fat accumulation, leptin, and hypercapnia in obstructive sleep apnea-hypopnea syndrome. Chest 2005;127:543–9.
24. Berger KI, Goldring RM, Rapoport DM. Obesity hypoventilation syndrome. Semin Respir Crit Care Med 2009;30:253–61.
25. Ayappa I, Berger KI, Norman RG, et al. Hypercapnia and ventilatory periodicity in obstructive sleep apnea syndrome. Am J Respir Crit Care Med 2002;166: 1112–5.
26. Norman R, Goldring RM, Clain JM, et al. Transition from acute to chronic hypercapnia in patients with periodic breathing: predictions from a computer model. J Appl Physiol 2006;100:1733–41.
27. Lin C, Wu KM, Chou CS, et al. Oral airway resistance during wakefulness in eucapnic and hypercapnic sleep apnea syndrome. Respir Physiol Neurobiol 2004; 139:215–24.
28. Adesanya A, Lee W, Greilich NB, et al. Perioperative management of obstructive sleep apnea. Chest 2010;138:1489–98.
29. Seet E, Chung F. Management of sleep apnea in adults - functional algorithms for the perioperative period. Can J Anaesth 2010;57:849–64.
30. Lee M, Lin CC, Shen SY, et al. Work of breathing in eucapnic and hypercapnic sleep apnea syndrome. Respiration 2009;77:146–53.
31. Sharp J, Henry JP, Sweany SK, et al. The total work of breathing in normal and obese men. J Clin Invest 1964;43:728–39.

32. Steier J, Jolley CJ, Seymour J, et al. Neural respiratory drive in obesity. Thorax 2009;64:719–25.
33. Lopata M, Onal E. Mass loading, sleep apnea, and the pathogenesis of obesity hypoventilation. Am Rev Respir Dis 1982;126:640–5.
34. Sampson M, Grassino K. Neuromechanical properties in obese patients during carbon dioxide rebreathing. Am J Med 1983;75:81–90.
35. Zwillich CW, Sutton FD, Pierson DJ, et al. Decreased hypoxic ventilatory drive in the obesity-hypoventilation syndrome. Am J Med 1975;59:343–8.
36. Kessler R, Chaouat A, Schinkewitch P, et al. The obesity-hypoventilation syndrome revisited: a prospective study of 34 consecutive cases. Chest 2001; 120:369–76.
37. Marik P, Desai H. Characteristics of patients with the "malignant obesity hypoventilation syndrome" admitted to an ICU. J Intensive Care Med 2012. http://dx.doi.org/10.1177/0885066612444261.
38. Sugerman HJ, Baron PL, Fairman RP, et al. Hemodynamic dysfunction in obesity hypoventilation syndrome and the effects of treatment with surgically induced weight loss. Ann Surg 1988;207:604–13.
39. de Divitiis O, Fazio S, Petitto M, et al. Obesity and cardiac function. Circulation 1981;64:477–82.
40. Arzt M, Young T, Finn L, et al. Association of sleep-disordered breathing and the occurrence of stroke. Am J Respir Crit Care Med 2005;172:1447–51.
41. Coughlin S, Mawdsley L, Mugarza JA, et al. Obstructive sleep apnoea is independently associated with an increased prevalence of metabolic syndrome. Eur Heart J 2004;25:735–41.
42. Peker Y, Kraiczi H, Hedner J, et al. An independent association between obstructive sleep apnoea and coronary artery disease. Eur Respir J 1999;14: 179–84.
43. Sin D, Fitzgerald F, Parker JD, et al. Relationship of systolic BP to obstructive sleep apnea in patients with heart failure. Chest 2003;123:1536–43.
44. Tung A. Anaesthetic considerations with the metabolic syndrome. Br J Anaesth 2010;105:24–33.
45. Chung S, Yuan H, Chung F. A systemic review of obstructive sleep apnea and its implications for anesthesiologists. Anesth Analg 2008;107:1543–63.
46. Kaw R, Pasupuleti V, Walker E, et al. Postoperative complications in patients with obstructive sleep apnea. Chest 2011;141:436–41.
47. Liao P, Yegneswaran B, Vairavanathan S, et al. Postoperative complications in patients with obstructive sleep apnea: a retrospective matched cohort study. Can J Anaesth 2009;56:819–28.
48. Nowbar S, Burkart KM, Gonzales R, et al. Obesity-associated hypoventilation in hospitalized patients: prevalence, effects, and outcome. Am J Med 2004;116:1–7.
49. Perez de Llano LA, Golpe R, Ortiz Piquer M, et al. Short-term and long-term effects of nasal intermittent positive pressure ventilation in patients with obesity-hypoventilation syndrome. Chest 2005;128:587–94.
50. Sugerman HJ, Fairman RP, Sood RK, et al. Long-term effects of gastric surgery for treating respiratory insufficiency of obesity. Am J Clin Nutr 1992;55: 597S–601S.
51. Efthimiou E, Sampalis J, Christou N. Validation of obesity surgery mortality risk score in patients undergoing gastric bypass in a Canadian center. Surg Obes Relat Dis 2009;5:643–7.
52. Lin C. Effect of nasal CPAP on ventilatory drive in normocapnic and hypercapnic patients with obstructive sleep apnoea syndrome. Eur Respir J 1994;7:2005–10.

53. Perez de Llano LA, Golpe R, Piquer MO, et al. Clinical heterogeneity among patients with obesity hypoventilation syndrome: therapeutic implications. Respiration 2008;75:34–9.

54. Piper AJ, Sullivan CE. Effects of short-term NIPPV in the treatment of patients with severe obstructive sleep apnea and hypercapnia. Chest 1994;105:434–40.

55. Banerjee D, Yee BJ, Piper AJ, et al. Obesity hypoventilation syndrome: hypoxemia during continuous positive airway pressure. Chest 2007;131:1678–84.

56. Chouri-Pontarollo N, Borel JC, Tamisier R, et al. Impaired objective daytime vigilance in obesity-hypoventilation syndrome: impact of noninvasive ventilation. Chest 2007;131:148–55.

57. Budweiser S, Riedl SG, Jörres RA, et al. Mortality and prognostic factors in patients with obesity-hypoventilation syndrome undergoing noninvasive ventilation. J Intern Med 2007;261:375–83.

58. de Lucas-Ramos P, de Miguel-Díez J, Santacruz-Siminiani A, et al. Benefits at 1 year of nocturnal intermittent positive pressure ventilation in patients with obesity-hypoventilation syndrome. Respir Med 2004;98:961–7.

59. Heinemann F, Budweiser S, Dobroschke J, et al. Non-invasive positive pressure ventilation improves lung volumes in the obesity hypoventilation syndrome. Respir Med 2007;101:1229–35.

60. Han F, Chen E, Wei H, et al. Treatment effects on carbon dioxide retention in patients with obstructive sleep apnea-hypopnea syndrome. Chest 2001;119:1814–9.

61. Priou P, Hamel JF, Person C, et al. Long-term outcome of noninvasive positive pressure ventilation for obesity hypoventilation syndrome. Chest 2010;138: 84–90.

62. Schafer H, Ewig S, Hasper E, et al. Failure of CPAP therapy in obstructive sleep apnoea syndrome: predictive factors and treatment with bilevel-positive airway pressure. Respir Med 1998;92:208–15.

63. Piper A, Wang D, Yee BJ, et al. Randomised trial of CPAP versus bilevel support in the treatment of obesity hypoventilation syndrome without severe nocturnal desaturation. Thorax 2008;63:395–401.

64. American Academy of Sleep Medicine. Clinical guidelines for the manual titration of positive airway pressure in patients with obstructive sleep apnea. J Clin Sleep Med 2008;4:157–71.

65. Contal O, Adler D, Borel JC, et al. Impact of different back-up respiratory rates on the efficacy of non-invasive positive pressure ventilation in obesity hypoventilation syndrome: a randomized trial. Chest 2012. http://dx.doi.org/10.1378/chest.11-2848.

66. Storre JH, Seuthe B, Fiechter R, et al. Average volume-assured pressure support in obesity hypoventilation: a randomized crossover trial. Chest 2006;130: 815–21.

67. Murphy P, Davidson C, Hind MD, et al. Volume targeted versus pressure support non-invasive ventilation in patients with super obesity and chronic respiratory failure: a randomised controlled trial. Thorax 2012;67:727–34.

68. Berry RB, Chediak A, Brown LK, et al. Best clinical practices for the sleep center adjustment of noninvasive positive pressure ventilation (NPPV) in stable chronic alveolar hypoventilation syndromes. J Clin Sleep Med 2010;6:491–509.

69. Aubier M, Murciano D, Milic-Emili J, et al. Effects of the administration of O2 on ventilation and blood gases in patients with chronic obstructive pulmonary disease during acute respiratory failure. Am Rev Respir Dis 1980;122:747–54.

70. Robinson T, Freiberg DB, Regnis JA, et al. The role of hypoventilation and ventilation-perfusion redistribution in oxygen-induced hypercapnia during acute

exacerbations of chronic obstructive pulmonary disease. Am J Respir Crit Care Med 2000;161:1524–9.

71. Wijesinghe M, Williams M, Perrin K, et al. The effect of supplemental oxygen on hypercapnia in subjects with obesity-associated hypoventilation: a randomized, crossover, clinical study. Chest 2011;139:1018–24.

72. Mokhlesi B, Tulaimat A, Parthasarathy S. Oxygen for obesity hypoventilation syndrome: a double-edged sword? Chest 2011;139:975–7.

73. Marti-Valeri C, Sabate A, Masdevall C, et al. Improvement of associated respiratory problems in morbidly obese patients after open Roux-en-Y gastric bypass. Obes Surg 2007;17:1102–10.

74. Greenburg D, Lettieri CJ, Eliasson AH. Effects of surgical weight loss on measures of obstructive sleep apnea: a meta-analysis. Am J Med 2009;122:535–42.

75. Buchwald H, Avidor Y, Braunwald E, et al. Bariatric surgery: a systematic review and meta-analysis. JAMA 2004;292:1724–37.

76. Fernandez AJ, Demaria EJ, Tichansky DS, et al. Multivariate analysis of risk factors for death following gastric bypass for treatment of morbid obesity. Ann Surg 2004;239:698–702.

77. Flum D, Belle SH, King WC, et al. Perioperative safety in the longitudinal assessment of bariatric surgery. N Engl J Med 2009;361:445–54.

78. Bayliss D, Millhorn DE. Central neural mechanisms of progesterone action: application to the respiratory system. J Appl Physiol 1992;73:393–404.

79. Sutton FJ, Zwillich CW, Creagh CE, et al. Progesterone for outpatient treatment of Pickwickian syndrome. Ann Intern Med 1975;83:476–9.

80. Poulter N, Chang CL, Farley TM, et al. Risk of cardiovascular diseases associated with oral progestagen preparations with therapeutic indications [letter]. Lancet 1999;354:1610.

81. Tojima H, Kunitomo F, Kimura H, et al. Effects of acetazolamide in patients with the sleep apnoea syndrome. Thorax 1988;43:113–9.

82. Whyte K, Gould GA, Airlie MA, et al. Role of protriptyline and acetazolamide in the sleep apnea/hypopnea syndrome. Sleep 1988;11:463–72.

83. Raurich J, Rialp G, Ibáñez J, et al. Hypercapnic respiratory failure in obesity-hypoventilation syndrome: CO2 response and acetazolamide treatment effects. Respir Care 2010;55:1442–8.

84. Pedersen T, Møller AM, Pedersen BD. Pulse oximetry for perioperative monitoring: systematic review of randomized, controlled trials. Anesth Analg 2003; 96:426–31.

85. Kaw R, Hernandez AV, Walker E, et al. Determinants of hypercapnia in obese patients with obstructive sleep apnea: a systematic review and meta-analysis of cohort studies. Chest 2009;136:787–96.

86. Chung F, Yegneswaran B, Liao P, et al. STOP questionnaire: a tool to screen patients for obstructive sleep apnea. Anesthesiology 2008;108:812–21.

87. Chung F, Yegneswaran B, Liao P, et al. Validation of the Berlin questionnaire and American Society of Anesthesiologists checklist as screening tools for obstructive sleep apnea in surgical patients. Anesthesiology 2008;108:822–30.

88. Abrishami A, Khajehdehi A, Chung F. A systematic review of screening questionnaires for obstructive sleep apnea. Can J Anaesth 2010;57:423–38.

89. Chung F, Subramanyam R, Liao P, et al. High STOP-Bang score indicates a high probability of obstructive sleep apnoea. Br J Anaesth 2012;108:768–75.

90. Lee T, Marcantonio ER, Mangione CM, et al. Derivation and prospective validation of a simple index for prediction of cardiac risk of major noncardiac surgery. Circulation 1999;100:1043–9.

91. Fleisher LA, Beckman JA, Brown KA, et al. ACC/AHA 2007 guidelines on perioperative cardiovascular evaluation and care for noncardiac surgery: a report of the American College of Cardiology/American Heart Association Task Force on Practice Guidelines (Writing Committee to Revise the 2002 Guidelines on Perioperative Cardiovascular Evaluation for Noncardiac Surgery): developed in collaboration with the American Society of Echocardiography, American Society of Nuclear Cardiology, Heart Rhythm Society, Society of Cardiovascular Anesthesiologists, Society for Cardiovascular Angiography and Interventions, Society for Vascular Medicine and Biology, and Society for Vascular Surgery. Circulation 2007;116:418–99.
92. Gallagher M, Franklin BA, Ehrman JK, et al. Comparative impact of morbid obesity vs heart failure on cardiorespiratory fitness. Chest 2005;127: 2197–203.
93. McCullough P, Gallagher MJ, Dejong AT, et al. Cardiorespiratory fitness and short-term complications after bariatric surgery. Chest 2006;130:517–25.
94. Smetana G. Preoperative pulmonary evaluation. N Engl J Med 1999;340: 937–44.
95. Memtsoudis S, Liu SS, Ma Y, et al. Perioperative pulmonary outcomes in patients with sleep apnea after noncardiac surgery. Anesth Analg 2011;112:113–21.
96. Qaseem A, Snow V, Fitterman N, et al. Risk assessment for and strategies to reduce perioperative pulmonary complications for patients undergoing noncardiothoracic surgery: a guideline from the American College of Physicians. Ann Intern Med 2006;144:575–80.
97. Siyam M, Benhamou D. Difficult endotracheal intubation in patients with sleep apnea syndrome. Anesth Analg 2002;95:1098–102.
98. Kim J, Lee JJ. Preoperative predictors of difficult intubation in patients with obstructive sleep apnea syndrome. Can J Anaesth 2006;53:393–7.
99. Langeron O, Masso E, Huraux C, et al. Prediction of difficult mask ventilation. Anesthesiology 2000;92:1229–36.
100. Rose D, Cohen MM. The airway: problems and predictions in 18,500 patients. Can J Anaesth 1994;41:372–83.
101. Brodsky J, Lemmens HJ, Brock-Utne JG, et al. Morbid obesity and tracheal intubation. Anesth Analg 2002;94:732–6.
102. Mashour G, Kheterpal S, Vanaharam V, et al. The extended Mallampati score and a diagnosis of diabetes mellitus are predictors of difficult laryngoscopy in the morbidly obese. Anesth Analg 2008;107:1919–23.
103. Kheterpal S, Han R, Tremper KK, et al. Incidence and predictors of difficult and impossible mask ventilation. Anesthesiology 2006;105:885–91.
104. Cattano D, Melnikov V, Khalil Y, et al. An evaluation of the rapid airway management positioner in obese patients undergoing gastric bypass or laparoscopic gastric banding surgery. Obes Surg 2010;20:1436–41.
105. Murgu S, Pecson J, Colt HG. Bronchoscopy during noninvasive ventilation: indications and technique. Respir Care 2010;55:595–600.
106. Wong D, Wang J, Venkatraghavan L. Awake bronchoscopic intubation through an air-Q® with the application of BIPAP. Can J Anaesth 2012;59:915–6.
107. Rothfleisch R, Davis LL, Kuebel DA, et al. Facilitation of fiberoptic nasotracheal intubation in a morbidly obese patient by simultaneous use of nasal CPAP. Chest 1994;106:287–8.
108. Gander S, Frascarolo P, Suter M, et al. Positive end-expiratory pressure during induction of general anesthesia increases duration of nonhypoxic apnea in morbidly obese patients. Anesth Analg 2005;100:580–4.

109. Gupta A, Stierer T, Zuckerman R, et al. Comparison of recovery profile after ambulatory anesthesia with propofol, isoflurane, sevoflurane and desflurane: a systematic review. Anesth Analg 2004;98:632–41.
110. Cashman J, Dolin SJ. Respiratory and haemodynamic effects of acute postoperative pain management: evidence from published data. Br J Anaesth 2004;93: 212–23.
111. Gali B, Whalen FX, Schroeder DR, et al. Identification of patients at risk for postoperative respiratory complications using a preoperative obstructive sleep apnea screening tool and postanesthesia care assessment. Anesthesiology 2009;110:869–77.
112. Macintyre P, Loadsman JA, Scott DA. Opioids, ventilation and acute pain management. Anaesth Intensive Care 2011;39:545–58.
113. Ready L, Oden R, Chadwick HS, et al. Development of an anesthesiology-based postoperative pain management service. Anesthesiology 1988;68:100–6.
114. Vila HJ, Smith RA, Augustyniak MJ, et al. The efficacy and safety of pain management before and after implementation of hospital-wide pain management standards: is patient safety compromised by treatment based solely on numerical pain ratings? Anesth Analg 2005;101:474–80.
115. American Society of Anesthesiologists Task Force on Neuraxial Opioids, Horlocker TT, Burton AW, Connis RT, et al. Practice guidelines for the prevention, detection, and management of respiratory depression associated with neuraxial opioid administration. Anesthesiology 2009;110:218–30.
116. Rennotte M, Baele P, Aubert G, et al. Nasal continuous positive airway pressure in the perioperative management of patients with obstructive sleep apnea submitted to surgery. Chest 1995;107:367–74.
117. El-Solh A, Aquilina A, Pineda L, et al. Noninvasive ventilation for prevention of post-extubation respiratory failure in obese patients. Eur Respir J 2006;28: 588–95.
118. Carr G, Mokhlesi B, Gehlbach BK. Acute cardiopulmonary failure from sleep-disordered breathing. Chest 2012;141:798–808.

Obesity and Diabetic Kidney Disease

Christine Maric-Bilkan, PhD

KEYWORDS

- Kidney • Obesity • Diabetes • Proteinuria • Hyperfiltration • Hypertension
- Glomerulopathy • Diabetic nephropathy

KEY POINTS

- The prevalence of obesity has risen to epidemic proportions and continues to be a major health problem worldwide.
- The high prevalence of obesity is closely linked to the increased incidence of several chronic diseases, including type 2 diabetes, hypertension, and cardiovascular disease.
- Obesity, type 2 diabetes, hypertension, and cardiovascular disease are all risk factors for chronic kidney disease (CKD) and end-stage renal disease (ESRD).
- The mechanisms by which obesity independently, or in concert with type 2 diabetes and hypertension, contributes to the development and/or progression of ESRD are not completely understood.

INTRODUCTION

The prevalence of obesity (body mass index [BMI] $\geq$30 kg/m^2) has risen to epidemic proportions and continues to be a major health problem worldwide.[1–3] The high prevalence of obesity is closely linked to the increased incidence of several chronic diseases, including type 2 diabetes, hypertension, and cardiovascular disease.[2,4–8] Obesity, type 2 diabetes, hypertension, and cardiovascular disease are all risk factors for chronic kidney disease (CKD) and end-stage renal disease (ESRD),[9–13] inasmuch as the presence of 1 or more of these risk factors multiplies the overall risk for disease development and progression (**Fig. 1**). In addition, evidence suggests that obesity may also increase the risk of ESRD independently of type 2 diabetes and hypertension.[14–16] However, the precise mechanisms by which obesity independently, or in concert with type 2 diabetes and hypertension, contributes to the development and/or progression of CKD and ESRD are not completely understood.

This article originally appeared in Medical Clinics of North America, Volume 97, Issue 1, January 2013.

The authors acknowledge the financial support of NIH/NIDDK (RO1DK075832 to C. Maric-Bilkan.

Department of Physiology and Biophysics, University of Mississippi Medical Center, 2500 North State Street, Jackson, MS 39216-4505, USA

E-mail address: cmaric@umc.edu

Clinics Collections 3 (2014) 165–180
http://dx.doi.org/10.1016/j.ccol.2014.09.038
2352-7986/14/$ – see front matter © 2014 Elsevier Inc. All rights reserved.

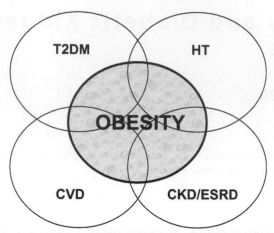

Fig. 1. Clustering of risk factors for obesity-related renal disease. Obesity, type 2 diabetes (T2DM), hypertension (HT), and cardiovascular disease (CVD) are all risk factors for chronic kidney disease (CKD) and end-stage renal disease (ESRD). The presence of 1 or more of these risk factors multiplies the overall risk for disease development and progression.

The two leading causes of ESRD are type 2 diabetes and hypertension, which together account for more than 70% of patients with ESRD.[17,18] Because the growing prevalence of obesity is a major driving force for the continued increase in the prevalence of type 2 diabetes,[7,19] it is often difficult to separate out the individual contribution of either obesity, type 2 diabetes, or hypertension to the development of ESRD. The pathophysiology of type 2 diabetes–related renal disease (ie, diabetic nephropathy) and obesity-related renal disease is almost identical. They both evolve in a sequence of stages beginning with initial increases in glomerular filtration rate (GFR) and intraglomerular capillary pressure (P_{Gc}), glomerular hypertrophy, and microalbuminuria.[20,21] Increased systolic blood pressure further exacerbates the disease progression to proteinuria, nodular glomerulosclerosis, and tubulointerstitial injury and a decrease in GFR leading to ESRD.[22,23] Diabetes-related and obesity-related renal disease also have common initiating events, which include interactions among multiple metabolic and hemodynamic factors that activate common intracellular signaling pathways that in turn trigger the production of cytokines and growth factors, leading to renal disease. The purpose of this review is to provide perspectives regarding the mechanisms by which obesity may lead to ESRD and to discuss prevention strategies and the treatment of obesity-related renal disease.

EPIDEMIOLOGY OF OBESITY AND DIABETES-RELATED KIDNEY DISEASE
Prevalence of Obesity and Type 2 Diabetes

Based on the most recent report from the National Health and Nutrition Examination Survey (NHANES) examining obesity prevalence among US adults, adolescents, and children, more than one-third of adults and almost 17% of children and adolescents were obese in 2009/2010.[24,25] Although there has been a significant increase in obesity prevalence among men and boys over the last decade, no changes were seen among women and girls. The prevalence of obesity is 35.5% among adult men, 35.8% among adult women, and 16.9% amongst children and adolescents of both sexes. Thus, the Healthy People 2010 goals of 15% obesity among adults and 5% obesity among children are far from being met.

Similar to obesity, the global prevalence of type 2 diabetes has more than doubled in the last 30 years and is predicted to continue to increase at an alarming rate. According to the World Health Organization, in 2008, almost 350 million people worldwide have diabetes, 90% of whom have type 2 diabetes.[26] Although the major driving force for the increase in the prevalence of type 2 diabetes is obesity, other factors, including genetic and environmental factors, are also important contributors to the development of type 2 diabetes. Accumulating evidence suggests that this markedly high prevalence of both obesity and type 2 diabetes contributes to the increased incidence of chronic diseases, including CKD and ESRD.[9–13]

Obesity, Diabetes, and CKD

Obesity is a well-recognized risk factor for both type 2 diabetes and hypertension, which are leading causes of CKD and ESRD.[27] Analysis of data from the Framingham Heart Study, which included more than 2600 patients with no CKD at baseline, showed an increased risk of developing stage 3 CKD in obese (BMI $\geq$30 kg/m^2) but not overweight (BMI 25–30 kg/m^2) patients after 18.5 years of follow-up.[9] However, this relationship was no longer significant after adjustment for known cardiovascular disease risk factors, including diabetes and hypertension. Numerous other studies have also demonstrated that the association between obesity and CKD is mediated through risk factors including diabetes, hypertension, and other elements of the metabolic syndrome.[10,16,28–30]

Although studies clearly indicate that the high risk of obesity-related CKD is driven by diabetes and hypertension, there are several other studies that suggest that obesity can lead to the development of CKD independently of either diabetes or hypertension. Specifically, the data from the Hypertension Detection and Follow-Up Program show that, in a cohort of 5897 patients with hypertension and no CKD at baseline, the incidence of CKD after a 5-year follow-up was 28% in patients with normal BMI, 31% in overweight patients, and 34% in obese patients.[16] This risk for CKD persisted in the overweight and obese patients even after adjustment for covariates, including type 2 diabetes, suggesting that obesity increases the risk of CKD independently of type 2 diabetes. Also supporting the notion that obesity increases the risk of CKD independently of diabetes and hypertension is the Physician's Health Study, a large cohort of initially healthy men, in which BMI was associated with increased risk for CKD over 14 years.[31] Furthermore, in 74,986 prehypertensive individuals participating in the first Health Study in Nord-Trøndelag in Norway, the risk of CKD over 21 years was shown to increase dramatically with obesity.[32] In addition to increasing the risk of CKD, obesity has also been suggested to have a higher rate of decline of GFR and progress faster to ESRD.[33]

Obesity, Diabetes, and ESRD

Several studies have shown that increased BMI is an independent risk factor for ESRD. In a cohort of 320,252 adult patients of Kaiser Permanente who were followed for 15 to 35 years, BMI was found to be a strong and common risk factor for ESRD.[10] This relationship between BMI and ESRD persisted even after controlling for baseline blood pressure and diabetes. Similarly, in a population-based, case-control study in Sweden, obesity was shown to be an important and potentially preventable risk factor for ESRD.[11] This study also showed that the coexistence of obesity and diabetes doubled the risk of new onset kidney disease. One study compared the temporal trends in mean BMI and obesity prevalence among incident ESRD by year of dialysis initiated between 1995 and 2002, and these trends were compared with those in the US population during this same period.[34] This study found that among incident patients with ESRD, mean BMI at the start of dialysis increased from 25.7 to 27.5 kg/m^2, and total obesity and stage 2 obesity increased by 33 and 63%, respectively. The slope of mean BMI at initiation of dialysis over the 8 years of follow-up was ~2-fold higher in the incident ESRD population compared with the US population for all age groups.[34]

In contrast to most of the studies suggesting that obesity is a risk factor for CKD and ESRD, some studies have reported that high BMI is associated with greater survival in patients on maintenance hemodialysis.[35,36] This phenomenon, commonly referred to as the obesity paradox, reasons that in patients receiving long-term hemodialysis, larger body size (ie, larger BMI) with more muscle mass (ie, higher serum creatinine concentration) is associated with greater survival. These observations indicate that it is the increase in muscle mass rather than increase in total body weight that confers protection, suggesting that BMI may not always be the most reliable index of CKD risk, at least in certain patient populations. Other studies indicate that visceral or central obesity, but not BMI, is associated with incident CKD[37] and increased cardiovascular disease in patients with CKD.[38] Thus, it is conceivable that overall weight loss with a concomitant increase in muscle mass may be an effective treatment strategy in preventing obesity-associated CKD and ESRD.

PATHOPHYSIOLOGY OF OBESITY AND DIABETES-RELATED KIDNEY DISEASE

Obesity-related renal disease, similar to diabetes-related renal disease, is associated with physiologic, anatomic, and pathologic changes in the kidney (**Fig. 2**). Both obesity and diabetes renal disease evolve in a sequence of stages beginning with initial increases in GFR and P_{Gc}, glomerular hypertrophy, and microalbuminuria.[20,21] Increased systolic blood pressure further exacerbates the disease progression to proteinuria, nodular glomerulosclerosis and tubulointerstitial injury, and a decline in GFR leading to ESRD.[22,23] Obesity-related and diabetes-related renal disease also share

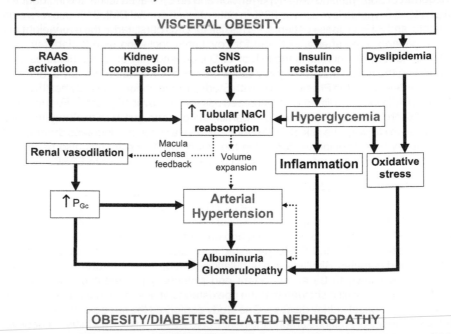

Fig. 2. Interaction between metabolic and hemodynamic pathways in the pathophysiology of obesity-related and diabetes-related renal disease. P_{Gc}, intraglomerular capillary pressure; RAAS, renin angiotensin aldosterone system; SNS, sympathetic nervous system.

common initiating events, which include interactions among multiple metabolic and hemodynamic factors that activate common intracellular signaling pathways that in turn trigger the production of cytokines and growth factors, leading to renal disease (**Fig. 3**).

Obesity, Diabetes, and Glomerular Hemodynamics

Experimental studies in diet-induced obese dogs and genetically induced obese rats show that one of the earliest changes in renal hemodynamics in response to the obese state is glomerular hyperfiltration. Specifically, dogs fed a high-fat diet for only 5 to 6 weeks and obese Zucker rats show an increase in GFR.[39,40] These changes in GFR are reversible, at least in the obese Zucker rats, in which food restriction was associated with attenuation of glomerular hyperfiltration, possibly due to decreased protein intake or overall weight loss.[40] These observations in experimental models have also been confirmed in obese humans. Studies have shown that obese individuals have around 50% higher GFR compared with lean individuals.[41] Although there is still some debate about the mechanisms underlying obesity-related glomerular hyperfiltration, the most likely explanation is increased sodium reabsorption by the proximal tubule or loop of Henle, leading to tubuloglomerular feedback (TGF)–mediated reduction in afferent arteriolar resistance, increased P_{Gc}, and thus increased GFR.[42] This TGF-driven dilation of afferent arterioles and resultant impairment of renal autoregulation, in turn, allows increases in blood pressure to be transmitted to the glomerulus causing further increases in P_{Gc} and subsequent glomerular injury.[43] This may be especially important in individuals with a reduced number of nephrons in whom there is a greater risk of enhanced glomerular blood pressure transmission due to the substantially greater preglomerular vasodilation.[43] There is also evidence for increased activation of the renin-angiotensin-aldosterone system (RAAS) and increased renal sympathetic tone as important stimuli for increased sodium reabsorption exacerbating the renal hemodynamic changes associated with obesity.[44–46]

It is generally believed that the initial increase in GFR associated with obesity likely serves as an early compensatory response that allows for restoration of salt balance despite continued increases in tubular reabsorption. However, in the long term, glomerular hyperfiltration may contribute to the development of renal injury, especially

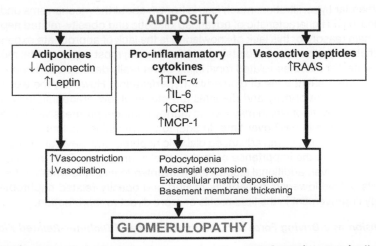

Fig. 3. Mechanisms of obesity-related glomerulopathy. CRP, C-reactive protein; IL-6, interleukin-6; MCP-1, monocyte chemoattractant protein-1; RAAS, renin angiotensin aldosterone system; TNF-α, tumor necrosis factor α.

if combined with hypertension. Studies supporting this notion show that weight loss reduces glomerular hyperfiltration and subsequent renal injury.[41,47]

Similar to obesity-associated glomerular hyperfiltration, renal vasodilation and increases in GFR and P_{Gc} also characterize the early stages of diabetes-associated renal disease.[48] Although the precise mechanisms underlying diabetes-associated glomerular hyperfiltration remain inconclusive, it is believed that mechanisms similar to those occurring in obesity drive the initial increase in GFR. Specifically, reduced delivery of salt to the macula densa, as a consequence of increased proximal reabsorption of glucose and sodium, reduces afferent arteriolar resistance leading to increased P_{Gc} and GFR via attenuated TGF.[49–51] In addition, afferent vasodilation and efferent vasoconstriction in response to circulating or locally formed vasoactive factors (eg, angiotensin II (Ang II) and endothelin) produced in response to hyperglycemia or shear stress are also believed to contribute to the development of diabetes-associated glomerular hyperfiltration.[52,53]

Although most studies suggest that the mechanisms underlying glomerular hyperfiltration due to obesity and diabetes are similar, there is some evidence to suggest that hyperglycemia and obesity may have at least partially additive effects on glomerular hemodynamics. Because obesity and diabetes coexist with elements of the metabolic syndrome, including hypertension, it is often difficult to separate the effects of each element on glomerular hemodynamics and progression of renal injury, at least in humans. However, experimental studies provide some mechanistic insights. Specifically, mice lacking the gene for the melanocortin-4 receptor are obese, hyperinsulinemic, and hyperleptinemic but normotensive at 55 weeks of age and exhibit moderately increased GFR compared with their wild-type counterparts.[54] However, when rendered hypertensive via treatment with N(G)-nitro-L-arginine methyl ester (L-NAME), they develop prominent glomerular hyperfiltration, suggesting that increases in blood pressure may exacerbate obesity-related increases in GFR. These data support the concept of a synergistic effect of various components of obesity, metabolic syndrome, diabetes, and hypertension on glomerular hemodynamics.

Although the early stages of obesity-related and diabetes-related renal disease are characterized by glomerular hyperfiltration, one of the hallmarks of the advanced stages of the disease is the decline in GFR. Unlike studies examining the mechanisms underlying glomerular hyperfiltration, much less is known about the mechanisms underlying the decline in GFR characteristic of advanced diabetic and obesity-related nephropathy. The main reason for this lack of knowledge is the lack of appropriate experimental models that mimic the advanced stages of the disease; most experimental models of obesity-related or diabetes-related renal injury never really develop overt nephropathy and are in a permanent state of glomerular hyperfiltration. However, the existing evidence suggests that obesity and diabetes are states of low-grade inflammation and oxidative stress, both of which may lead to kidney damage, progressive loss of nephrons, and decrease in GFR over time. In addition, hyperlipidemia has been linked to reduced GFR associated with advanced diabetic nephropathy. Several clinical studies have demonstrated the importance of lipid control in preserving GFR in patients with diabetes.[55] However, additional studies are warranted to examine whether the beneficial effects of lipid lowering in diabetes-related and obesity-related nephropathy are caused by improvement in the lipid profile or more direct renoprotection.

Hypertension as a Driving Force for Obesity-Related and Diabetes-Related Kidney Disease

The nearly linear relationship between BMI and blood pressure in diverse populations throughout the world[35,56–58] has led to the notion that obesity contributes to the development of hypertension. Numerous clinical, population, and basic research studies have shown that visceral obesity, the main driver of type 2 diabetes, increases blood pressure.[59,60] Data from the Framingham Heart Study and other population-based studies indicate that excess weight gain may account for as much as 78% of primary (essential) hypertension in men and 65% in women.[61,62] In addition, obese individuals have a 3.5-fold increase in the risk for developing hypertension.[56,63] Clinical studies also indicate that weight loss reduces blood pressure in most patients with hypertension and is effective in the primary prevention of hypertension.[60] Discussing the mechanisms underlying obesity-driven hypertension is beyond the scope of this review, but accumulating evidence suggests that physiologic, environmental, and genetic factors all contribute to obesity-related hypertension.[64] Given that the focus of this review is the contribution of obesity to the development of renal disease, the question to be asked is how does obesity-related hypertension lead to the development of renal disease?

Several studies have suggested that visceral (but not subcutaneous) obesity induces hypertension, initially by increasing renal tubular sodium reabsorption and causing a hypertensive shift of renal-pressure natriuresis via activation of multiple pathways including the sympathetic nervous system and the RAAS.[39,64,65] In addition, physical compression of the kidneys caused by visceral obesity has also been suggested to contribute to the increase in blood pressure, at least in some experimental models.[39] This increase in blood pressure, alongside increases in P_{Gc} and GFR (discussed later), and other metabolic abnormalities (eg, dyslipidemia, hyperglycemia) all likely interact to contribute to the initial renal insult. A similar sequence of events has been proposed to contribute to renal injury in the setting of type 2 diabetes, independent of obesity, suggesting that hypertension plays a major role in obesity as well as diabetes-associated renal disease. Hypertension, in addition to contributing to the initial development of renal injury is also an important factor in the disease progression. Progressive renal injury only occurs when hypertension is superimposed on obesity or diabetes.[54] The importance of tight blood pressure control for treating diabetic nephropathy is recognized in current guidelines, with a recommended target blood pressure of less than 130/80 mm Hg.[66] Several studies have shown clear renoprotection with respect to slowing progression of nephropathy in patients with type 2 diabetes by lowering blood pressure.[67–71]

Obesity, Diabetes, and Albuminuria

The earliest clinical manifestation of obesity-related and diabetes-related renal injury is microalbuminuria (30–300 mg/d) which, over time, can progresses to overt proteinuria (300–3000 mg/d).[72–74] Microalbuminuria, in turn, signifies increased risk of progression to ESRD and cardiovascular disease.[74] Studies in nondiabetic and diabetic overweight individuals have shown that increases in urine albumin excretion strongly correlate with increases in body weight and other markers of obesity, including BMI, waist circumference, and waist-to-hip ratio.[75–78] In the Prevention of Renal and Vascular End stage Disease (PREVEND) study, the prevalence of microalbuminuria in lean and obese individuals correlated with central obesity even after correction for confounding variables.[79] Retrospective analysis of the database of a population study showing that the prevalence of microalbuminuria increased from 9.5% in men with normal BMI to 18.3% in overweight men, and 29.3% in obese men further supports the notion of a direct correlation between BMI and microalbuminuria.[77] In a cross-sectional study of a cohort of African Americans, microalbuminuria was most prevalent in patients with newly diagnosed type 2 diabetes and was independently associated with BMI.[78] Others have shown that even moderate weight reduction in patients with type 2 diabetes with proteinuria reduces urine protein excretion by approximately 30%.[80] Furthermore, weight reduction achieved by either dietary caloric restriction or bariatric surgery has been shown to attenuate progression of proteinuria in obese nondiabetic individuals.[81,82]

The development of microalbuminuria in either nondiabetic or diabetic individuals was traditionally believed to result from damage to the glomerular filtration barrier as a consequence of an increase in blood pressure which is transmitted to the glomeruli, increasing P_{Gc} and GFR. In addition, in the setting of diabetes, hyperglycemia-associated inflammation and oxidative stress have been shown to contribute to the damage to the glomerular filtration barrier, contributing to increased leakage of protein across the membrane leading to the development of albuminuria.[72] In the setting of obesity, cytokines including adiponectin have been suggested to play a role in the development of albuminuria. Specifically, the adiponectin knockout mouse exhibits increased baseline albuminuria and podocyte foot process effacement, suggesting that adiponectin regulates podocyte function and thus contributes to the initial development of albuminuria.[83] Apart from the glomerulocentric view of the origin of albuminuria, a more recent theory on the mechanisms of albuminuria, especially in the setting of diabetes, is that the diabetic milieu also impairs proximal tubular reabsorption of albumin leading to increased urine albumin excretion.[84]

Obesity, Diabetes, and Glomerulopathy

Accompanying the hemodynamic changes, the early stage of obesity is associated with up to a 40% increase in kidney weight.[39,85] Histologically, the obese kidney is characterized by glomerulomegaly, mesangial expansion, and podocytopenia, leading to focal segmental glomerulosclerosis.[43,86,87] These features, which precede overt renal insufficiency, have been observed in biopsies from obese humans[88] and experimental models of obesity-related kidney disease, namely the obese Zucker rat[89,90] and dogs fed a high-fat diet.[39] However, the degree of glomerulosclerosis seems to be highly variable amongst different experimental models and obese individuals,[91] and some studies indicate that some obese individuals do not even develop glomerulosclerosis, despite the glomerulomegaly.[87] A review of native 6818 renal biopsies indicated that obesity-related glomerulopathy is characterized by lesser segmental sclerosis, less podocyte effacement, but more glomerulomegaly compared with idiopathic glomerulosclerosis.[91] However, despite the less pronounced glomerular lesions in obesity-related glomerulopathy, the long-term prognosis of the disease is just as poor. It has been reported that the probabilities of renal survival are 77% and 51% at 5 and 10 years, respectively,[92] and that nephron number may play a significant role in the renal prognosis.[93] Specifically, in patients with unilateral renal agenesis, the decline in renal function is most pronounced in obese patients, suggesting that obesity accelerates renal dysfunction in patients with severe reductions in renal mass.[93]

Similar to obesity-related glomerulopathy, early diabetic nephropathy is accompanied by hyperfiltration and microalbuminuria. Histologically, the diabetic kidney exhibits glomerular hypertrophy, widening of the glomerular basement membrane, mesangial expansion, podocytopenia leading to nodular (Kimmelstiel-Wilson) glomerulosclerosis, and tubulointerstitial fibrosis.[22] Thus, given the similarities in the histologic appearance of the renal lesions from diabetic and obese individuals, it is not surprising that the mechanisms underlying these changes have many similarities.

Mechanisms of Obesity-Related and Diabetes-Related Glomerulopathy

Obesity (ie, visceral adiposity) and diabetes (hyperglycemia) both promote a low-grade inflammatory state and are associated with infiltration of macrophages into the kidney.

The infiltrated macrophages, in turn, become a source of a whole host of proinflammatory mediators such as tumor necrosis factor-α (TNF-α), interleukin-6 (IL-6), C-reactive protein, monocyte chemoattractant protein-1, and macrophage migration inhibitory factor.[94,95] In addition, visceral fat releases adipokines such as adiponectin and leptin into the circulation which also play a role in the pathophysiology of renal injury.[95] Apart from adipokines and inflammatory mediators, vasoactive peptides such as Ang II also contribute to obesity-associated and diabetes-associated glomerulopathy.

Adiponectin

Obese humans are characterized by consistently low levels of circulating adiponectin. However, in patients with CKD and ESRD due to obesity or diabetes, adiponectin levels are increased, possibly because of impaired renal function.[96,97] Experimental studies have shown that genetic deletion of adiponectin is associated with albuminuria and podocyte effacement, which are further exacerbated by diabetes.[98] Treatment of these mice with exogenous adiponectin results in normalization of albuminuria, improvement of podocyte foot process effacement, increased activation of glomerular AMP-activated kinase, and reduced urinary and glomerular markers of oxidative stress.[83] These observations suggest that adiponectin may have a renoprotective effect.

Leptin

Although the primary action of leptin is to act on the satiety center to limit food intake, leptin has also been linked to renal disease. Circulating leptin levels are increased in CKD and in patients on hemodialysis.[99,100] Leptin levels are also typically increased in obese individuals. Mice overexpressing leptin have more renal disease than leptin-deficient mice.[101] Long-term infusion of recombinant leptin in rats is associated with proteinuria, increased expression of extracellular matrix proteins (collagen type IV), transforming growth factor-beta (TGF-β) and other proinflammatory cytokines, macrophage infiltration, and glomerulosclerosis.[102] These observations suggest that, unlike adiponectin, leptin promotes the development of renal injury in both obese and lean individuals.

Inflammatory markers

Both obesity and diabetes are characterized by increased levels of circulating cytokines, including TNF-α and IL-6,[103,104] and markers of inflammation are inversely associated with measures of kidney function and positively with albuminuria. It is believed that the major source of proinflammatory cytokines in obese and diabetic individuals that directly contribute to renal injury are infiltrated macrophages.[101] In addition, renal parenchyma has also been shown to release proinflammatory cytokines in response to hyperglycemia or locally active vasoactive peptides, such as Ang II.[105] Once released, these proinflammatory mediators contribute to a low-grade chronic inflammatory state that contributes to obesity-associated and diabetes-associated glomerulopathy. In particular, TNF-α has been shown to reduce the expression of key components of the slit diaphragm, nephrin and podocin, thus contributing to podocytopathy.[106] Similarly, IL-6 promotes the expression of adhesion molecules and subsequent oxidative stress,[107] whereas blocking the IL-6 receptor prevents progression of proteinuria, renal lipid deposition, and mesangial cell proliferation associated with severe hyperlipoproteinemia.[108] Thus, there is strong evidence for the contribution of inflammation in obesity-associated and diabetes-associated renal disease.

Other factors

Although several vasoactive peptides have been implicated in the pathogenesis of obesity-associated and diabetes-associated glomerulopathy, the most prominent, and certainly the best described vasoactive hormonal pathway is the RAAS; Ang II is the most biologically active component. Both obesity and persistent hyperglycemia are associated with upregulation of the intrarenal RAAS.[109,110] Activation of the RAAS leads to both hemodynamic and cellular effects. Ang II leads to increases in efferent arteriolar vasoconstriction and glomerular pressure, sodium retention, and cell proliferation.[111–113] On a cellular level, Ang II activates protein kinase C and mitogen-activated protein kinase, and transcription factors such as nuclear factor-κB that lead to alteration in the gene expression of several growth factors and cytokines including TGF-β. TGF-β, in turn, promotes podocyte apoptosis, mesangial cell proliferation, and extracellular matrix synthesis, cellular events that are important in the development of obesity-associated and diabetes-associated glomerulopathy.[114]

Although there are many similarities between the obese and diabetic kidney, there are some features unique to obesity in the absence of diabetes. Glomerular/mesangial lipid deposits (foam cells) are frequently seen in the kidneys of obese individuals, supporting the concept of lipotoxicity (ie, lipid-induced renal injury). This lipid accumulation in the glomerulus then leads to upregulation of the sterol-regulatory element-binding proteins (SREBP-1 and -2), which, in turn, promote podocyte apoptosis and mesangial cell proliferation and cytokine synthesis.[115]

SUMMARY

Obesity and diabetes are major causes of CKD and ESRD, and are thus enormous health concerns worldwide. Both obesity and diabetes, along with other elements of the metabolic syndrome including hypertension, are highly interrelated and contribute to the development and progression of renal disease. Studies show that multiple factors act in concert to initially cause renal vasodilation, glomerular hyperfiltration, and albuminuria, leading to the development of glomerulopathy. The coexistence of hypertension contributes to the disease progression, which, if not treated, may lead to ESRD. Although early intervention and management of body weight, hyperglycemia, and hypertension are imperative, novel therapeutic approaches are also necessary to reduce the high morbidity and mortality associated with both obesity-related and diabetes-related renal disease.

REFERENCES

1. Yanovski SZ, Yanovski JA. Obesity prevalence in the United States–up, down, or sideways? N Engl J Med 2011;364(11):987–9.
2. Flegal KM, Carroll MD, Ogden CL, et al. Prevalence and trends in obesity among US adults, 1999-2008. JAMA 2010;303(3):235–41.
3. World Health Organization. Obesity and overweight fact sheet. 2012. Available at: http://www.who.int/mediacentre/factsheets/fs311/en/index.html. Accessed on October 2nd, 2012.
4. Kopelman P. Health risks associated with overweight and obesity. Obes Rev 2007;8(Suppl 1):13–7.
5. Eknoyan G. Obesity, diabetes, and chronic kidney disease. Curr Diab Rep 2007;7(6):449–53.
6. Hall JE, Crook ED, Jones DW, et al. Mechanisms of obesity-associated cardiovascular and renal disease. Am J Med Sci 2002;324(3):127–37.
7. Ogden CL, Carroll MD, Curtin LR, et al. Prevalence of overweight and obesity in the United States, 1999-2004. JAMA 2006;295(13):1549–55.
8. Neeland IJ, Turer AT, Ayers CR, et al. Dysfunctional adiposity and the risk of prediabetes and type 2 diabetes in obese adults. JAMA 2012;308(11):1150–9.

9. Foster MC, Hwang SJ, Larson MG, et al. Overweight, obesity, and the development of stage 3 CKD: the Framingham Heart Study. Am J Kidney Dis 2008; 52(1):39–48.

10. Hsu CY, McCulloch CE, Iribarren C, et al. Body mass index and risk for end-stage renal disease. Ann Intern Med 2006;144(1):21–8.

11. Ejerblad E, Fored CM, Lindblad P, et al. Obesity and risk for chronic renal failure. J Am Soc Nephrol 2006;17(6):1695–702.

12. Praga M, Morales E. Obesity, proteinuria and progression of renal failure. Curr Opin Nephrol Hypertens 2006;15(5):481–6.

13. Wang Y, Chen X, Song Y, et al. Association between obesity and kidney disease: a systematic review and meta-analysis. Kidney Int 2008;73(1):19–33.

14. Ogden CL, Yanovski SZ, Carroll MD, et al. The epidemiology of obesity. Gastroenterology 2007;132(6):2087–102.

15. Coresh J, Selvin E, Stevens LA, et al. Prevalence of chronic kidney disease in the United States. JAMA 2007;298(17):2038–47.

16. Kramer H, Luke A, Bidani A, et al. Obesity and prevalent and incident CKD: the hypertension detection and follow-up program. Am J Kidney Dis 2005;46(4): 587–94.

17. de Zeeuw D, Ramjit D, Zhang Z, et al. Renal risk and renoprotection among ethnic groups with type 2 diabetic nephropathy: a post hoc analysis of RENAAL. Kidney Int 2006;69(9):1675–82.

18. Remuzzi G, Macia M, Ruggenenti P. Prevention and treatment of diabetic renal disease in type 2 diabetes: the BENEDICT study. J Am Soc Nephrol 2006; 17(4 Suppl 2):S90–7.

19. US Renal Data System. USRDS 2009 annual data report: atlas of chronic kidney disease and end-stage renal disease in the United States. Bethesda (MD): National Institutes of Health, National Institute of Diabetes and Digestive and Kidney Diseases; 2009.

20. Thomson SC, Vallon V, Blantz RC. Kidney function in early diabetes: the tubular hypothesis of glomerular filtration. Am J Physiol Renal Physiol 2004;286(1):F8–15.

21. Hostetter TH. Hyperfiltration and glomerulosclerosis. Semin Nephrol 2003;23(2): 194–9.

22. Caramori ML, Mauer M. Diabetes and nephropathy. Curr Opin Nephrol Hypertens 2003;12(3):273–82.

23. Leon CA, Raij L. Interaction of haemodynamic and metabolic pathways in the genesis of diabetic nephropathy. J Hypertens 2005;23(11):1931–7.

24. Ogden CL, Carroll MD, Kit BK, et al. Prevalence of obesity and trends in body mass index among US children and adolescents, 1999-2010. JAMA 2012; 307(5):483–90.

25. Flegal KM, Carroll MD, Kit BK, et al. Prevalence of obesity and trends in the distribution of body mass index among US adults, 1999-2010. JAMA 2012;307(5): 491–7.

26. Danaei G, Finucane MM, Lin JK, et al. National, regional, and global trends in systolic blood pressure since 1980: systematic analysis of health examination surveys and epidemiological studies with 786 country-years and 5.4 million participants. Lancet 2011;377(9765):568–77.

27. US Renal Data System. USRDS 2006 annual data report: atlas of end-stage renal disease in the United States. Bethesda (MD): National Institutes of Health, National Institute of Diabetes and Digestive and Kidney Diseases; 2006.

28. Kurella M, Lo JC, Chertow GM. Metabolic syndrome and the risk for chronic kidney disease among nondiabetic adults. J Am Soc Nephrol 2005;16(7):2134–40.

29. Chen J, Muntner P, Hamm LL, et al. The metabolic syndrome and chronic kidney disease in U.S. adults. Ann Intern Med 2004;140(3):167–74.
30. Stengel B, Tarver-Carr ME, Powe NR, et al. Lifestyle factors, obesity and the risk of chronic kidney disease. Epidemiology 2003;14(4):479–87.
31. Gelber RP, Kurth T, Kausz AT, et al. Association between body mass index and CKD in apparently healthy men. Am J Kidney Dis 2005;46(5):871–80.
32. Munkhaugen J, Lydersen S, Wideroe TE, et al. Prehypertension, obesity, and risk of kidney disease: 20-year follow-up of the HUNT I study in Norway. Am J Kidney Dis 2009;54(4):638–46.
33. Iseki K, Ikemiya Y, Kinjo K, et al. Body mass index and the risk of development of end-stage renal disease in a screened cohort. Kidney Int 2004;65(5):1870–6.
34. Kramer HJ, Saranathan A, Luke A, et al. Increasing body mass index and obesity in the incident ESRD population. J Am Soc Nephrol 2006;17(5):1453–9.
35. Kalantar-Zadeh K, Kopple JD. Obesity paradox in patients on maintenance dialysis. Contrib Nephrol 2006;151:57–69.
36. Kalantar-Zadeh K, Streja E, Kovesdy CP, et al. The obesity paradox and mortality associated with surrogates of body size and muscle mass in patients receiving hemodialysis. Mayo Clin Proc 2010;85(11):991–1001.
37. Elsayed EF, Sarnak MJ, Tighiouart H, et al. Waist-to-hip ratio, body mass index, and subsequent kidney disease and death. Am J Kidney Dis 2008;52(1):29–38.
38. Elsayed EF, Tighiouart H, Weiner DE, et al. Waist-to-hip ratio and body mass index as risk factors for cardiovascular events in CKD. Am J Kidney Dis 2008;52(1):49–57.
39. Henegar JR, Bigler SA, Henegar LK, et al. Functional and structural changes in the kidney in the early stages of obesity. J Am Soc Nephrol 2001;12(6):1211–7.
40. Maddox DA, Alavi FK, Santella RN, et al. Prevention of obesity-linked renal disease: age-dependent effects of dietary food restriction. Kidney Int 2002;62(1):208–19.
41. Chagnac A, Weinstein T, Herman M, et al. The effects of weight loss on renal function in patients with severe obesity. J Am Soc Nephrol 2003;14(6):1480–6.
42. Hall JE. The kidney, hypertension, and obesity. Hypertension 2003;41(3 Pt 2):625–33.
43. Griffin KA, Kramer H, Bidani AK. Adverse renal consequences of obesity. Am J Physiol Renal Physiol 2008;294(4):F685–96.
44. Hall JE, Kuo JJ, da Silva AA, et al. Obesity-associated hypertension and kidney disease. Curr Opin Nephrol Hypertens 2003;12(2):195–200.
45. Esler M, Rumantir M, Wiesner G, et al. Sympathetic nervous system and insulin resistance: from obesity to diabetes. Am J Hypertens 2001;14(11 Pt 2):304S–9S.
46. Blanco S, Bonet J, Lopez D, et al. ACE inhibitors improve nephrin expression in Zucker rats with glomerulosclerosis. Kidney Int Suppl 2005;(93):S10–4.
47. Chagnac A, Herman M, Zingerman B, et al. Obesity-induced glomerular hyperfiltration: its involvement in the pathogenesis of tubular sodium reabsorption. Nephrol Dial Transplant 2008;23(12):3946–52.
48. Yip JW, Jones SL, Wiseman MJ, et al. Glomerular hyperfiltration in the prediction of nephropathy in IDDM: a 10-year follow-up study. Diabetes 1996;45(12):1729–33.
49. Vallon V, Schroth J, Satriano J, et al. Adenosine A(1) receptors determine glomerular hyperfiltration and the salt paradox in early streptozotocin diabetes mellitus. Nephron Physiol 2009;111(3):p30–8.
50. Woods LL, Mizelle HL, Hall JE. Control of renal hemodynamics in hyperglycemia: possible role of tubuloglomerular feedback. Am J Physiol 1987;252(1 Pt 2):F65–73.

51. Persson P, Hansell P, Palm F. Tubular reabsorption and diabetes-induced glomerular hyperfiltration. Acta Physiol (Oxf) 2010;200(1):3–10.
52. Cherney DZ, Scholey JW, Miller JA. Insights into the regulation of renal hemodynamic function in diabetic mellitus. Curr Diabetes Rev 2008;4(4):280–90.
53. Carmines PK. The renal vascular response to diabetes. Curr Opin Nephrol Hypertens 2010;19(1):85–90.
54. do Carmo JM, Tallam LS, Roberts JV, et al. Impact of obesity on renal structure and function in the presence and absence of hypertension: evidence from melanocortin-4 receptor-deficient mice. Am J Physiol Regul Integr Comp Physiol 2009;297(3):R803–12.
55. Fried LF, Orchard TJ, Kasiske BL. Effect of lipid reduction on the progression of renal disease: a meta-analysis. Kidney Int 2001;59(1):260–9.
56. Must A, Spadano J, Coakley EH, et al. The disease burden associated with overweight and obesity. JAMA 1999;282(16):1523–9.
57. Wilson PW, D'Agostino RB, Sullivan L, et al. Overweight and obesity as determinants of cardiovascular risk: the Framingham experience. Arch Intern Med 2002;162(16):1867–72.
58. Doll S, Paccaud F, Bovet P, et al. Body mass index, abdominal adiposity and blood pressure: consistency of their association across developing and developed countries. Int J Obes Relat Metab Disord 2002;26(1):48–57.
59. Hall JE, Jones DW, Kuo JJ, et al. Impact of the obesity epidemic on hypertension and renal disease. Curr Hypertens Rep 2003;5(5):386–92.
60. Neter JE, Stam BE, Kok FJ, et al. Influence of weight reduction on blood pressure: a meta-analysis of randomized controlled trials. Hypertension 2003; 42(5):878–84.
61. Garrison RJ, Kannel WB, Stokes J 3rd, et al. Incidence and precursors of hypertension in young adults: the Framingham Offspring Study. Prev Med 1987;16(2): 235–51.
62. Kannel WB, Zhang T, Garrison RJ. Is obesity-related hypertension less of a cardiovascular risk? The Framingham Study. Am Heart J 1990;120(5): 1195–201.
63. Mokdad AH, Ford ES, Bowman BA, et al. Prevalence of obesity, diabetes, and obesity-related health risk factors, 2001. JAMA 2003;289(1):76–9.
64. Kotchen TA. Obesity-related hypertension: epidemiology, pathophysiology, and clinical management. Am J Hypertens 2010;23(11):1170–8.
65. Hall JE, Henegar JR, Dwyer TM, et al. Is obesity a major cause of chronic kidney disease? Adv Ren Replace Ther 2004;11(1):41–54.
66. Van Buren PN, Toto R. Hypertension in diabetic nephropathy: epidemiology, mechanisms, and management. Adv Chronic Kidney Dis 2011;18(1):28–41.
67. Mancia G. Effects of intensive blood pressure control in the management of patients with type 2 diabetes mellitus in the Action to Control Cardiovascular Risk in Diabetes (ACCORD) trial. Circulation 2010;122(8):847–9.
68. Heerspink HJ, de Zeeuw D. The kidney in type 2 diabetes therapy. Rev Diabet Stud 2011;8(3):392–402.
69. Rayner HC, Hollingworth L, Higgins R, et al. Systematic kidney disease management in a population with diabetes mellitus: turning the tide of kidney failure. BMJ Qual Saf 2011;20(10):903–10.
70. Williams ME. The goal of blood pressure control for prevention of early diabetic microvascular complications. Curr Diab Rep 2011;11(4):323–9.
71. Grossman E, Messerli FH. Management of blood pressure in patients with diabetes. Am J Hypertens 2011;24(8):863–75.

72. Jauregui A, Mintz DH, Mundel P, et al. Role of altered insulin signaling pathways in the pathogenesis of podocyte malfunction and microalbuminuria. Curr Opin Nephrol Hypertens 2009;18(6):539–45.

73. de Boer IH, Sibley SD, Kestenbaum B, et al. Central obesity, incident microalbuminuria, and change in creatinine clearance in the epidemiology of diabetes interventions and complications study. J Am Soc Nephrol 2007;18(1):235–43.

74. Eijkelkamp WB, Zhang Z, Remuzzi G, et al. Albuminuria is a target for renoprotective therapy independent from blood pressure in patients with type 2 diabetic nephropathy: post hoc analysis from the Reduction of Endpoints in NIDDM with the Angiotensin II Antagonist Losartan (RENAAL) trial. J Am Soc Nephrol 2007; 18(5):1540–6.

75. Klausen KP, Parving HH, Scharling H, et al. Microalbuminuria and obesity: impact on cardiovascular disease and mortality. Clin Endocrinol (Oxf) 2009; 71(1):40–5.

76. Savage S, Nagel NJ, Estacio RO, et al. Clinical factors associated with urinary albumin excretion in type II diabetes. Am J Kidney Dis 1995;25(6):836–44.

77. de Jong PE, Verhave JC, Pinto-Sietsma SJ, et al. Obesity and target organ damage: the kidney. Int J Obes Relat Metab Disord 2002;26(Suppl 4):S21–4.

78. Kohler KA, McClellan WM, Ziemer DC, et al. Risk factors for microalbuminuria in black Americans with newly diagnosed type 2 diabetes. Am J Kidney Dis 2000; 36(5):903–13.

79. Pinto-Sietsma SJ, Navis G, Janssen WM, et al. A central body fat distribution is related to renal function impairment, even in lean subjects. Am J Kidney Dis 2003;41(4):733–41.

80. Morales E, Valero MA, Leon M, et al. Beneficial effects of weight loss in overweight patients with chronic proteinuric nephropathies. Am J Kidney Dis 2003;41(2):319–27.

81. Praga M, Morales E. Obesity-related renal damage: changing diet to avoid progression. Kidney Int 2010;78(7):633–5.

82. Mohan S, Tan J, Gorantla S, et al. Early improvement in albuminuria in non-diabetic patients after Roux-en-Y bariatric surgery. Obes Surg 2012;22(3): 375–80.

83. Sharma K, Ramachandrarao S, Qiu G, et al. Adiponectin regulates albuminuria and podocyte function in mice. J Clin Invest 2008;118(5):1645–56.

84. Comper WD, Russo LM. The glomerular filter: an imperfect barrier is required for perfect renal function. Curr Opin Nephrol Hypertens 2009;18(4):336–42.

85. Kasiske BL, Cleary MP, O'Donnell MP, et al. Effects of genetic obesity on renal structure and function in the Zucker rat. J Lab Clin Med 1985;106(5):598–604.

86. Tran HA. Obesity-related glomerulopathy. J Clin Endocrinol Metab 2004;89(12): 6358.

87. Ritz E, Koleganova N, Piecha G. Is there an obesity-metabolic syndrome related glomerulopathy? Curr Opin Nephrol Hypertens 2011;20(1):44–9.

88. Kasiske BL, Napier J. Glomerular sclerosis in patients with massive obesity. Am J Nephrol 1985;5(1):45–50.

89. Coimbra TM, Janssen U, Grone HJ, et al. Early events leading to renal injury in obese Zucker (fatty) rats with type II diabetes. Kidney Int 2000;57(1):167–82.

90. O'Donnell MP, Kasiske BL, Cleary MP, et al. Effects of genetic obesity on renal structure and function in the Zucker rat. II. Micropuncture studies. J Lab Clin Med 1985;106(5):605–10.

91. Kambham N, Markowitz GS, Valeri AM, et al. Obesity-related glomerulopathy: an emerging epidemic. Kidney Int 2001;59(4):1498–509.

92. Praga M, Hernandez E, Morales E, et al. Clinical features and long-term outcome of obesity-associated focal segmental glomerulosclerosis. Nephrol Dial Transplant 2001;16(9):1790–8.
93. Praga M. Synergy of low nephron number and obesity: a new focus on hyperfiltration nephropathy. Nephrol Dial Transplant 2005;20(12):2594–7.
94. King GL. The role of inflammatory cytokines in diabetes and its complications. J Periodontol 2008;79(Suppl 8):1527–34.
95. Tang J, Yan H, Zhuang S. Inflammation and oxidative stress in obesity-related glomerulopathy. Int J Nephrol 2012;2012:608397.
96. Guebre-Egziabher F, Bernhard J, Funahashi T, et al. Adiponectin in chronic kidney disease is related more to metabolic disturbances than to decline in renal function. Nephrol Dial Transplant 2005;20(1):129–34.
97. Saraheimo M, Forsblom C, Thorn L, et al. Serum adiponectin and progression of diabetic nephropathy in patients with type 1 diabetes. Diabetes Care 2008; 31(6):1165–9.
98. Ma K, Cabrero A, Saha PK, et al. Increased beta-oxidation but no insulin resistance or glucose intolerance in mice lacking adiponectin. J Biol Chem 2002; 277(38):34658–61.
99. Kastarinen H, Kesaniemi YA, Ukkola O. Leptin and lipid metabolism in chronic kidney failure. Scand J Clin Lab Invest 2009;69(3):401–8.
100. Sharma K, Considine RV, Michael B, et al. Plasma leptin is partly cleared by the kidney and is elevated in hemodialysis patients. Kidney Int 1997;51(6):1980–5.
101. Mathew AV, Okada S, Sharma K. Obesity related kidney disease. Curr Diabetes Rev 2011;7(1):41–9.
102. Wolf G, Ziyadeh FN. Leptin and renal fibrosis. Contrib Nephrol 2006;151: 175–83.
103. Park HS, Park JY, Yu R. Relationship of obesity and visceral adiposity with serum concentrations of CRP, TNF-alpha and IL-6. Diabetes Res Clin Pract 2005;69(1): 29–35.
104. Gupta J, Mitra N, Kanetsky PA, et al. Association between albuminuria, kidney function, and inflammatory biomarker profile. Clin J Am Soc Nephrol 2012. http://dx.doi.org/10.2215/CJN.03500412.
105. Ruiz-Ortega M, Ruperez M, Lorenzo O, et al. Angiotensin II regulates the synthesis of proinflammatory cytokines and chemokines in the kidney. Kidney Int Suppl 2002;(82):S12–22.
106. Ikezumi Y, Suzuki T, Karasawa T, et al. Activated macrophages down-regulate podocyte nephrin and podocin expression via stress-activated protein kinases. Biochem Biophys Res Commun 2008;376(4):706–11.
107. Patel NS, Chatterjee PK, Di Paola R, et al. Endogenous interleukin-6 enhances the renal injury, dysfunction, and inflammation caused by ischemia/reperfusion. J Pharmacol Exp Ther 2005;312(3):1170–8.
108. Tomiyama-Hanayama M, Rakugi H, Kohara M, et al. Effect of interleukin-6 receptor blockage on renal injury in apolipoprotein E-deficient mice. Am J Physiol Renal Physiol 2009;297(3):F679–84.
109. Ahmed SB, Fisher ND, Stevanovic R, et al. Body mass index and angiotensin-dependent control of the renal circulation in healthy humans. Hypertension 2005;46(6):1316–20.
110. Kennefick TM, Anderson S. Role of angiotensin II in diabetic nephropathy. Semin Nephrol 1997;17(5):441–7.
111. Zhuo JL, Li XC. Novel roles of intracrine angiotensin II and signalling mechanisms in kidney cells. J Renin Angiotensin Aldosterone Syst 2007;8(1):23–33.

112. Griffin KA, Bidani AK. Progression of renal disease: renoprotective specificity of renin-angiotensin system blockade. Clin J Am Soc Nephrol 2006;1(5):1054–65.
113. Crowley SD, Gurley SB, Coffman TM. AT(1) receptors and control of blood pressure: the kidney and more. Trends Cardiovasc Med 2007;17(1):30–4.
114. Ziyadeh FN. Mediators of diabetic renal disease: the case for tgf-Beta as the major mediator. J Am Soc Nephrol 2004;15(Suppl 1):S55–7.
115. Jiang G, Li Z, Liu F, et al. Prevention of obesity in mice by antisense oligonucleotide inhibitors of stearoyl-CoA desaturase-1. J Clin Invest 2005;115(4):1030–8.

Obesity and Reproductive Function

Emily S. Jungheim, MD, MSCI[a],*, Jennifer L. Travieso, BS[a],
Kenneth R. Carson, MD[b,c], Kelle H. Moley, MD[a]

KEYWORDS

- Fertility • Obesity • Reproduction • Public health

KEY POINTS

- There is an epidemic of obesity among women and men of reproductive age.
- Numerous epidemiologic and translational studies demonstrate adverse effects of obesity on various stages of the reproductive process, although the underlying mechanisms are largely unknown.
- Of all the evidence linking obesity to adverse reproductive function and outcomes, the most concerning is the evidence demonstrating links between preconceptional maternal obesity and long-term disease in the offspring.
- Weight loss through lifestyle interventions or surgical therapy may improve reproductive function and outcomes, but data are limited.
- Given the epidemic of obesity in women and men of reproductive age, efforts to understand the impact of obesity on reproductive function and outcomes are an important component of future public health policy.

MEASURING OBESITY AND REPRODUCTIVE RISK

Disentangling the individual components of obesity associated with poor health outcomes is difficult.[1,2] Body mass index (BMI), calculated as the weight in kilograms divided by the height in meters squared, or overall body size adjusted for height, is

This article originally appeared in Obstetrics and Gynecology Clinics, Volume 39, Issue 4, December 2012.
Disclosures: This work was supported by grant K12HD063086 from the National Institutes of Health (NIH), Bethesda, Maryland. The contents of this work are the responsibility of the authors and do not necessarily represent the official views of the NIH.
[a] Division of Reproductive Endocrinology and Infertility, Department of Obstetrics and Gynecology, Washington University in St Louis, St Louis, MO, USA; [b] Division of Hematology and Oncology, Department of Internal Medicine, Washington University in St Louis, St Louis, MO, USA; [c] Division of Public Health Sciences, Department of Surgery, Washington University in St Louis, St Louis, MO, USA
* Corresponding author. Washington University in St Louis, Campus Box 8513, 4444 Forest Park Avenue, Suite 3100, St Louis, MO 63108.
E-mail address: jungheime@wustl.edu

obviously, the most accessible measure of obesity because tools for measuring BMI are readily available. On the other hand, adiposity (regional or total body fat), adipokine production, and lifestyle components may also contribute individually or together to the overall obesity-related health risk. The bulk of the work relating obesity to health risks has focused on chronic diseases; however, we are learning more about components of obesity that relate to reproductive risk.

Body Mass Index

In general, the risk of obesity-related reproductive morbidity is associated with increasing BMI. BMI categories are as follows:

- Overweight: 25 to 29.9 kg/m^2: increased disease risk
- Class I obesity: 30 to 34.9 kg/m^2: high disease risk
- Class II obesity: 30 to 34.9 kg/m^2: very high disease risk
- Class III obesity: 40 kg/m^{2}or more: extremely high disease risk[3]

These standard BMI categories are born out of associations made between obesity and risks of developing chronic conditions such as diabetes and cardiovascular disease. Although these conditions may exist in some obese women of reproductive age, many of them have not had long enough exposure time to manifest these diseases. Instead, signs of poor reproductive function such as anovulation and/or subfertility may be the first obesity-related morbidity that younger women experience. Standard BMI categories were not developed to relate the risk that young women face of poor reproductive function. Despite this, BMI is the measure used most often in counseling obese women regarding reproductive and pregnancy risks. In fact, some providers and practice organizations advocate for restricting fertility treatment to women based on BMI.[4]

There may be more specific measures associated with reproductive risk in obese women because BMI represents a measure of total body energy balance. Recent translational work has demonstrated that better predictors of metabolic risk and disease may exist such as quantity of visceral adipose tissue and intrahepatic triglyceride content.[5] Also, epidemiologic work has shown strong associations between lifestyle factors such as diet and physical activity and risk of cardiovascular disease, both of which influence energy balance and BMI but are independent factors.[6,7] Whether or not there are markers of obesity-related reproductive risk better than BMI is yet to be determined. Further study of relationships existing among adipokines, various measures of adiposity, and lifestyle factors such as diet and physical activity and reproductive outcomes may prove useful. In the meantime, studies of reproductive risk and obesity that categorize risk by BMI represent most of the data that can be used clinically in counseling obese women.

Adipokines

Adipokines are signaling molecules produced by adipose cells, and their production varies with adipose mass. Adipokines that may be important to obesity-related morbidity include leptin, tumor necrosis factor α (TNF-α), interleukin 6 (IL-6), free fatty acids, and adiponectin.[8–10] Abnormalities in adipokines may cause inflammation and abnormal cell signaling, which in turn leads to impaired cellular metabolism and function.

Emerging evidence links abnormalities in adipokines to abnormal reproductive function.[8] For example, leptin may affect reproductive function at the level of the hypothalamus, providing the signal both to initiate reproductive maturation and to maintain normal signaling of the hypothalamic-pituitary-ovarian axis.[8,11] This mechanism has been demonstrated in a mouse model of diet-induced obesity in which hyperleptine-mia causes central leptin resistance and hypogonadism.[11] Such a mechanism could explain findings of altered pulsatile luteinizing hormone (LH) amplitude in obese women.[12] Also, leptin and TNF-α levels vary between follicular and luteal phases of the menstrual cycle.[8] Although the significance of these variations in adipokines be-tween the stages of the menstrual cycle is unknown, it is possible that they may affect signaling within the hypothalamic-pituitary-ovarian axis required for normal oocyte recruitment and ovulation. Other work has demonstrated that adiponectin signaling may be important to preimplantation embryonic development and implantation.[13] The authors have recently shown that elevated free fatty acid levels are associated with impaired oocyte maturation and decreased chances of pregnancy.[14,15] The spe-cific role of various adipokines in reproductive function is largely unknown, but the aforementioned examples suggest that they may provide an important link between obesity and pathologic reproductive function.

Lifestyle: Dietary Factors

Dietary choices that contribute to obesity may also play a role in the adverse reproduc-tive outcomes associated with obesity. The potential role of diet in reproductive func-tion has been elegantly demonstrated through the Nurses Health Study II (NHSII), a prospective epidemiologic cohort study in which the lifestyle patterns of nurses are tracked and long-term health outcomes are followed up. In a series of publications, di-etary choices, such as vegetable sources of protein as against animal proteins, and limiting the intake of transfats and refined carbohydrates have been shown to be asso-ciated with decreased risks of ovulatory infertility independent of the BMI and total caloric intake.[16–18] Work demonstrating that dietary changes improve ovulatory func-tion in anovulatory obese women has yet to be done, but certainly, the prospective research that has come from NHSII on lifestyle and ovulatory infertility is intriguing and offers clinicians and their patients a place to institute lifestyle changes that may help with weight loss that does improve ovulatory function in obese women.[19]

Lipotoxicity is one mechanism by which fat intake may influence reproductive tis-sues.[20–24] This process is characterized by excess circulating long-chain saturated fatty acids, which are produced by adipocytes themselves and are also obtained through the diet. When the adipocytes can no longer store these fatty acids, other non-adipose cell types begin to store fat. This leads to an increase in the production of reactive oxygen species with subsequent mitochondrial dysfunction, endoplasmic re-ticulum stress, and ultimately, cell death.[25] The reproductive tissues affected include granulosa cells and oocytes, leading to impaired oocyte maturation and poor oocyte quality.[24,26] In a murine model, we have recently shown that brief preimplantation em-bryonic exposure to excess palmitic acid, a long-chain saturated fatty acid obtained from the diet and produced by adipocytes, can result in fetal growth restriction with subsequent postdelivery catch-up growth and a metabolic-like syndrome in adult-hood.[21] Whether or not this work is representative of what happens in the human con-dition is unknown; however, it does suggest that preconceptional and periconceptional diet and obesity have long-term impact on the offspring.

Lifestyle: Physical Activity

Lack of physical activity decreases energy expenditure and contributes to developing and continuing obesity. Whether or not lack of activity and exercise directly contribute to the pathophysiologic mechanisms linking obesity to disease is unclear.[27] On the other hand, in another analysis using NHSII data that controlled for BMI, women with the highest levels of physical activity were less likely to have ovulatory infertility than women who had low levels of physical activity.[19] In another recent study of physical activity and time to pregnancy, increased physical activity levels were associated with decreased time to pregnancy.[28] Altogether, poor dietary choices and decreased levels of physical activity contribute to the development and sustenance of obesity,[27] and therefore, physical activity may be an important component to improve reproductive function in the setting of obesity.

A Culmination of Risk Factors: Adverse Reproductive Outcomes in Obesity

Anovulation

Increasing BMI and obesity are associated with increased reproductive risks including menstrual irregularities, typically a result of anovulation.[29] Metabolic abnormalities induced by obesity, such as insulin resistance, may promote the development of polycystic ovary syndrome (PCOS), a condition diagnosed by the presence of oligomenorrhea and hyperandrogenism; however, not all anovulatory obese women meet these diagnostic criteria. As discussed, adipokines may have effects on hypothalamic-pituitary signaling and communication that inhibit ovulation and thus pose another mechanism by which obesity may increase the risk of irregular menses and anovulation.[11,12] Different women may have a different threshold for anovulation at various different body weights and overall adiposity as hypothalamic-pituitary signaling depending on other environmental exposures and genetic factors.[30]

Subfertility

While anovulation certainly contributes to subfertility among obese women, even in obese women with regular cycles, the time to pregnancy is increased in this group compared with women of normal weight.[31] It has been argued this increase is due to decreased frequency of sexual intercourse among obese women; however, in a research done through the NIH-sponsored Reproductive Medicine Network's Pregnancy in Polycystic Ovary Syndrome Trial, obesity was not associated with decreased frequency of sexual intercourse in couples trying to conceive.[32] Whether or not subfertility in ovulatory obese women is secondary to poorer oocyte or embryo quality, impairments in embryo implantation, or a combination of all these factors is unknown.

Miscarriage

It is difficult to get a true measure of the risk of miscarriage among obese women who conceive spontaneously because many women with early pregnancy loss may not realize that they are pregnant and therefore may never present to their physicians. This situation may be especially true for obese women with irregular menses. On the other hand, studies of women undergoing fertility treatments offer a unique opportunity to capture preconceptional exposures such as obesity and to relate these preconceptional exposures to reproductive outcomes such as miscarriage and others including ovulation, time to pregnancy, pregnancy risks, and neonatal outcomes.[33] Despite the opportunity for preconceptional exposures that infertile women and women undergoing assisted reproductive technology (ART) offer for such measures, data from a recent meta-analysis of obesity and miscarriage risk demonstrate that in general obesity is associated with an increased risk of miscarriage; however, the evidence linking obesity to increased risk of miscarriage in women undergoing ARTs is insufficient.[34] It is possible that ART may counter the increased risks of miscarriage in the setting of obesity by allowing for selection of better embryos and therefore lower risk of miscarriage, by improving endometrial conditions through the supraphysiologic doses of gonadotropin administered, or by allowing for correction of abnormal oocyte metabolism through in vitro culture out of the abnormal environment that obesity poses. Data supporting these hypotheses are lacking.

Adverse pregnancy outcomes

In pregnancy, obesity is associated with significant increased risk of maternal and fetal morbidity including increased risk of preeclampsia, gestational diabetes, fetal growth abnormalities, stillbirth, congenital abnormalities, and the need for cesarean delivery.[35] This is also true for obese women who conceive with in vitro fertilization (IVF).[36]

The reproductive phenotype of obesity varies in its severity, as some women conceive without difficulty and proceed through pregnancy without complication, whereas others may have some or a combination of the reproductive outcomes discussed. At present, beyond measurements of BMI and history of preexisting diabetes, there are few reliable risk factors to predict which obese women are going to have adverse reproductive and pregnancy outcomes. Regardless of how minor the reproductive phenotype an obese woman expresses, emerging evidence that children of obese mothers are at increased risk of obesity-related morbidity later in life is concerning because we may be propagating the obesity-related health problems that are already common today in this so-called "Fifth Phase of the Epidemiologic Transition: The Age of Obesity and Inactivity."[37–40] The mechanisms leading to this increased risk of obesity in the offspring are unknown, but laboratory data from animal models suggest that maternal obesity imposes epigenetic changes that lead to obesity in the offspring.[20,41] Anticipated findings from the National Children's Study, an ongoing prospective cohort study of 100,000 children that includes collection of data regarding pregnancy exposures and development of chronic disease, may shed more light on these concerns.[42]

OBESITY'S REPRODUCTIVE TARGETS
The Central Nervous System (CNS)

As mentioned previously, obese women exhibit decreased LH pulse amplitude and decreased excretion of progesterone metabolites.[12] In addition to causing anovulation, abnormal LH pulsatility may affect ovarian follicular steroidogenesis, leading to abnormal oocyte recruitment and poor oocyte quality and/or altered endometrial development, and it could affect the function of the corpus luteum in the luteal phase. How decreased LH pulse amplitude specifically affects subsequent reproductive function has yet to be discerned, but in any case, it does highlight the fact that mechanisms leading to anovulation in obese women may be different from those leading to anovulation in nonobese women with PCOS.[30] We have demonstrated that ART outcomes in morbidly obese women with PCOS are worse than those in women with PCOS who are not morbidly obese, suggesting that it is not chronic anovulation alone or abnormal central nervous system (CNS) signaling that affects the ovarian follicle and subsequent reproductive function, but perhaps some other component of obesity that is also important.[43]

The Ovary, Ovarian Follicle, and Oocytes

The authors recently investigated the effects of diet-induced obesity in a reproductive mouse model.[20] They isolated ovaries from obese mice and nonobese controls and stained them for apoptosis. Ovaries taken from the obese mice demonstrated increased apoptosis in the cells of the ovarian follicles. Oocytes isolated from the obese mice were smaller, and fewer oocytes from these mice were mature compared with control mice. In another study using a diet-induced obesity model, Igosheva and colleagues[44] found that preconceptional obesity is associated with altered mitochondria in mouse oocytes and zygotes, possibly the result of oxidative stress. Obese mice were less likely to support blastocyst development compared with lean mice. The authors concluded that abnormal oocyte and early embryonic mitochondrial metabolism contribute to poor reproductive outcomes in obese women.

It could be that abnormal signaling from the CNS alone results in abnormal ovarian follicular recruitment and development with poor-quality oocytes in obese women; however, work done by Robker and colleagues[45] suggests otherwise. Dr Robker has demonstrated that insulin levels are increased in the ovarian follicular fluid isolated from obese women undergoing IVF compared with women of moderate weight. In further work using a diet-induced obesity model, Dr Robker has shown that a high-fat diet is associated with lipid accumulation in oocytes along with markers of a lipotoxic response.[22] Similarly, in specimens isolated from women undergoing IVF, the authors have demonstrated that increased ovarian follicular fluid free fatty acid concentrations are associated with poor oocyte quality.[14] Supporting the theory that dietary factors, adipokines, or some other circulating factors directly affect the ovarian follicle, granulosa cells exposed to increasing concentrations of palmitic acid, a long-chain saturated fatty acid obtained from the diet and made by adipocytes, undergo apoptosis with decreased hormone steroidogenesis.[46]

In addition to abnormal endocrine and paracrine cues along with circulating adipokines, inflammatory factors, and metabolites, other factors may play a role in ovarian follicular health. Citing evidence from in vitro models of ovarian follicular development and unpublished work demonstrating increased rigidity in ovaries from obese versus nonobese mice, Woodruff and Shea[47] hypothesize that the physical environment of the ovary may also contribute to the pathologic features of polycystic ovaries.

The Embryo

Abnormal metabolism and other oocyte quality issues may carry over into abnormal embryonic metabolism and competence. This has been demonstrated in animal models of type 1 diabetes, and is suspected to be important in the setting of obesity based on maternal models of diet-induced obesity.[20,48] Poor embryo quality may originate with the oocyte, but an abnormal tubal or uterine environment may also influence embryo quality. In an in vitro model of obesity, the authors exposed preimplantation embryos to excess amounts of palmitic acid—a fatty acid that has been detected in uterine and tubal fluid.[21] This exposure resulted in abnormal embryonic expression of the insulinlike growth factor (IGF-1) receptor, which is responsible for insulin signaling in the embryo. When transferred back into normal recipient mice, the palmitic-acid-exposed embryos resulted in growth-restricted fetuses and the offspring demonstrated a metabolic-like syndrome.[21] Data from a similar model of type II diabetes demonstrate that embryonic insulin resistance is associated with increased risk of miscarriage and that metformin, an insulin sensitizer, reverses this risk.[49] Obesity also induces insulin resistance and could potentially cause similar issues of insulin resistance in preimplantation embryos.[20] Whether or not embryonic insulin resistance underlies the increased risk of miscarriage seen among obese women is unknown, but there is evidence to suggest that treating women with recurrent miscarriages with metformin improves the chances of a live birth.[50] Randomized controlled trials supporting the routine use of metformin in obese women with recurrent pregnancy loss are lacking.

The Endometrium

The endometrium is yet another potential target of the abnormal milieu created by obesity. One model that has been used to specifically address the endometrium is the donor oocyte model. In this model, oocytes from healthy donors are transferred into women who are typically unable to conceive with their own oocytes. Researchers have evaluated the impact of increasing BMI of recipients of donor oocyte on embryonic implantation rate, clinical pregnancy rate, miscarriage rate, and chances of live birth. These studies have yielded conflicting results with several studies demonstrating a BMI-related impact on measures of reproductive success[51,52] and others demonstrating no effect.[53,54] In any case, however, alterations in endometrial gene expression in the peri-implantation period have been noted to be different in obese versus nonobese women.[55]

IMPROVING REPRODUCTIVE FUNCTION IN OBESE WOMEN WITH SUBFERTILITY
An Opportunity for Intervention

Obesity-related anovulation and subfertility may provide an important opportunity for preconceptional intervention and improvements in reproductive function and outcomes. These opportunities go beyond interventions for obesity because they include opportunities to screen for pregestational diabetes mellitus and optimization of glucose control in women who are diabetic, opportunities to screen for preconceptional rubella and varicella vaccination, counseling regarding healthy diet and lifestyle preconceptionally and during pregnancy including the use of prenatal vitamins, and screening for any other previously undiagnosed medical issues important to healthy pregnancy outcome such as thyroid disease.

Pregnancy has been referred to as a "teachable moment" for weight control and obesity prevention because it may motivate women to adopt improved lifestyle habits that may lead to better weight control.[56] It is agreed that efforts should be made to educate and counsel pregnant women about weight gain and a healthy lifestyle during pregnancy; however, for obese women, preconception interventions may offer more potential for an impact on subsequent reproductive and pregnancy outcomes than intragestational interventions.

Weight Loss Through Lifestyle Changes

There are little data regarding lifestyle changes in subfertile obese women and improvements in spontaneous conception and other reproductive outcomes. Most data that exist examine lifestyle changes in women with PCOS, and even these data are limited. In a recent Cochrane review on lifestyle intervention and PCOS, the effectiveness of lifestyle intervention in improving reproductive outcomes in women with PCOS was investigated.[57] The investigators limited their search to randomized controlled trials comparing lifestyle intervention to minimal or no treatment in women with PCOS and concluded that there were no existing data demonstrating an effect of lifestyle on clinical reproductive outcomes. The authors performed a systematic review of the literature to include observational studies eliminated by the Cochrane review and to include studies of obese women without PCOS. They searched Medline up to June 2012 using the keywords "weight loss" and "reproduction." The search was limited to studies in women published in English in the past 5 years. With this search,8 studies were identified. Of these, 6 studies investigated reproductive function after treatment with medical therapies including metformin, orlistat, sibutramine, and myo-inositol.[58–63] One study outlined the strategy of an ongoing trial evaluating the costs and effects of a structured lifestyle program in overweight and obese subfertile women in Norway, but no result was available.[64] Only 1 study reported specifically on the effects of a lifestyle intervention on reproductive function in obese women, and this was in obese women preparing to undergo IVF.[65] This study by Moran and colleagues[65] randomized 38 overweight and obese women to active dietary modification and exercise or standard treatment before IVF. The investigators found a significant effect of the intervention on BMI and weight but no difference in pregnancy or live births between the intervention group and control group. The sample size was small, which limited the outcomes investigated.

Clearly, further work investigating preconceptional weight loss and reproductive function is needed, particularly translational work investigating specific steps in the reproductive process so that improved treatments and evidence-based management can be developed for obese women hoping to conceive.

Weight Loss Through Bariatric Surgery

Clinically meaningful weight loss through lifestyle changes may be difficult for some women. Bariatric surgery may offer greater and more sustainable weight loss. In 2008, Maggard and colleagues[66] published a systematic review of pregnancy and fertility after bariatric surgery. The investigators found that women of reproductive age accounted for 49% of all patients undergoing bariatric surgery. Overall, they concluded that the data support improved pregnancy outcomes in women who have undergone bariatric surgery compared with obese women who have not undergone bariatric surgery. These outcomes included decreased risk of gestational diabetes and preeclampsia and improved neonatal outcomes. In their search, studies regarding fertility were limited. The investigators identified 6 observational studies published between 1988 and 2004. All these studies demonstrated improvement of menstrual cycles in women who underwent bariatric surgery, but none of the studies investigated fertility as a primary outcome.

To determine if additional studies had been published since the JAMA review regarding bariatric procedures and fertility, the authors performed a review of Medline up to June 2012, limiting studies to those performed in women and published in English in the past 5 years. Keywords searched were "bariatric surgery and reproduction." A total of 40 articles were identified, but 15 articles were reviews,[67–82] 16 were on pregnancy outcomes after bariatric surgery,[83–98] 3 were commentaries or author replies,[99–101] 2 investigated contraceptive use postbariatric surgery,[102,103] 1 was a cross-sectional assessment of reproductive health in women undergoing bariatric surgery,[104] 1 was a case report of empty follicle syndrome in a woman postbariatric surgery undergoing IVF,[105] and 1 article was a case series of IVF in women who had previously undergone bariatric surgery.[106] In these last two articles, special considerations were outlined for IVF in women with previous bariatric surgery.[106] Only 1 of the articles identified investigated reproductive function after bariatric surgery. In this article, Rochester and colleagues[107] discuss improvements in LH and progesterone metabolite excretion after weight loss in obese women who have undergone bariatric surgery.

COMPETING RISKS IN THE SETTING OF INFERTILITY: OBESITY VERSUS AGE

As discussed, for obese women with infertility, weight loss may offer improved fertility. On the other hand, after the age of 35 years, there may be less of an effect of obesity on fertility rates with IVF,[108,109] although the obstetric risks that obesity poses remain. Furthermore, after the age of 35 years, there is a decrease in success of IVF in all women undergoing IVF, regardless of the infertility diagnosis or BMI.[109] These issues make for a difficult clinical scenario because age and obesity become competing risks in treating women with infertility. Also, neither does preconceptional weight loss guarantee pregnancy nor does it guarantee a pregnancy and delivery free of complication. For these reasons, some women with infertility may choose to accept obesity-related risks and proceed with fertility treatment instead.

FERTILITY TREATMENT OF OBESE WOMEN

Numerous studies have demonstrated decreased efficacy of fertility treatments in obese women.[33,43] As a result, some centers offering fertility treatments have put BMI limits on who they will treat and what types of treatment they will offer. In fact, in New Zealand, where fertility treatments are covered under the national health care plan, there is a BMI cutoff of 32 kg/m^2 that limits access to IVF. In the United States, some fertility treatment centers have BMI restrictions; however, these restrictions vary from center to center and are not universally enforced.[110] Furthermore, despite decreased efficacy of fertility treatments, the success of various fertility treatment strategies still offer a reasonable chance of success in obese women.[43,111] Subsequently, members of the Ethics Committee of the American Society for Reproductive Medicine recently proposed that restricting access to fertility treatment based on BMI is discriminatory.[112]

THE NEED FOR TRANSDISCIPLINARY RESEARCH AND NOVEL APPROACHES

The authors propose that obesity research as it relates to reproduction requires a transdisciplinary approach because both obesity and reproduction are complex systems affected by social, environmental, biologic, economic, and genetic influences to name a few. Tackling the problem of reproduction in obese women will require cooperative efforts among experts in all these fields of study. Ultimately, this type of research may help inform models of shared decision making in which physicians and patients mutually decide how to proceed with strategies for fertility. These models may be especially helpful because there is a significant degree of uncertainty that exists in treating obese women with infertility.[113] Such models would likely include consideration of the potential risks and benefits an individual (at a given age and weight) would gain from fertility treatment with or without a strategy for weight loss before or during treatment.

SUMMARY

There are many components of obesity that may affect the different steps of the reproductive process leading to adverse reproductive outcomes. Clearly, there is good data demonstrating that weight loss improves ovulatory function in obese women and improves pregnancy outcomes. On the other hand, female fertility is limited by time, the reproductive phenotype of obesity is variable, and current measures of obesity are not reliable predictors of these phenotypes. Because of the complex nature of obesity and reproduction, when an obese woman with subfertility presents for fertility treatment, an individualized yet systematic approach is needed.

REFERENCES

1. Luke DA, Stamatakis KA. Systems science methods in public health: dynamics, networks, and agents. Annu Rev Public Health 2012;33:357–76.
2. Hammond RA. Complex systems modeling for obesity research. Prev Chronic Dis 2009;6(3):A97.
3. Clinical guidelines on the identification, evaluation, and treatment of overweight and obesity in adults–the evidence report. National Institutes of Health. Obes Res 1998;6(Suppl 2):51S–209S.
4. Balen AH, Anderson RA. Impact of obesity on female reproductive health: British Fertility Society, Policy and Practice Guidelines. Hum Fertil (Camb) 2007;10(4):195–206.

5. Fabbrini E, Magkos F, Mohammed BS, et al. Intrahepatic fat, not visceral fat, is linked with metabolic complications of obesity. Proc Natl Acad Sci U S A 2009; 106(36):15430–5.

6. Stampfer MJ, Hu FB, Manson JE, et al. Primary prevention of coronary heart disease in women through diet and lifestyle. N Engl J Med 2000;343(1):16–22.

7. Hu FB, Stampfer MJ, Manson JE, et al. Trends in the incidence of coronary heart disease and changes in diet and lifestyle in women. N Engl J Med 2000;343(8): 530–7.

8. Gosman GG, Katcher HI, Legro RS. Obesity and the role of gut and adipose hormones in female reproduction. Hum Reprod Update 2006;12(5):585–601.

9. Hampton T. Scientists study fat as endocrine organ. JAMA 2006;296(13): 1573–5.

10. Shuldiner AR, Yang R, Gong DW. Resistin, obesity and insulin resistance–the emerging role of the adipocyte as an endocrine organ. N Engl J Med 2001; 345(18):1345–6.

11. Tortoriello DV, McMinn J, Chua SC. Dietary-induced obesity and hypothalamic infertility in female DBA/2J mice. Endocrinology 2004;145(3):1238–47.

12. Jain A, Polotsky AJ, Rochester D, et al. Pulsatile luteinizing hormone amplitude and progesterone metabolite excretion are reduced in obese women. J Clin Endocrinol Metab 2007;92(7):2468–73.

13. Kim ST, Marquard K, Stephens S, et al. Adiponectin and adiponectin receptors in the mouse preimplantation embryo and uterus. Hum Reprod 2011;26(1):82–95.

14. Jungheim ES, Macones GA, Odem RR, et al. Associations between free fatty acids, cumulus oocyte complex morphology and ovarian function during in vitro fertilization. Fertil Steril 2011;95(6):1970–4.

15. Jungheim ES, Macones GA, Odem RR, et al. Elevated serum alpha-linolenic acid levels are associated with decreased chance of pregnancy after in vitro fertilization. Fertil Steril 2011;96(4):880–3.

16. Chavarro JE, Rich-Edwards JW, Rosner BA, et al. Dietary fatty acid intakes and the risk of ovulatory infertility. Am J Clin Nutr 2007;85(1):231–7.

17. Chavarro JE, Rich-Edwards JW, Rosner BA, et al. Protein intake and ovulatory infertility. Am J Obstet Gynecol 2008;198(2):210.e1–7.

18. Chavarro JE, Rich-Edwards JW, Rosner BA, et al. A prospective study of dietary carbohydrate quantity and quality in relation to risk of ovulatory infertility. Eur J Clin Nutr 2009;63(1):78–86.

19. Chavarro JE, Rich-Edwards JW, Rosner BA, et al. Diet and lifestyle in the prevention of ovulatory disorder infertility. Obstet Gynecol 2007;110(5):1050–8.

20. Jungheim ES, Schoeller EL, Marquard KL, et al. Diet-induced obesity model: abnormal oocytes and persistent growth abnormalities in the offspring. Endocrinology 2010;151(8):4039–46.

21. Jungheim ES, Louden ED, Chi MM, et al. Preimplantation exposure of mouse embryos to palmitic acid results in fetal growth restriction followed by catch-up growth in the offspring. Biol Reprod 2011;85(4):678–83.

22. Wu LL, Dunning KR, Yang X, et al. High-fat diet causes lipotoxicity responses in cumulus-oocyte complexes and decreased fertilization rates. Endocrinology 2010;151(11):5438–45.

23. Robker RL, Wu LL, Yang X. Inflammatory pathways linking obesity and ovarian dysfunction. J Reprod Immunol 2011;88(2):142–8.

24. Yang X, Wu LL, Chura LR, et al. Exposure to lipid-rich follicular fluid is associated with endoplasmic reticulum stress and impaired oocyte maturation in cumulus-oocyte complexes. Fertil Steril 2012;97(6):1438–43.

25. Schaffer JE. Lipotoxicity: when tissues overeat. Curr Opin Lipidol 2003;14(3): 281–7.
26. Wu LL, Norman RJ, Robker RL. The impact of obesity on oocytes: evidence for lipotoxicity mechanisms. Reprod Fertil Dev 2011;24(1):29–34.
27. Wolin KY, Carson K, Colditz GA. Obesity and cancer. Oncologist 2010;15(6): 556–65.
28. Wise LA, Rothman KJ, Mikkelsen EM, et al. A prospective cohort study of physical activity and time to pregnancy. Fertil Steril 2012;97(5):1136–42.e1–4.
29. Obesity and reproduction: an educational bulletin. Fertil Steril 2008;90(Suppl 5): S21–9.
30. Fritz M, Speroff L. Clincal gynecologic endocrinology and infertility. 8th edition. Philadelphia: Lippincott Williams & Wilkins; 2011.
31. Wise LA, Rothman KJ, Mikkelsen EM, et al. An internet-based prospective study of body size and time-to-pregnancy. Hum Reprod 2010;25(1):253–64.
32. Pagidas K, Carson SA, McGovern PG, et al. Body mass index and intercourse compliance. Fertil Steril 2010;94(4):1447–50.
33. Jungheim ES, Moley KH. Current knowledge of obesity's effects in the pre- and periconceptional periods and avenues for future research. Am J Obstet Gynecol 2010;203(6):525–30.
34. Metwally M, Ong KJ, Ledger WL, et al. Does high body mass index increase the risk of miscarriage after spontaneous and assisted conception? A meta-analysis of the evidence. Fertil Steril 2008;90(3):714–26.
35. Catalano PM, Ehrenberg HM. The short- and long-term implications of maternal obesity on the mother and her offspring. BJOG 2006;113(10):1126–33.
36. Dokras A, Baredziak L, Blaine J, et al. Obstetric outcomes after in vitro fertilization in obese and morbidly obese women. Obstet Gynecol 2006;108(1):61–9.
37. Gaziano JM. Fifth phase of the epidemiologic transition: the age of obesity and inactivity. JAMA 2010;303(3):275–6.
38. Laitinen J, Jaaskelainen A, Hartikainen AL, et al. Maternal weight gain during the first half of pregnancy and offspring obesity at 16 years: a prospective cohort study. BJOG 2012;119(6):716–23.
39. Catalano PM, Hauguel-De Mouzon S. Is it time to revisit the Pedersen hypothesis in the face of the obesity epidemic? Am J Obstet Gynecol 2011;204(6):479–87.
40. Dabelea D, Crume T. Maternal environment and the transgenerational cycle of obesity and diabetes. Diabetes 2011;60(7):1849–55.
41. Dunn GA, Bale TL. Maternal high-fat diet effects on third-generation female body size via the paternal lineage. Endocrinology 2011;152(6):2228–36.
42. Landrigan PJ, Trasande L, Thorpe LE, et al. The National Children's Study: a 21-year prospective study of 100,000 American children. Pediatrics 2006;118(5): 2173–86.
43. Jungheim ES, Lanzendorf SE, Odem RR, et al. Morbid obesity is associated with lower clinical pregnancy rates after in vitro fertilization in women with polycystic ovary syndrome. Fertil Steril 2009;92(1):256–61.
44. Igosheva N, Abramov AY, Poston L, et al. Maternal diet-induced obesity alters mitochondrial activity and redox status in mouse oocytes and zygotes. PloS One 2010;5(4):e10074.
45. Robker RL, Akison LK, Bennett BD, et al. Obese women exhibit differences in ovarian metabolites, hormones, and gene expression compared with moderate-weight women. J Clin Endocrinol Metab 2009;94(5):1533–40.
46. Mu YM, Yanase T, Nishi Y, et al. Saturated FFAs, palmitic acid and stearic acid, induce apoptosis in human granulosa cells. Endocrinology 2001;142(8):3590–7.

47. Woodruff TK, Shea LD. A new hypothesis regarding ovarian follicle development: ovarian rigidity as a regulator of selection and health. J Assist Reprod Genet 2011;28(1):3–6.
48. Jungheim ES, Moley KH. The impact of type 1 and type 2 diabetes mellitus on the oocyte and the preimplantation embryo. Semin Reprod Med 2008;26(2): 186–95.
49. Eng GS, Sheridan RA, Wyman A, et al. AMP kinase activation increases glucose uptake, decreases apoptosis, and improves pregnancy outcome in embryos exposed to high IGF-I concentrations. Diabetes 2007;56(9):2228–34.
50. Moll E, Korevaar JC, Bossuyt PM, et al. Does adding metformin to clomifene citrate lead to higher pregnancy rates in a subset of women with polycystic ovary syndrome? Hum Reprod 2008;23(8):1830–4.
51. DeUgarte DA, DeUgarte CM, Sahakian V. Surrogate obesity negatively impacts pregnancy rates in third-party reproduction. Fertil Steril 2010;93(3):1008–10.
52. Bellver J, Melo MA, Bosch E, et al. Obesity and poor reproductive outcome: the potential role of the endometrium. Fertil Steril 2007;88(2):446–51.
53. Styne-Gross A, Elkind-Hirsch K, Scott RT Jr. Obesity does not impact implantation rates or pregnancy outcome in women attempting conception through oocyte donation. Fertil Steril 2005;83(6):1629–34.
54. Wattanakumtornkul S, Damario MA, Stevens Hall SA, et al. Body mass index and uterine receptivity in the oocyte donation model. Fertil Steril 2003;80(2):336–40.
55. Bellver J, Martinez-Conejero JA, Labarta E, et al. Endometrial gene expression in the window of implantation is altered in obese women especially in association with polycystic ovary syndrome. Fertil Steril 2011;95(7):2335–41, 2341.e1–8.
56. Phelan S. Pregnancy: a "teachable moment" for weight control and obesity prevention. Am J Obstet Gynecol 2010;202(2):135.e1–8.
57. Moran LJ, Hutchison SK, Norman RJ, et al. Lifestyle changes in women with polycystic ovary syndrome. Cochrane Database Syst Rev 2011;(7):CD007506.
58. Metwally M, Amer S, Li TC, et al. An RCT of metformin versus orlistat for the management of obese anovulatory women. Hum Reprod 2009;24(4):966–75.
59. Ghandi S, Aflatoonian A, Tabibnejad N, et al. The effects of metformin or orlistat on obese women with polycystic ovary syndrome: a prospective randomized open-label study. J Assist Reprod Genet 2011;28(7):591–6.
60. Ladson G, Dodson WC, Sweet SD, et al. The effects of metformin with lifestyle therapy in polycystic ovary syndrome: a randomized double-blind study. Fertil Steril 2011;95(3):1059–66.e1–7.
61. Gerli S, Papaleo E, Ferrari A, et al. Randomized, double blind placebo-controlled trial: effects of myo-inositol on ovarian function and metabolic factors in women with PCOS. Eur Rev Med Pharmacol Sci 2007;11(5):347–54.
62. Florakis D, Diamanti-Kandarakis E, Katsikis I, et al. Effect of hypocaloric diet plus sibutramine treatment on hormonal and metabolic features in overweight and obese women with polycystic ovary syndrome: a randomized, 24-week study. Int J Obes (Lond) 2008;32(4):692–9.
63. Panidis D, Farmakiotis D, Rousso D, et al. Obesity, weight loss, and the polycystic ovary syndrome: effect of treatment with diet and orlistat for 24 weeks on insulin resistance and androgen levels. Fertil Steril 2008;89(4):899–906.
64. Mutsaerts MA, Groen H, ter Bogt NC, et al. The LIFESTYLE study: costs and effects of a structured lifestyle program in overweight and obese subfertile women to reduce the need for fertility treatment and improve reproductive outcome. A randomised controlled trial. BMC Womens Health 2010;10:22.

65. Moran L, Tsagareli V, Norman R, et al. Diet and IVF pilot study: short-term weight loss improves pregnancy rates in overweight/obese women undertaking IVF. Aust N Z J Obstet Gynaecol 2011;51(5):455–9.
66. Maggard MA, Yermilov I, Li Z, et al. Pregnancy and fertility following bariatric surgery: a systematic review. JAMA 2008;300(19):2286–96.
67. Sarwer DB, Lavery M, Spitzer JC. A review of the relationships between extreme obesity, quality of life, and sexual function. Obes Surg 2012;22(4):668–76.
68. Conrad K, Russell AC, Keister KJ. Bariatric surgery and its impact on child-bearing. Nurs Womens Health 2011;15(3):226–33 [quiz: 234].
69. Wax JR, Cartin A, Wolff R, et al. Pregnancy following gastric bypass surgery for morbid obesity: maternal and neonatal outcomes. Obes Surg 2008;18(5):540–4.
70. Ginsburg ES. Reproductive endocrinology: pregnancy and fertility after bariatric surgery. Nat Rev Endocrinol 2009;5(5):251–2.
71. Guelinckx I, Devlieger R, Vansant G. Reproductive outcome after bariatric surgery: a critical review. Hum Reprod Update 2009;15(2):189–201.
72. Merhi ZO. Impact of bariatric surgery on female reproduction. Fertil Steril 2009; 92(5):1501–8.
73. Shah DK, Ginsburg ES. Bariatric surgery and fertility. Curr Opin Obstet Gynecol 2010;22(3):248–54.
74. Wax JR, Pinette MG, Cartin A, et al. Female reproductive issues following bariatric surgery. Obstet Gynecol Surv 2007;62(9):595–604.
75. Merhi ZO, Pal L. Effect of weight loss by bariatric surgery on the risk of miscarriage. Gynecol Obstet Invest 2007;64(4):224–7.
76. Kominiarek MA. Pregnancy after bariatric surgery. Obstet Gynecol Clin North Am 2010;37(2):305–20.
77. ACOG practice bulletin no. 105: bariatric surgery and pregnancy. Obstet Gynecol 2009;113(6):1405–13.
78. Shekelle PG, Newberry S, Maglione M, et al. Bariatric surgery in women of reproductive age: special concerns for pregnancy. Evid Rep Technol Assess 2008;(169):1–51.
79. Beard JH, Bell RL, Duffy AJ. Reproductive considerations and pregnancy after bariatric surgery: current evidence and recommendations. Obes Surg 2008; 18(8):1023–7.
80. Karmon A, Sheiner E. Pregnancy after bariatric surgery: a comprehensive review. Arch Gynecol Obstet 2008;277(5):381–8.
81. Abodeely A, Roye GD, Harrington DT, et al. Pregnancy outcomes after bariatric surgery: maternal, fetal, and infant implications. Surg Obes Relat Dis 2008;4(3): 464–71.
82. Landsberger EJ, Gurewitsch ED. Reproductive implications of bariatric surgery: pre- and postoperative considerations for extremely obese women of child-bearing age. Curr Diab Rep 2007;7(4):281–8.
83. Lesko J, Peaceman A. Pregnancy outcomes in women after bariatric surgery compared with obese and morbidly obese controls. Obstet Gynecol 2012; 119(3):547–54.
84. Stone RA, Huffman J, Istwan N, et al. Pregnancy outcomes following bariatric surgery. J Womens Health (Larchmt) 2011;20(9):1363–6.
85. Josefsson A, Blomberg M, Bladh M, et al. Bariatric surgery in a national cohort of women: sociodemographics and obstetric outcomes. Am J Obstet Gynecol 2011;205(3):206.e1–8.
86. Dell'Agnolo CM, Carvalho MD, Pelloso SM. Pregnancy after bariatric surgery: implications for mother and newborn. Obes Surg 2011;21(6):699–706.

87. Sheiner E, Edri A, Balaban E, et al. Pregnancy outcome of patients who conceive during or after the first year following bariatric surgery. Am J Obstet Gynecol 2011;204(1):50.e1–6.
88. Bebber FE, Rizzolli J, Casagrande DS, et al. Pregnancy after bariatric surgery: 39 pregnancies follow-up in a multidisciplinary team. Obes Surg 2011;21(10): 1546–51.
89. Carelli AM, Ren CJ, Youn HA, et al. Impact of laparoscopic adjustable gastric banding on pregnancy, maternal weight, and neonatal health. Obes Surg 2011;21(10):1552–8.
90. Santulli P, Mandelbrot L, Facchiano E, et al. Obstetrical and neonatal outcomes of pregnancies following gastric bypass surgery: a retrospective cohort study in a French referral centre. Obes Surg 2010;20(11):1501–8.
91. Lapolla A, Marangon M, Dalfra MG, et al. Pregnancy outcome in morbidly obese women before and after laparoscopic gastric banding. Obes Surg 2010;20(9): 1251–7.
92. Smith J, Cianflone K, Biron S, et al. Effects of maternal surgical weight loss in mothers on intergenerational transmission of obesity. J Clin Endocrinol Metab 2009;94(11):4275–83.
93. Sheiner E, Balaban E, Dreiher J, et al. Pregnancy outcome in patients following different types of bariatric surgeries. Obes Surg 2009;19(9):1286–92.
94. Dias MC, Fazio Ede S, de Oliveira FC, et al. Body weight changes and outcome of pregnancy after gastroplasty for morbid obesity. Clin Nutr 2009;28(2):169–72.
95. Weintraub AY, Levy A, Levi I, et al. Effect of bariatric surgery on pregnancy outcome. Int J Gynaecol Obstet 2008;103(3):246–51.
96. Wax JR, Cartin A, Wolff R, et al. Pregnancy following gastric bypass for morbid obesity: effect of surgery-to-conception interval on maternal and neonatal outcomes. Obes Surg 2008;18(12):1517–21.
97. Patel JA, Patel NA, Thomas RL, et al. Pregnancy outcomes after laparoscopic Roux-en-Y gastric bypass. Surg Obes Relat Dis 2008;4(1):39–45.
98. Ducarme G, Revaux A, Rodrigues A, et al. Obstetric outcome following laparoscopic adjustable gastric banding. Int J Gynaecol Obstet 2007;98(3):244–7.
99. Macones GA, Stamilio DM, Odibo A, et al. Discussion: 'bariatric surgery and obstetric outcomes' by Josefsson. Am J Obstet Gynecol 2011;205(3):e1–2.
100. Rinaldi AP, Kral JG. Comments on Sheiner et al's "Pregnancy outcome of patients who conceive during or after the first year following bariatric surgery". Am J Obstet Gynecol 2011;205(4):e11 [author reply: e11–2].
101. Devlieger R, Vansant G, Guelinckx I. Bariatric surgery. Am J Obstet Gynecol 2011;205(3):e7 [author reply: e7–8].
102. Mody SK, Hacker MR, Dodge LE, et al. Contraceptive counseling for women who undergo bariatric surgery. J Womens Health (Larchmt) 2011;20(12): 1785–8.
103. Paulen ME, Zapata LB, Cansino C, et al. Contraceptive use among women with a history of bariatric surgery: a systematic review. Contraception 2010;82(1): 86–94.
104. Gosman GG, King WC, Schrope B, et al. Reproductive health of women electing bariatric surgery. Fertil Steril 2010;94(4):1426–31.
105. Hirshfeld-Cytron J, Kim HH. Empty follicle syndrome in the setting of dramatic weight loss after bariatric surgery: case report and review of available literature. Fertil Steril 2008;90(4):1199.e21–3.
106. Doblado MA, Lewkowksi BM, Odem RR, et al. In vitro fertilization after bariatric surgery. Fertil Steril 2010;94(7):2812–4.

107. Rochester D, Jain A, Polotsky AJ, et al. Partial recovery of luteal function after bariatric surgery in obese women. Fertil Steril 2009;92(4):1410–5.

108. Sneed ML, Uhler ML, Grotjan HE, et al. Body mass index: impact on IVF success appears age-related. Hum Reprod 2008;23(8):1835–9.

109. Luke B, Brown MB, Stern JE, et al. Female obesity adversely affects assisted reproductive technology (ART) pregnancy and live birth rates. Hum Reprod 2011;26(1):245–52.

110. Harris ID, Python J, Roth L, et al. Physicians' perspectives and practices regarding the fertility management of obese patients. Fertil Steril 2011;96(4): 991–2.

111. Koning AM, Mutsaerts MA, Kuchenbecher WK, et al. Complications and outcome of assisted reproduction technologies in overweight and obese women. Hum Reprod 2012;27(2):457–67.

112. Bryzyski R, Fox J, Zera C, et al. Weight limits for access to fertility services: discriminatory or nonmaleficence? 2011.

113. Politi MC, Han PK, Col NF. Communicating the uncertainty of harms and benefits of medical interventions. Med Decis Making 2007;27(5):681–95.

The Impact of Obesity and Metabolic Syndrome on Chronic Hepatitis C

Nicolas Goossens, MD, MSc[a], Francesco Negro, MD[a,b],*

KEYWORDS

- Liver • Hypertension • Steatosis • Fibrosis • Insulin resistance • Diabetes

KEY POINTS

- The interplay between the metabolic syndrome and hepatitis C virus (HCV) infection is complex and multilayered.
- HCV alters glucose metabolism and can lead to insulin resistance (IR) or overt diabetes in susceptible individuals, whereas in the case of IR and/or diabetes, the clinical outcome of HCV-infected individuals worsen.
- The strong relationship between HCV, especially genotype 3 HCV, and steatosis is also clear; however, its clinical consequences, if any, need further study.
- Insulin sensitizers seem to be a logical target to try and improve IR, however clinical trials in the context of antiviral treatment did not document a clear benefit in virologic outcomes.
- The optimal management of HCV-infected individuals with the metabolic syndrome should focus on lifestyle interventions, treatment of diabetes, and aggressive management of cofactors.

INTRODUCTION

Approximately 2.35% of the world's population, or 185 million people, are infected with the hepatitis C virus (HCV).[1] HCV is a major cause of chronic liver disease, culminating in cirrhosis, hepatocellular carcinoma (HCC), and increased mortality from both

This article originally appeared in Clinics in Liver Disease, Volume 18, Issue 1, February 2014.
The authors' quoted work is supported by Swiss National Science Foundation grant numbers 314730-130498 and 314730-146991 and by the Foundation for Liver and Gut Studies, Geneva, Switzerland.
Conflicts of Interest: F. Negro is advising Roche, MSD, Gilead, Janssen Novartis, and Boehringer Ingelheim and has received unrestricted research grants from Roche, Novartis, and Gilead. N. Goossens has nothing to disclose.
[a] Division of Gastroenterology and Hepatology, Geneva University Hospital, 4 rue Gabrielle-Perret-Gentil, 1211 Geneva 4, Switzerland; [b] Division of Clinical Pathology, Geneva University Hospital, 4 rue Gabrielle-Perret-Gentil, 1211 Geneva 4, Switzerland
* Corresponding author. Division of Clinical Pathology, Geneva University Hospital, 4 rue Gabrielle-Perret-Gentil, 1211 Geneva 4, Switzerland.
E-mail address: Francesco.Negro@hcuge.ch

Clinics Collections 3 (2014) 197–206
http://dx.doi.org/10.1016/j.ccol.2014.09.040
2352-7986/14/$ – see front matter © 2014 Elsevier Inc. All rights reserved.

hepatic and extrahepatic disease.[2] On the other hand, the metabolic syndrome is a global health burden associated with increased cardiovascular disease and diabetes.[3,4] Its prevalence varies from 23.7% of adults in the United States in one cross-sectional survey and 9.8% to 17.8% of Chinese adults in another study.[5,6]

In view of their high prevalence, there is bound to be significant interaction between these 2 conditions. However, it is becoming clear that their relationship is complex. First, HCV is associated with insulin resistance (IR), a fundamental characteristic of the metabolic syndrome.[7,8] Second, the metabolic syndrome and especially IR and/or diabetes play a role on the progression of HCV and on clinically relevant endpoints such as liver-related mortality[9] or the development of HCC.[10,11] Third, HCV has a very peculiar relationship with lipid metabolism: HCV virions circulate bound to lipoproteins, lipids modulate the HCV life cycle, and HCV is associated, in a distinct subgroup of patients, with severe steatosis.[12]

In this review therefore the relationship between the metabolic syndrome and HCV infection, its clinical impact, and potential management strategies are discussed.

DEFINITIONS

The metabolic syndrome is a cluster of risk factors for cardiovascular disease and type 2 diabetes mellitus. Its definition has gradually evolved from the initial definition by the World Health Organization[13] to the latest harmonized definition from the International Diabetes Federation Task Force on Epidemiology and Prevention, the National Heart, Lung, and Blood Institute, the American Heart Association, the World Heart Federation, the International Atherosclerosis Society, and the International Association for the Study of Obesity.[14] Essentially, to qualify for metabolic syndrome, a patient should have 3 or more abnormal findings of the 5 criteria, namely, raised blood pressure, dyslipidemia (elevated triglycerides or low high-density lipoprotein cholesterol [HDL-C]), elevated waist circumference, and raised fasting glucose (**Table 1**). Defining thresholds for abdominal obesity is difficult due to a lack of clear clinical thresholds and ethnic differences, but in common practice the thresholds defined by the International Diabetes Federation are used (ie, more than 94 cm waist circumference for men and more than 80 cm for women).[14]

Table 1 Criteria for the clinical diagnosis of the metabolic syndrome	
Clinical Parameter	**Threshold**
Abdominal obesity	Population-specific. In general ≥94 cm waist circumference in men, ≥80 cm in women
Dyslipidemia	
Low HDL-C	<40 mg/dL (1.0 mmol/L) in men <50 mg/dL (1.3 mmol/L) in women or Treated for low HDL-C
Raised triglycerides	≥150 mg/dL (1.7 mmol/L) or Treated for raised triglycerides
Raised blood pressure	Systolic ≥130 mm Hg and/or Diastolic ≥85 mm Hg or Treated for hypertension
Impaired fasting glucose	≥100 mg/dL (5.6 mmol/L) or Treated for diabetes

Three or more positive criteria qualify a patient for the metabolic syndrome.
Abbreviation: HDL-C, high-density lipoprotein cholesterol.

Over the years, an international expert committee has been assessing and adapting guidelines to diagnose diabetes by measuring blood glucose (in the fasting state or after a glucose challenge, see **Table 2**).[15] Due to recent, improved standardization of glycated hemoglobin (HbA$_{1c}$), this biochemical test has been implemented in the diagnosis of diabetes. Importantly, the expert committee recognized a group of patients with higher than normal glucose levels, without reaching the criteria for diabetes, due to either high fasting glucose levels (impaired fasting glucose) or raised glucose levels after an oral glucose challenge (impaired glucose tolerance) (see **Table 2**).[15] These patients, sometimes referred to as having "prediabetes," have a higher risk of developing diabetes as well as cardiovascular disease and often have other components of the metabolic syndrome as mentioned above.[4,16]

Finally, IR is defined as a condition in which higher than normal insulin concentrations are needed to achieve normal metabolic responses or, alternatively, normal insulin concentrations are unable to achieve normal metabolic responses.[17] IR is often measured using the homeostasis model assessment of IR, or HOMA-IR, although its in vivo gold-standard measurement is the hyperinsulinemic-euglycemic clamp.[18]

HCV AND IR

Evidence from clinical, epidemiologic, and experimental fields concurs to suggest that there is a link between HCV infection and IR, an important feature of the metabolic syndrome.[7,8] Population-based cross-sectional studies have found an increased proportion of diabetics in HCV-positive patients compared with HCV-negative controls.[19–21] This association was verified in longitudinal, prospective studies comparing the incidence of diabetes in HCV-positive and HCV-negative individuals. In one trial of 1084 adults, HCV-positive patients at high risk of developing diabetes (based on body mass index and age) were 11 times more likely to develop diabetes than HCV-negative individuals, although this effect was not found in patients at low risk of developing diabetes.[22] Similar results were found in a Taiwanese cohort with a

Table 2
Definition of diabetes and prediabetic states according to the American Diabetes Association guidelines

		Prediabetes		
Test	Normal	IFG	IGT	Diabetes
Fasting plasma glucose	<100 mg/dL (5.6 mmol/L)	100 mg/dL (5.6 mmol/L) to 125 mg/dL (6.9 mmol/L)	—	≥126 mg/dL (7.0 mmol/L)
2 h values of plasma glucose in the 75 g OGTT	<140 mg/dL (7.8 mmol/L)	—	140 mg/dL (7.8 mmol/L) to 199 mg/dL (11.0 mmol/L)	≥200 mg/dL (11.1 mmol/L)
HbA$_{1c}$	<5.7%	5.7%–6.4%		≥6.5%

In patients without classic symptoms of hyperglycemia, the diagnostic test must be repeated to confirm the diagnosis of diabetes, but in patients with classic symptoms, a random plasma glucose of ≥200 mg/dL (11.1 mmol/L) is sufficient to diagnose diabetes. Note that there is not 100% concordance between the different tests (fasting glucose, 2 h post oral glucose load and HbA$_{1c}$), and it is not yet clear how to characterise patients clinically with differing glycemic statuses according to these tests.

Abbreviations: HbA$_{1c}$, glycosylated hemoglobin; IFG, impaired fasting glucose; IGT, impaired glucose tolerance; OGTT, oral glucose tolerance test.

hazard ratio of 1.7 of developing diabetes for HCV-positive patients; alternatively, a recent study from Southern Italy with a follow-up of 20 years of 2472 subjects only found such an association in HCV-infected patients with elevated alanine transaminase levels.[23,24] To define the epidemiologic interaction between IR and HCV further, a systematic review pooled all studies analyzing the risk of diabetes in patients with HCV.[25] In this review, combining 34 studies and a total of more than 300,000 patients, the pooled estimate of type 2 diabetes in HCV patients was an adjusted odds ratio of approximately 1.68 (95% confidence interval [CI] 1.15–2.20), significant in both prospective and retrospective meta-analyses.[25] Therefore, there is a clear epidemiologic association between HCV and the development of diabetes.

The mechanism by which HCV infection alters glucose metabolism seems to be related to an increase in IR rather than a change in β-cell function.[7] In a study of 260 HCV-positive subjects, IR, as measured by HOMA-IR, was increased as compared with healthy matched controls, even in subjects with minimal fibrosis.[26] This increase was confirmed in other studies, where IR was more frequent in HCV patients than in matched HCV-negative patients with or without chronic HBV, also suggesting a role of HCV on glucose metabolism.[27,28] However, not all studies have reproduced this finding[29] and further longitudinal, prospective studies are warranted to clarify this point of debate.

If HCV plays a role in glucose metabolism, then its eradication should improve IR. Two independent studies show that sustained viral response (SVR) is associated with a reduction in the risk of type 2 diabetes development in patients with HCV[30,31]; however, other studies did not show a significant difference in IR after SVR.[32,33] A recent large study, presented in abstract form, including 20,486 veterans treated for HCV noted a reduced incidence of diabetes (hazard ratio 0.76, 95% CI 0.70–0.82) in patients achieving SVR.[34] Therefore, overall data tend to show a reduction of the incidence of diabetes, and possibly IR, in HCV-positive patients achieving SVR.

Taken together, this data suggest that HCV affects glucose metabolism at early stages of the natural course of the disease by inducing IR. HCV seems to increase the progression from IR to overt diabetes in susceptible patients and curing HCV seems to improve IR and decrease the risk of diabetes. Below, the effect of IR on the natural history of HCV infection is discussed.

HCV AND STEATOSIS

Although steatosis is not a component of the metabolic syndrome definition per se, these 2 conditions interact closely and potentiate each other's effect.[35,36] Steatosis occurs in up to 80% of hepatitis C patients and was used in the preserology era as a diagnostic tool to identify non-A, non-B hepatitis patients.[37,38] Even when controlling for other factors known to induce a fatty liver, the prevalence of steatosis is still double that seen in chronic hepatitis B patients, suggesting a role for viral factors in the development of steatosis.[39,40]

The major piece of evidence arguing in favor of HCV-induced fatty liver is the strong association with genotype 3, where steatosis is more frequent and severe and its severity correlates with HCV replication, in both serum and liver,[41,42] whereas in non-3 genotypes, steatosis seems to correlate with traditional metabolic factors associated with a fatty liver.[43] Furthermore, in genotype 3, steatosis disappears after successful antiviral therapy in patients, while in most patients with other genotypes it is largely unaffected even in case of SVR.[42,44,45]

Therefore, there is a strong epidemiologic link between steatosis and HCV, although the clinical consequences of this link have yet to be completely unraveled.

HCV AND OTHER COMPONENTS OF THE METABOLIC SYNDROME

Although there is a close relationship between IR and HCV infection, the other components of the metabolic syndrome are not as clearly associated with HCV. The metabolic syndrome is characterized by hypertriglyceridemia and low HDL-C concentrations, whereas the lipid profile in patients with HCV, especially genotype 3, is characterized by low levels of total cholesterol and triglycerides.[12] On the other hand, recent data show an association between HCV infection and hypertension (odds ratio of 2.06) in a cohort of 19,741 participants of whom 0.88% were HCV-positive.[46] This data must be confirmed in further longitudinal studies.

HCV AND THE METABOLIC SYNDROME: DOES IT MATTER?

Although there seems to be a clear association between HCV and the metabolic syndrome, especially IR, what is the clinical consequence of this interaction and how does it affect patients? The clinical impact of this association and its relevance on patient-relevant outcomes such as mortality, incidence of HCC, and influence on HCV cure rates, are discussed.

In a large NHANES III population-based study, an association was demonstrated between IR or type 2 diabetes and all-cause mortality in chronic HBV-infected patients, nonalcoholic fatty liver disease, and alcoholic liver disease but not in patients with HCV. However, diabetes and IR were independent predictors of liver-related mortality in HCV in the same study,[9] suggesting that IR and diabetes act together with HCV infection to increase liver-related mortality, possibly by favoring progression of liver fibrosis and increasing incidence of HCC (see below).

Due to the close link between HCV, type 2 diabetes, and other metabolic factors, one of the first legitimate questions is whether the interaction of all these factors is reflected in an increased cardiovascular morbidity and mortality in patients with HCV. A large retrospective cohort study showed an increase in cardiovascular mortality among HCV-positive blood donors (hazard ratio 2.21, 95% CI: 1.41, 3.46) and another study showed larger carotid intima-media thickness (IMT), an index of early atherosclerosis, in HCV-positive patients when compared with controls.[47,48] A further, more recent, study demonstrated an association between HCV infection and congestive heart failure subtype of cardiovascular diseases but not ischemic heart disease and stroke.[46] In another prospective cohort, the REVEAL study based in Taiwan, anti-HCV seropositivity was associated, in multivariable analysis, with multiple extrahepatic complications, including mortality from circulatory diseases (adjusted hazard ratio 1.50, 95% CI 1.10–2.33).[2] In this study, showing that HCV-infected patients had a higher mortality from hepatic and extrahepatic disease, HCV was associated with mortality from circulatory disease only if HCV patients had detectable HCV RNA levels, suggesting that patients with undetectable HCV RNA levels return to their baseline cardiovascular risk.[2] Other studies, however, did not confirm this association; for example, a large German cross-sectional study failed to find an association between HCV positivity and IMT or other cardiovascular endpoints.[49] In a more recent Egyptian cross-sectional study, IMT and number of patients with carotid plaques did not seem increased in patients with HCV compared with healthy controls, although there was an association after complete adjustment for other cardiovascular risk factors.[50] A weakness of many of these studies is a lack of liver biopsies to exclude superimposed NAFLD. Whether the weak association between cardiovascular diseases and HCV infection may be related to the favorable lipid profile in HCV-infected individuals, namely low LDL cholesterol, is open to debate.[12]

A series of recent studies and meta-analyses confirmed that the risk of several types of malignancies, including HCC, is increased in the setting of type 2 diabetes.[51] In population-based data of 19,349 diabetic patients and 77,396 controls in Taiwan, Lai and colleagues[52] found that diabetes was associated with a doubled incidence of HCC and that HCV increased that risk with a hazard ratio of 5.61. A systematic review pooled 13 case-control studies and cohort studies and showed a significant association between diabetes and HCC in both cases.[53] A recent retrospective study of 4302 Japanese HCV-positive patients treated with interferon found that type 2 diabetes was associated with a 1.73-fold increase in the risk of development of HCC or other malignancies, but this risk decreased when HbA1c levels were maintained less than 7.0%, suggesting a role for improved glycemic control as a strategy to decrease HCC occurrence.[54] Other factors associated with HCC development in this study were advanced fibrosis, lack of SVR, male sex, age of $\geq$50 years, and alcohol abuse.[54] Another meta-analysis showed that HCC is increased by 17% in overweight subjects and by 89% in obese individuals, but the combined risk factors of diabetes, obesity, and HBV or HCV infection increased the risk more than 100 times in one follow-up study of 23,820 Taiwan residents,[10,11] which underlines the importance of the synergistic links between features of the metabolic syndrome and viral factors in the pathogenesis of HCC. Interestingly, pathologic data studying HCV-positive liver explants and retrospective clinical data of HCV-positive individuals suggest that steatosis is also associated with increased HCC incidence.[55,56] Unfortunately, the relative contribution of viral versus metabolic steatosis was not assessed in these studies and must be further studied.

IR also seems to accelerate fibrosis progression rates in patients with HCV. For instance, in 260 HCV-infected patients HOMA-IR was an independent predictor for the degree of fibrosis (P<.001) and the rate of fibrosis progression (P = .03).[26] However, a matter of debate is whether hepatic steatosis or IR mediates the increased fibrosis progression rate, although IR seems to be the best predictor for advanced fibrosis.[57]

IR also seems to affect the rate of virologic response to anti-HCV interferon-based therapy. In a systematic review of 14 studies, SVR was less frequent in patients with IR (as assessed with baseline HOMA-IR) with a mean difference of −13.0% (95% CI: −22.6% to −3.4%, P = .008).[58] Speculative pathogenic mechanisms include increased viral replication, impairment of interferon-α, and insulin signaling or increased liver fibrosis.[8] Interestingly, similarly to what is reported for liver steatosis, it seems to be host-induced IR (rather than IR caused by HCV) that affects the response to viral therapy, although this remains speculative and must be confirmed in further research.[59,60] In the meantime, it remains to be seen whether IR will continue to predict treatment response in the era of newer direct-acting antivirals. Recent data in genotype 1-infected patients show that virologic response was not affected by IR in treatment-naïve or experienced HCV patients treated with telaprevir-based therapy.[61,62]

Of all the factors in the metabolic syndrome, IR and type 2 diabetes seem to have the greatest importance in the clinical consequence of the metabolic syndrome on HCV infection. Fibrosis progression rate is increased and liver-related mortality is higher. HCC incidence is also increased and these patients seem to respond less well to interferon-based therapy. As discussed above, curing HCV may be associated with reduced incidence of diabetes and possibly an improved cardiovascular risk profile.[2,30] Therefore, although longer term studies are warranted, achieving SVR in these patients could lead to reduced morbidity and mortality linked to cardiovascular disease and diabetes.

SUMMARY

The interplay between the metabolic syndrome and HCV infection is complex and multilayered. HCV alters glucose metabolism and can lead to IR or overt diabetes in susceptible individuals, whereas in the case of IR and/or diabetes the clinical outcome of HCV-infected individuals worsen. The relationship between genotype 3 HCV and steatosis is also clear; however, its clinical consequences, if any, need further studies.

Insulin sensitizers seem to be a logical target to try and improve IR especially in the setting of antiviral therapy for HCV. Unfortunately, results involving pioglitazone and metformin are discouraging without a clear improvement in virologic outcomes.[60,63–65]

Therefore, for the time being, the optimal management of HCV-infected individuals with the metabolic syndrome should focus on lifestyle interventions, treatment of diabetes, and aggressive management of cofactors.

REFERENCES

1. Mohd Hanafiah K, Groeger J, Flaxman AD, et al. Global epidemiology of hepatitis C virus infection: new estimates of age-specific antibody to HCV seroprevalence. Hepatology 2013;57(4):1333–42.
2. Lee MH, Yang HI, Lu SN, et al. Chronic hepatitis C virus infection increases mortality from hepatic and extrahepatic diseases: a community-based long-term prospective study. J Infect Dis 2012;206:469–77.
3. Ford ES. Risks for all-cause mortality, cardiovascular disease, and diabetes associated with the metabolic syndrome: a summary of the evidence. Diabetes Care 2005;28(7):1769–78.
4. Ford ES, Zhao G, Li C. Pre-diabetes and the risk for cardiovascular disease: a systematic review of the evidence. J Am Coll Cardiol 2010;55(13):1310–7.
5. Ford ES, Giles WH, Dietz WH. Prevalence of the metabolic syndrome among US adults: findings from the third National Health and Nutrition Examination Survey. JAMA 2002;287(3):356–9.
6. Gu D, Reynolds K, Wu X, et al. Prevalence of the metabolic syndrome and overweight among adults in China. Lancet 2005;365(9468):1398–405.
7. Kaddai V, Negro F. Current understanding of insulin resistance in hepatitis C. Expert Rev Gastroenterol Hepatol 2011;5(4):503–16.
8. Bugianesi E, Salamone F, Negro F. The interaction of metabolic factors with HCV infection: does it matter? J Hepatol 2012;56(Suppl 1):S56–65.
9. Stepanova M, Rafiq N, Younossi ZM. Components of metabolic syndrome are independent predictors of mortality in patients with chronic liver disease: a population-based study. Gut 2010;59(10):1410–5.
10. Chen CL, Yang HI, Yang WS, et al. Metabolic factors and risk of hepatocellular carcinoma by chronic hepatitis B/C infection: a follow-up study in Taiwan. Gastroenterology 2008;135(1):111–21.
11. Larsson SC, Wolk A. Overweight, obesity and risk of liver cancer: a meta-analysis of cohort studies. Br J Cancer 2007;97(7):1005–8.
12. Negro F. Abnormalities of lipid metabolism in hepatitis C virus infection. Gut 2010; 59(9):1279–87.
13. Alberti KG, Zimmet PZ. Definition, diagnosis and classification of diabetes mellitus and its complications. Part 1: diagnosis and classification of diabetes mellitus provisional report of a WHO consultation. Diabet Med 1998;15(7):539–53.
14. Alberti KG, Eckel RH, Grundy SM, et al. Harmonizing the metabolic syndrome: a joint interim statement of the International Diabetes Federation Task Force on Epidemiology and Prevention; National Heart, Lung, and Blood Institute;

American Heart Association; World Heart Federation; International Atherosclerosis Society; and International Association for the Study of Obesity. Circulation 2009;120(16):1640–5.

15. American Diabetes Association. Diagnosis and classification of diabetes mellitus. Diabetes Care 2013;36(Suppl 1):S67–74.

16. Tabak AG, Herder C, Rathmann W, et al. Prediabetes: a high-risk state for diabetes development. Lancet 2012;379(9833):2279–90.

17. Bugianesi E, McCullough AJ, Marchesini G. Insulin resistance: a metabolic pathway to chronic liver disease. Hepatology 2005;42(5):987–1000.

18. Matthews DR, Hosker JP, Rudenski AS, et al. Homeostasis model assessment: insulin resistance and beta-cell function from fasting plasma glucose and insulin concentrations in man. Diabetologia 1985;28(7):412–9.

19. Allison ME, Wreghitt T, Palmer CR, et al. Evidence for a link between hepatitis C virus infection and diabetes mellitus in a cirrhotic population. J Hepatol 1994; 21(6):1135–9.

20. Negro F, Alaei M. Hepatitis C virus and type 2 diabetes. World J Gastroenterol 2009;15(13):1537–47.

21. Mehta SH, Brancati FL, Sulkowski MS, et al. Prevalence of type 2 diabetes mellitus among persons with hepatitis C virus infection in the United States. Ann Intern Med 2000;133(8):592–9.

22. Mehta SH, Brancati FL, Strathdee SA, et al. Hepatitis C virus infection and incident type 2 diabetes. Hepatology 2003;38(1):50–6.

23. Wang CS, Wang ST, Yao WJ, et al. Hepatitis C virus infection and the development of type 2 diabetes in a community-based longitudinal study. Am J Epidemiol 2007;166(2):196–203.

24. Montenegro L, De Michina A, Misciagna G, et al. Virus C hepatitis and type 2 diabetes: a cohort study in southern Italy. Am J Gastroenterol 2013;108(7):1108–11.

25. White DL, Ratziu V, El-Serag HB. Hepatitis C infection and risk of diabetes: a systematic review and meta-analysis. J Hepatol 2008;49(5):831–44.

26. Hui JM, Sud A, Farrell GC, et al. Insulin resistance is associated with chronic hepatitis C virus infection and fibrosis progression [corrected]. Gastroenterology 2003;125(6):1695–704.

27. Dai CY, Yeh ML, Huang CF, et al. Chronic hepatitis C infection is associated with insulin resistance and lipid profiles. J Gastroenterol Hepatol 2013. [Epub ahead of print].

28. Moucari R, Asselah T, Cazals-Hatem D, et al. Insulin resistance in chronic hepatitis C: association with genotypes 1 and 4, serum HCV RNA level, and liver fibrosis. Gastroenterology 2008;134(2):416–23.

29. Tanaka N, Nagaya T, Komatsu M, et al. Insulin resistance and hepatitis C virus: a case-control study of non-obese, non-alcoholic and non-steatotic hepatitis virus carriers with persistently normal serum aminotransferase. Liver Int 2008;28(8): 1104–11.

30. Arase Y, Suzuki F, Suzuki Y, et al. Sustained virological response reduces incidence of onset of type 2 diabetes in chronic hepatitis C. Hepatology 2009; 49(3):739–44.

31. Romero-Gomez M, Fernandez-Rodriguez CM, Andrade RJ, et al. Effect of sustained virological response to treatment on the incidence of abnormal glucose values in chronic hepatitis C. J Hepatol 2008;48(5):721–7.

32. Brandman D, Bacchetti P, Ayala CE, et al. Impact of insulin resistance on HCV treatment response and impact of HCV treatment on insulin sensitivity using direct measurements of insulin action. Diabetes Care 2012;35(5):1090–4.

33. Giordanino C, Bugianesi E, Smedile A, et al. Incidence of type 2 diabetes mellitus and glucose abnormalities in patients with chronic hepatitis C infection by response to treatment: results of a cohort study. Am J Gastroenterol 2008; 103(10):2481–7.
34. Hyder SM, Krishnan S, Promrat K. #608 Sustained virological response prevents the development of new type 2 diabetes in patients with chronic hepatitis C. Gastroenterology 2013;144(5):S951.
35. Marchesini G, Brizi M, Bianchi G, et al. Nonalcoholic fatty liver disease: a feature of the metabolic syndrome. Diabetes 2001;50(8):1844–50.
36. Marchesini G, Bugianesi E, Forlani G, et al. Nonalcoholic fatty liver, steatohepatitis, and the metabolic syndrome. Hepatology 2003;37(4):917–23.
37. Dienes HP, Popper H, Arnold W, et al. Histologic observations in human hepatitis non-A, non-B. Hepatology 1982;2(5):562–71.
38. Wiese M, Haupt R. Histomorphologic picture of chronic non-A, non-B hepatitis. Dtsch Z Verdau Stoffwechselkr 1985;45(3):101–10 [in German].
39. Czaja AJ, Carpenter HA, Santrach PJ, et al. Host- and disease-specific factors affecting steatosis in chronic hepatitis C. J Hepatol 1998;29(2):198–206.
40. Peng D, Han Y, Ding H, et al. Hepatic steatosis in chronic hepatitis B patients is associated with metabolic factors more than viral factors. J Gastroenterol Hepatol 2008;23(7 Pt 1):1082–8.
41. Fartoux L, Poujol-Robert A, Guechot J, et al. Insulin resistance is a cause of steatosis and fibrosis progression in chronic hepatitis C. Gut 2005;54(7):1003–8.
42. Rubbia-Brandt L, Quadri R, Abid K, et al. Hepatocyte steatosis is a cytopathic effect of hepatitis C virus genotype 3. J Hepatol 2000;33(1):106–15.
43. Adinolfi LE, Gambardella M, Andreana A, et al. Steatosis accelerates the progression of liver damage of chronic hepatitis C patients and correlates with specific HCV genotype and visceral obesity. Hepatology 2001;33(6):1358–64.
44. Kumar D, Farrell GC, Fung C, et al. Hepatitis C virus genotype 3 is cytopathic to hepatocytes: reversal of hepatic steatosis after sustained therapeutic response. Hepatology 2002;36(5):1266–72.
45. Poynard T, Ratziu V, McHutchison J, et al. Effect of treatment with peginterferon or interferon alfa-2b and ribavirin on steatosis in patients infected with hepatitis C. Hepatology 2003;38(1):75–85.
46. Younossi ZM, Stepanova M, Nader F, et al. Associations of chronic hepatitis C with metabolic and cardiac outcomes. Aliment Pharmacol Ther 2013;37(6):647–52.
47. Guiltinan AM, Kaidarova Z, Custer B, et al. Increased all-cause, liver, and cardiac mortality among hepatitis C virus-seropositive blood donors. Am J Epidemiol 2008;167(6):743–50.
48. Targher G, Bertolini L, Padovani R, et al. Differences and similarities in early atherosclerosis between patients with non-alcoholic steatohepatitis and chronic hepatitis B and C. J Hepatol 2007;46(6):1126–32.
49. Volzke H, Schwahn C, Wolff B, et al. Hepatitis B and C virus infection and the risk of atherosclerosis in a general population. Atherosclerosis 2004;174(1):99–103.
50. Mostafa A, Mohamed MK, Saeed M, et al. Hepatitis C infection and clearance: impact on atherosclerosis and cardiometabolic risk factors. Gut 2010;59(28): 1135–40.
51. Vigneri P, Frasca F, Sciacca L, et al. Diabetes and cancer. Endocr Relat Cancer 2009;16(4):1103–23.
52. Lai SW, Chen PC, Liao KF, et al. Risk of hepatocellular carcinoma in diabetic patients and risk reduction associated with anti-diabetic therapy: a population-based cohort study. Am J Gastroenterol 2012;107(1):46–52.

53. El-Serag HB, Hampel H, Javadi F. The association between diabetes and hepatocellular carcinoma: a systematic review of epidemiologic evidence. Clin Gastroenterol Hepatol 2006;4(3):369–80.
54. Arase Y, Kobayashi M, Suzuki F, et al. Effect of type 2 diabetes on risk for malignancies includes hepatocellular carcinoma in chronic hepatitis C. Hepatology 2013;57(3):964–73.
55. Ohata K, Hamasaki K, Toriyama K, et al. Hepatic steatosis is a risk factor for hepatocellular carcinoma in patients with chronic hepatitis C virus infection. Cancer 2003;97(12):3036–43.
56. Pekow JR, Bhan AK, Zheng H, et al. Hepatic steatosis is associated with increased frequency of hepatocellular carcinoma in patients with hepatitis C-related cirrhosis. Cancer 2007;109(12):2490–6.
57. Bugianesi E, Marchesini G, Gentilcore E, et al. Fibrosis in genotype 3 chronic hepatitis C and nonalcoholic fatty liver disease: role of insulin resistance and hepatic steatosis. Hepatology 2006;44(6):1648–55.
58. Deltenre P, Louvet A, Lemoine M, et al. Impact of insulin resistance on sustained response in HCV patients treated with pegylated interferon and ribavirin: a meta-analysis. J Hepatol 2011;55(6):1187–94.
59. Fattovich G, Covolo L, Pasino M, et al. The homeostasis model assessment of the insulin resistance score is not predictive of a sustained virological response in chronic hepatitis C patients. Liver Int 2011;31(1):66–74.
60. Negro F. Steatosis and insulin resistance in response to treatment of chronic hepatitis C. J Viral Hepat 2012;19(Suppl 1):42–7.
61. Serfaty L, Forns X, Goeser T, et al. Insulin resistance and response to telaprevir plus peginterferon alpha and ribavirin in treatment-naive patients infected with HCV genotype 1. Gut 2012;61(10):1473–80.
62. Younossi Z, Negro F, Serfaty L, et al. The homeostasis model assessment of insulin resistance does not seem to predict response to telaprevir in chronic hepatitis C in the REALIZE trial. Hepatology 2013. in press.
63. Overbeck K, Genne D, Golay A, et al. Pioglitazone in chronic hepatitis C not responding to pegylated interferon-alpha and ribavirin. J Hepatol 2008;49(2):295–8.
64. Harrison SA, Hamzeh FM, Han J, et al. Chronic hepatitis C genotype 1 patients with insulin resistance treated with pioglitazone. Hepatology 2012;56:464–73.
65. Romero-Gomez M, Diago M, Andrade RJ, et al. Treatment of insulin resistance with metformin in naive genotype 1 chronic hepatitis C patients receiving peginterferon alfa-2a plus ribavirin. Hepatology 2009;50(6):1702–8.

The Insulin-Like Growth Factors in Adipogenesis and Obesity

Antje Garten, PhD, Susanne Schuster, Wieland Kiess, MD*

KEYWORDS

- Insulin-like growth factors • Growth hormone • Adipogenesis • Obesity

KEY POINTS

- Growth hormone (GH) treatment induces a reduction in adipocyte size and enhances lipolysis in patients with untreated growth hormone deficiency (GHD).
- GH acts directly via activation of the GH receptor or indirectly via insulin-like growth factor (IGF)-I.
- Insulin-like growth factor (IGF)-I is a critical mediator of preadipocyte proliferation, differentiation, and survival.
- Results from clinical studies on GH treatment in patients with GH deficiency or GH insensitivity syndrome can be used to dissect GH and IGF as well as IGF-binding protein (IGFBP) actions in vivo.

First evidence for the importance of growth hormone (GH) and insulin-like growth factor (IGF)-I in adipocyte differentiation and metabolism came from patients with untreated GH deficiency that generally are obese and have enlarged adipocytes. GH treatment induced a reduction in adipocyte size and enhanced lipolysis (reviewed in Ref.[1]). Therefore, adipose tissue was recognized as a major target of GH action (reviewed in Ref.[2]).

GH is a 191-amino-acid, single-chain polypeptide that is synthesized, stored, and secreted in various molecular forms by the somatotroph cells within the lateral wings of the anterior pituitary gland in a pulsatile manner. GH release is mainly regulated by growth hormone–releasing hormone (GHRH) and somatotropin release-inhibiting factor (somatostatin), both of which are secreted by neurosecretory nuclei within the hypothalamus. Several other factors have an impact on GH balance. Circulating GH and IGF-I decrease GH release via a negative feedback mechanism. Ghrelin, a 28-kDa polypeptide, stimulates both food intake and GH secretion. In the central nervous

This article originally appeared in Endocrinology and Metabolism Clinics of North America, Volume 41, Issue 2, June 2012.

Department of Women and Child Health, Hospital for Children and Adolescents, Center for Pediatric Research Leipzig (CPL), University Hospitals, Liebigstraße 20a, 04103 Leipzig, Germany

* Corresponding author.

E-mail address: Wieland.Kiess@medizin.uni-leipzig.de

2352-7986/14/$ – see front matter © 2014 Elsevier Inc. All rights reserved.

system, ghrelin stimulates appetite and is therefore an important link between the regulation of energy homeostasis and the activity of the GH/IGF-I axis (reviewed in Ref.[3]). Physiologic stimulators include exercise and deep sleep, while GH secretion is negatively influenced by free fatty acids. An overview of the regulation of GH secretion is given in **Fig. 1**.

GH circulates partially bound to growth hormone–binding protein (GHBP), which is a truncated part of the GH receptor (GHR).

GH acts directly via activation of the GHR, mainly during periods of fuel shortage (fasting, prolonged exercise). The indirect actions of GH are mediated by IGF-I. Circulating IGF-I is predominately stimulated by GH, and is mainly produced in the liver in the presence of sufficient nutrient intake and elevated portal insulin levels (reviewed in Ref.[4]). IGF-I circulates as a ternary complex bound to IGF-binding proteins (IGFBPs) and acid-labile subunit (ALS). In addition, many other tissues and cell types are able to synthesize IGF-I (reviewed in Ref.[5]).

In in vitro studies on primary preadipocytes, GH inhibited adipocyte differentiation but stimulated preadipocyte proliferation.[6,7] The mechanism by which GH inhibits the differentiation of primary preadipocytes to adipocytes is not well understood. Whereas GH treatment of preadipocytes leads to stimulation of cell proliferation via upregulation of IGF-I secretion, the inhibition of glucose uptake and lipogenesis as well as the stimulation of lipolysis by GH in mature adipocytes seem to be independent of IGF-I.[6,7] No influence of GH on the expression of the classic lipolytic enzymes such as adipocyte triglyceride lipase, hormone-sensitive lipase (HSL), or monoglyceride lipase has been shown in humans,[8] although GH has been demonstrated to increase HSL activity.[9]

In contrast to earlier studies, adipose tissue is now regarded as a major source of circulating IGF-I.[10] IGF-I is a critical mediator of preadipocyte proliferation, differentiation, and survival. Apart from systemic effects, IGF-I activates the IGF-I receptor

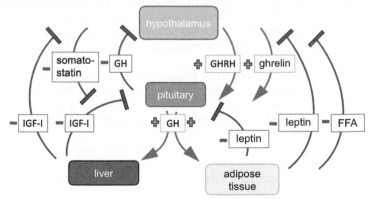

Fig. 1. An overview of the regulation of growth hormone (GH) and insulin-like growth factor I (IGF-I) secretion. Green arrows and plus-signs indicate a stimulatory effect, while red lines and minus-signs show inhibitory actions. GH is released from the pituitary upon stimulation with growth hormone–releasing hormone (GHRH) or ghrelin, which originate from the hypothalamus. There are numerous inhibitory effectors of GH release: somatostatin from the hypothalamus, leptin and free fatty acids (FFA) from adipose tissue. Negative feedback loops are elicited by GH itself or IGF-I from the liver or adipose tissue. IGF-I is released upon stimulation of hepatocytes or adipocytes by GH. (*Adapted from* Ahima RS, Saper CB, Flier JS, et al. Leptin regulation of neuroendocrine systems. Front Neuroendocrinol 2000;21:263–307; and Veldhuis JD. A tripeptidyl ensemble perspective of interactive control of growth hormone secretion. Horm Res 2003;60(Suppl 1):86–101.)

(IGF1R) in an autocrine or paracrine fashion in neighboring adipocytes, with a feedback mechanism regulating *IGF-I* mRNA expression.[11] IGF-I also activates the insulin receptor (IR) in preadipocytes. In addition, the formation of insulin/IGF-I hybrid receptors has been described.[12] IGF-I and insulin seem to act synergistically to induce adipocyte differentiation. IGF-I alone can induce CCAAT/enhancer binding protein α (C/EBPα) and adipocyte lipid binding protein (aP2) mRNA expression, but not lipid droplet accumulation associated with maturation.[13]

IGF-II is known to regulate fetal growth. Less is known about IGF-II action on adipocytes. Studies of *igf2* gene polymorphisms in pigs implicated an influence of IGF-II on fat deposition.[14] In an in vitro model of rat adipocyte progenitor cells, IGF-II stimulated adipocyte differentiation.[15]

The bioavailability of IGF-I is modulated by IGFBP-3 and other IGFBPs. The secretion of IGFBP-2, -3, and -4 is upregulated during adipocyte differentiation.[16,17] IGFBP-3 is thought to act by both binding to and sequestering IGF-I, and to exert IGF-I–independent effects. In adipocytes from visceral adipose tissue, IGFBP-3 was found to reduce insulin-stimulated 2-deoxyglucose uptake.[18] IGFBP-3 also blocks in vitro differentiation of the mouse preadipocyte cell line 3T3-L1 in an IGF-I–independent manner. By contrast, both IGF-I and IGFBP-3 stimulated glycerol-3-phosphate dehydrogenase activity during differentiation of visceral and subcutaneous preadipocytes isolated from adipose tissue of children (reviewed in Ref.[19]).

IGFBP-1 inhibits in vitro adipose differentiation by IGF-I, probably by preventing IGF-I binding to the IGF1R.[20] Systemic overexpression of IGFBP-1 or IGFBP-2 was found to protect mice from diet-induced or age-induced obesity and insulin resistance.[21,22]

EXPERIMENTAL/IN VITRO EVIDENCE
Changes in the IGF System During Adipose Differentiation In Vitro

The GH/IGF system changes during adipocyte differentiation. GHR mRNA expression is upregulated during adipogenesis of the murine adipocyte cell line 3T3-L1[23] and binding of GH to adipocyte precursors increases during differentiation.[7] The ratio of IR to IGF1R expression increases approximately 10-fold during differentiation, due to an increased IR expression. Preadipocytes express IGF1R and IR isoform A, whereas mature adipocytes express predominantly both isoform A and isoform B of the IR.[24] The increased IR expression is reflected by an increase in insulin sensitivity, with an EC_{50} for the stimulation of glucose uptake at 10^{-11} M insulin in adipocytes, compared with 10^{-9} M insulin in preadipocytes.[12]

The secretion of IGF-I and IGFBP-3 was shown to increase during adipocyte differentiation. GH was a positive regulator only in preadipocytes, whereas insulin stimulated the release of both proteins also in mature adipocytes.[17] By contrast, IGF-II and IGFBP-5 expression was shown to decrease in differentiating porcine adipocytes.[25]

Signaling Pathways of GH/IGF in Adipocytes

GH signaling
By binding to and activating its receptor, GH initiates multiple signaling pathways. On receptor activation, the GHR-associated Janus kinase 2 (JAK2) is activated, phosphorylates itself and the GHR, and can recruit several signaling molecules. In turn, this leads to the activation of signal transducers and activators of transcription (STATs), ERK1/2 or phosphatidylinositol-3 (PI3)-kinase.[26] Whereas some studies suggest PI3-kinase or protein kinase C to be essential for the activation of ERK1/2 by GH,[27,28] others show that the adapter proteins Shc and Grb2 initiate the signaling cascade leading to ERK1/2 activation.[29]

The growth-promoting action of GH is mediated by the JAK2-STAT5a/b pathway, the activity of which is terminated by the suppressor of cytokine signaling (SOCS) proteins. SOCS2 is a key regulator of GHR sensitivity, regulating cellular GHR levels through direct ubiquitination.[30]

A potential effector of GH is Sirt1, a nicotinamide adenine dinucleotide (NAD)-dependent deacetylase that is implicated in the regulation of differentiation, energy metabolism, and stress responses. In preadipocytes, Sirt1 represses adipocyte differentiation via repression of peroxisome proliferator-activated receptor γ (PPARγ). In differentiated adipocytes, upregulation of Sirt1 triggers lipolysis and decreases lipogenesis.[31,32] GH has already been shown to increase the expression of Sirt1 and activation of adenosine-monophosphate kinase in other cellular contexts.[33,34] The activity of Sirt1 is regulated by Nampt, the key enzyme in NAD biosynthesis starting from nicotinamide. GH has been shown to downregulate *Nampt* expression in 3T3-L1 adipocytes.[35]

Mammalian target of rapamycin complex 1 (mTORC1) is another metabolic regulator that has recently been shown to regulate triglyceride storage. Inhibition of mTORC1 by rapamycin induces lipolysis and increases plasma free fatty acid levels in humans.[36] It has been shown that GH acutely activates protein synthesis through signaling via mTORC1.[37] GH can modulate mTOR signaling by increasing the tyrosine phosphorylation of upstream signaling molecules insulin receptor substrate (IRS)-1, IRS-2, JAK2, and Shc.[38]

Insulin/IGF signaling

Insulin/IGF signaling is very complex, because there are 3 ligands (IGF-I, IGF-II, and insulin) binding to at least 3 receptors (IGF1R, IR isoform A, and IR isoform B) with different affinities. The formation of hybrid receptors adds even more complexity and variability to the IGF system. IGF1R has a higher affinity for IGFs, but can be activated by high insulin concentrations (eg, during differentiation of adipocyte cell culture models). Of the insulin receptor isoforms, IR B has a highly preferential affinity for insulin compared with the IGFs, and IR A, which differs from IR B only by the deletion of 12 amino acids, is predominantly a receptor for insulin and IGF-II. IR–IGF1R hybrids appear to behave more like IGF1R, with preferential affinity for IGF-I over insulin. IGF-II also has a specific receptor (IGF2R), which is structurally distinct from the IGF1R or IR. The IGF2R regulates intracellular trafficking of mannose-6-phosphate proteins such as lysosomal enzymes, and influences IGF signaling by sequestering IGF-II.[19]

To make matters even more complicated, Huang and colleagues[39] found that GH induces the formation of a complex that includes GHR, JAK2, and IGF1R in the preadipocyte cell lines 3T3-L1 and 3T3-F442A. Complex formation does not appear to be dependent on GH-induced activation of the ERK or PI3-kinase signaling pathways or on the tyrosine phosphorylation of GHR, JAK2, or IGF1R. Furthermore, GH and IGF-I act synergistically to induce ERK activation and IGF-I enhances GH-induced assembly of conformationally active GHRs.

IGF-I and insulin act through multiple signaling pathways. Several studies performed with cultivated adipocytes from various animals demonstrated that IGF-I is implicated in the regulation of adipocyte differentiation and cell cycle by activation of the PI3-kinase/AKT pathway. This activation is initiated by receptor autophosphorylation and subsequent phosphorylation of IRS-1 or IRS-2. PI3-kinase associates with IRS-1 or -2 and produces the phospholipid messenger phosphatidylinositol-3,4,5-trisphosphate (PI-3,4,5-P3), which in turn recruits 3′-phosphoinosite-dependent protein kinase-1 (PDK1) and AKT to the cell membrane. AKT is activated by Thr308-phosphorylation through PDK1. AKT can phosphorylate several substrates relevant to insulin-like signaling. The mTORC1 is activated via AKT-mediated phosphorylation and inhibition of tuberous sclerosis complex 2. Recent work suggests that mTORC1 also plays an important role in lipid biosynthesis by promoting the cleavage and activation of sterol response element binding protein 1 (SREBP1). Cleaved SREBP1 is a transcription factor that promotes the expression of diverse genes with important roles in lipid synthesis, including fatty acid synthase (FASN), glycerol-3-phosphate acyltransferases (GPAT), ATP citrate lyase (ACLY), acetyl-CoA carboxylase (ACC), stearoyl-CoA desaturase 1 (SCD1), and glucokinase (GK).[40]

IGF-I stimulates proliferation of 3T3-L1 preadipocytes through activation of mitogen-activated protein kinase (MAPK), which is mediated through the Src family of nonreceptor tyrosine kinases.[41] Another study found that insulin stimulation of 3T3-L1 led to phosphorylation of the atypical protein kinase WNK1, which is a negative regulator of preadipocyte proliferation.[42]

A fundamental function of insulin is the maintenance of glucose homeostasis by increasing the rate of glucose uptake into myocytes and adipocytes. Both GH and IGF-I have been shown to inhibit insulin-stimulated glucose uptake. Chronic GH pretreatment of the 3T3-L1 preadipocyte cell line inhibits insulin-induced glucose uptake without affecting glucose transporter 4 (GLUT4) translocation, through the reduction of IRS-2–associated PI3-kinase activity.[43] IGF-I administration has the same effect in 3T3-L1 adipocytes. However, IGF-I was shown to stimulate the production of reactive oxygen species and thereby disturb insulin-mediated tyrosine phosphorylation of IRS-1.[44]

IGFBP-3 signaling

Apart from specific and high-affinity binding of IGFs, IGFBP-3 can modulate proliferation and cell survival in an IGF-independent manner. IGFBP-3 can translocate to the nucleus and bind to retinoid X receptor α and PPARγ, thereby inhibiting adipose differentiation.[45] By reducing GLUT4 translocation to the plasma membrane and Thr308 phosphorylation of AKT, IGFBP-3 attenuated insulin-stimulated glucose uptake.[18] In other cell types, IGFBP-3 was shown to activate PI3-kinase. This effect was inhibited by pertussis toxin, indicating the involvement of a pertussis toxin–sensitive G protein.[46]

A summary of the effects of GH, IGF-I, and IGFBP-3 on (pre)adipocytes in vitro is given in **Table 1**.

CLINICAL CONSIDERATIONS
Regulation of Adipose Mass

Adipose mass is determined by both the volume and number of adipocytes. Adipocyte number may increase through proliferation and differentiation of preadipocytes.[50] Adults with severe obesity exhibit an increased total fat cell number independent of the onset of obesity. Adipose tissue of adults contains a remarkable number of specific precursor cells that are able to differentiate into mature fat cells under appropriate conditions.[1]

Because GH induces secretion of IGF-I and IGFBP-3, it is difficult to separate the effects of GH, IGF-I, and IGFBP-3 in vivo. Much of the information on the effects of GH in vivo comes from treatment of patients with GH deficiency (GHD). By systematically reviewing blinded, randomized, placebo-controlled trials of GH treatment in adult patients with GHD, Maison and colleagues[51] found a negative effect of GH treatment on fat mass and an improvement in low-density lipoprotein (LDL) and serum cholesterol levels. Adipose tissue of adult individuals with untreated GHD was shown to contain adipocytes with a very large diameter. Of importance is that this was accompanied by increased expression of proinflammatory markers and

Table 1
Effects of GH, IGF-I, and IGFBP-3 on (pre)adipocytes in vitro

Hormone	Effect	Adipocyte Model	Reference
GH	↑ Differentiation	Rodent cell lines (3T3-F442A)	47
	↓ Differentiation	Primary human	6
	↓ GAPDH activity		
	↓ Cellular glucose uptake, incorporation of glucose into lipids		
	↑ Lipolysis		
	↓ Differentiation	Primary rat	7
	↓ GAPDH activity		
	↓ Cellular glucose uptake		
	↓ Lipogenesis		
	↑ IGF-I synthesis		
	↑ Proliferation of precursor cells		
	↑ Lipolysis		
	↓ Insulin-stimulated glucose uptake	3T3-L1	43
IGF-I	↑ Proliferation	3T3-L1	41
	↓ Death-receptor–mediated induction of apoptosis	SGBS, primary human	48
	↑ Differentiation	Human mesenchymal stem cells (HMSCs)	49
	↑ Proliferation		
	↑ Expression of C/EBPα and aP2 mRNA	Rat mesenteric stromal vascular cells (mSVCs)	13
	↓ Insulin-stimulated glucose uptake	3T3-L1	44
IGFBP-3	↓ Insulin-stimulated glucose uptake	3T3-L1	18
	↓ Differentiation	3T3-L1	45

↓, decreasing effect; ↑, increasing effect.
Abbreviations: GAPDH, glyceraldehyde-3-phosphate dehydrogenase; SGBS, Simpson-Golabi-Behmel syndrome.

inflammatory cytokines as well as impaired insulin action in obese patients with GHD, whereas lean individuals with GHD had low protein levels in several cytokines and growth factors, indicating defective adipocyte differentiation and proliferation as well as attenuated angiogenesis and neurogenesis.[52] Children with GHD were described to be generally moderately obese. At the cellular level, an increased mean adipocyte volume but a reduced number of fat cells was detected, compared with healthy children. After GH substitution, these changes were shifted toward normal.[1]

GH treatment was shown to regulate several genes involved in triglyceride hydrolysis and storage, diacylglycerol synthesis, and the expression of components of extracellular matrix and transforming growth factor β signaling pathways, as has been shown in adipose tissue biopsies from male subjects with GHD. Moreover, GH was able to decrease hydroxysteroid-(11β)-dehydrogenase 1, which activates local cortisol production. Accordingly, GH may be able to reduce the amount of locally produced cortisol in adipose tissue.[8]

Individuals with obesity that is not associated with an endocrinopathy were shown to have a lower *GHR* mRNA expression in omental as well as subcutaneous adipose tissues, compared with lean subjects. This fact might offer one explanation as to why GH treatment is not effective in patients with idiopathic obesity.[53]

Body fat mass influences basal and stimulated GH release, both of which are attenuated by increased body fat (reviewed in Ref.[54]). Obese subjects were found to have lower bioactive GH and elevated GHBP serum concentrations in comparison with lean individuals after exercise.[55] Serum levels of GHBP were also found to be increased in obese children and adolescents, and correlated with waist circumference.[56] In addition, GH serum levels were reported to be decreased by short-term overeating without a concomitant increase in body weight. This reduction was due to a decreased amplitude of the GH pulse and was accompanied by a reduction in IGFBP-1 serum levels, which resulted in increased free IGF-I serum concentrations.[57] This finding is supported by results from an earlier study showing that despite GH hyposecretion in obesity, total IGF-I and IGFBP-3 serum concentrations did not differ between obese and lean male subjects. However, free IGF-I concentrations were higher in obese subjects, probably because of decreased hepatic IGFBP-1 and IGFBP-2 production.[58]

Effects of IGF-I alone can be evaluated in patients with GH insensitivity syndrome (GHIS) resulting from mutations in the GH receptor and consequent IGF-I deficiency. These patients have metabolic disturbances that include obesity and, particularly in young individuals, spontaneous hypoglycemia caused by lack of GH effects on lipolysis and hepatic glucose production. In elderly patients, fasting hyperinsulinemia is prevalent and the risk of type 2 diabetes is increased.[59,60] IGF-I treatment of adult patients with GHIS decreased body fat mass while lean body mass increased. Measures of lipolytic activity and fat oxidation increased as well, concomitant with an increase in plasma free fatty acid and β-hydroxybutyrate concentrations and a reduced plasma insulin concentration.[61]

Visceral Versus Subcutaneous Adipose Tissue

Clinical studies have shown that in visceral adipose depots, adipocytes are less sensitive to insulin than those found in subcutaneous sites, and they appear less able to differentiate into mature adipocytes,[62] indicating that impairment of adipocyte differentiation occurs in a site-specific manner. A current hypothesis argues that in people whose fat stores are unable to differentiate optimally, excess calories are more likely to be stored in sites other than fat, such as liver, skeletal muscle, and heart, thus contributing to metabolic dysregulation with insulin resistance (reviewed in Ref.[19]). A recent study supported the finding that visceral fat deposition is associated with insulin resistance while an increase in subcutaneous fat depots is associated with a protection from insulin resistance.[63]

Significant differences exist between the growth patterns of different adipose depots. In rats fed ad libitum it was shown that the cumulative growth of the 2 intraabdominal fat depots (mesenteric and epididymal) was due mostly to hypertrophy (increases in cell volume of 83% and 64%, respectively), whereas the growth of the other 2 depots (retroperitoneal and inguinal) was due predominantly to hyperplasia (increases in cell number of 58% and 65%, respectively).[64] This difference was found to be reflected by depot-specific expression patterns of the *IGF-I* and *leptin* genes. expression of both genes was highest in retroperitoneal and epididymal depots, followed by mesenteric and subcutaneous inguinal depots. Both *leptin* and *IGF-I* mRNAs, when expressed per 10^6 adipocytes, correlated with the adipocyte volume, suggesting that the autocrine/paracrine actions of these cytokines could modulate region-specific patterns of adipose tissue growth.[65] A more recent study reported that IGF-I–stimulated DNA synthesis was significantly lower in omental preadipocytes than in subcutaneous preadipocytes from obese subjects. IGF-I–mediated phosphorylation of the IGF1R and the ERK pathway was comparable in subcutaneous and omental cells. However, omental preadipocytes had decreased IRS-1 protein associated with increased IRS-1-degradation. Consequently, IGF-I–stimulated phosphorylation of AKT on serine (473) but not threonine (308) was decreased in omental cells, and activation of downstream targets, including p70 S6 kinase, glycogen synthase kinase 3, and the transcription factor Forkhead box O1, was also impaired. CyclinD1 abundance was decreased in omental cells because of increased degradation. These results propose an intrinsic defect in IGF-I activation of the AKT pathway in omental preadipocytes from obese subjects that involves IRS-1 and could contribute to the distinct growth phenotype of preadipocytes in visceral fat of obese subjects.[66] In contrast to these results, Bashan and colleagues[67] demonstrated that tyrosine phosphorylation and signal transduction to AKT after insulin stimulation of omental fat was not inferior to that detected in fragments of subcutaneous fat tissue. Instead a stronger activation of stress-related kinases such as p38 MAPK and JNK was observed.

In acromegaly, a state of GH and IGF-I excess, both visceral and subcutaneous adipose tissue, but most markedly visceral adipose tissue, were shown to be decreased whereas intramuscular visceral adipose was greater. This finding suggests that increased visceral adipose in muscle could be associated with GH-induced insulin resistance.[68]

Adipose Tissue and Glucose Homeostasis

An emerging function for adipose tissue is the regulation of whole-body glucose homeostasis and insulin sensitivity. Supporting evidence came from a mouse model overexpressing GLUT4 in adipose tissue, which displayed increased glucose tolerance.[69] Tightly linked to this important role of adipose tissue is the fact that individuals with low birth weight have an increased risk of developing type 2 diabetes and other features of the metabolic syndrome later in life. A study comparing the expression of insulin/IGF-signaling molecules in adipose tissue of low-birth-weight and normal-birth-weight young males found a lower expression of genes for GLUT4 and PI3-kinase p85 and p110 subunits, as well as for IRS-1.[70] These results were supported by findings from another study involving children born small for gestational age (SGA) and control subjects born appropriate for gestational age (AGA). The content of IGF1R, IR, ERK1/2, and AKT was lower in subcutaneous adipocytes from SGA compared with that from AGA children. ERK1/2 phosphorylation after stimulation of adipocytes with insulin or IGF-I was decreased in SGA.[71]

An overview of the effects of GH and IGF-I on adipose tissue–related responses in vivo is given in **Table 2**.

Table 2
Effects of GH and IGF-I on adipose tissue–related responses in vivo

Hormone	Effect	Subjects/Animal Models	Reference
GH/IGF-I	↓ Adipocyte size ↑ Adipocyte number	Human subjects with GHD	1
GH/IGF-I	↑ Lipolysis ↑ Lipid oxidation	Human male subjects with GHD, adipose tissue biopsies	8
GH	↓ Insulin sensitivity	Liver IGF-I–deficient mice	72
GH	↑ Lipolysis ↑ Circulating free fatty acid concentrations	Humans, abdominal and femoral adipose tissue	73
GH	↑ Circulating IGF-I levels	Insulin-dependent diabetics and healthy subjects	74

↓, decreasing effect; ↑, increasing effect.

OPEN QUESTIONS

Nowadays a wealth of information is available about the differentiation process of adipocytes, the multitude of factors influencing this process, and the clinical consequences of high or low circulating GH or IGFs. Sometimes it is difficult, however, to reconcile the results of different studies, especially when the effects seen in cell lines are the opposite of effects observed in primary cells. For example, GH has been described to stimulate differentiation in the murine adipocyte cell line 3T3-F442A,[47] whereas primary preadipocytes incubated with GH did not differentiate.[6] Results from preadipocyte cell lines have to be viewed cautiously, because the immortalization process might influence the signaling pathways and therefore the cellular responses to GH or IGF stimuli. IGF-I and IGFBP-3 are known to have antiapoptotic and proapoptotic effects, respectively, in cancer cell lines,[75,76] which might confound cell responses of immortalized preadipocyte cell lines.

Another experimental strategy is the use of primary adipocyte cultures of various animals (rat, pig, mouse). In addition to the uncertainty as to whether these adipocyte cultures behave like human adipocytes, there might be differences specific to adipose depot that have to be taken into account when interpreting the results.

When using primary human material, differing study outcomes do not only occur because of technical differences (the use of isolated adipocytes, in vivo biopsies, or tissue-fragment explants) but also as a result of patient selection.[67] In addition, in vivo it is difficult to decide whether the observed effects are caused by GH directly or by increased expression of IGF-I or IGFBPs.

Taken together, the available evidence suggests that GH and IGF-I are indeed important regulators of adipocyte survival and differentiation. In addition, in obese subjects a blunted GH/IGF-I response is being observed on a regular basis. GH and/or IGF-I are nevertheless unable to influence the development of obesity in healthy subjects.

REFERENCES

1. Wabitsch M, Hauner H, Heinze E, et al. The role of growth hormone/insulin-like growth factors in adipocyte differentiation. Metabolism 1995;44(10 Suppl 4):45–9.
2. Blüher S, Kratzsch J, Kiess W. Insulin-like growth factor I, growth hormone and insulin in white adipose tissue. Best Pract Res Clin Endocrinol Metab 2005;19:577–87.
3. Gahete MD, Durán-Prado M, Luque RM, et al. Understanding the multifactorial control of growth hormone release by somatotropes: lessons from comparative endocrinology. Ann N Y Acad Sci 2009;1163:137–53.
4. Møller N, Jørgensen JO. Effects of growth hormone on glucose, lipid, and protein metabolism in human subjects. Endocr Rev 2009;30:152–77.
5. Kaplan SA, Cohen P. The somatomedin hypothesis 2007: 50 years later. J Clin Endocrinol Metab 2007;92:4529–35.
6. Wabitsch M, Braun S, Hauner H, et al. Mitogenic and antiadipogenic properties of human growth hormone in differentiating human adipocyte precursor cells in primary culture. Pediatr Res 1996;40:450–6.
7. Wabitsch M, Heinze E, Hauner H, et al. Biological effects of human growth hormone in rat adipocyte precursor cells and newly differentiated adipocytes in primary culture. Metabolism 1996;45:34–42.
8. Zhao JT, Cowley MJ, Lee P, et al. Identification of novel GH-regulated pathway of lipid metabolism in adipose tissue: a gene expression study in hypopituitary men. J Clin Endocrinol Metab 2011;96:E1188–96.

9. Vijayakumar A, Novosyadlyy R, Wu Y, et al. Biological effects of growth hormone on carbohydrate and lipid metabolism. Growth Horm IGF Res 2010;20:1–7.
10. Möller C, Arner P, Sonnenfeld T, et al. Quantitative comparison of insulin-like growth factor mRNA levels in human and rat tissues analysed by a solution hybridization assay. J Mol Endocrinol 1991;7:213–22.
11. Klöting N, Koch L, Wunderlich T, et al. Autocrine IGF-1 action in adipocytes controls systemic IGF-1 concentrations and growth. Diabetes 2008;57:2074–82.
12. Bäck K, Brännmark C, Strålfors P, et al. Differential effects of IGF-I, IGF-II and insulin in human preadipocytes and adipocytes—role of insulin and IGF-I receptors. Mol Cell Endocrinol 2011;339:130–5.
13. Sato T, Nagafuku M, Shimizu K, et al. Physiological levels of insulin and IGF-1 synergistically enhance the differentiation of mesenteric adipocytes. Cell Biol Int 2008;32:1397–404.
14. Nezer L, Moreau B, Brouwers W, et al. An imprinted QTL with major effect on muscle mass and fat deposition maps to the IGF2 locus in pigs. Nat Genet 1999;21:155–6.
15. Bellows CG, Jia D, Jia Y, et al. Different effects of insulin and insulin-like growth factors I and II on osteoprogenitors and adipocyte progenitors in fetal rat bone cell populations. Calcif Tissue Int 2006;79:57–65.
16. Boney CM, Moats-Staats BM, Stiles AD, et al. Expression of insulin-like growth factor-I (IGF-I) and IGF-binding proteins during adipogenesis. Endocrinology 1994;135:1863–8.
17. Wabitsch M, Heinze E, Debatin KM, et al. IGF-I and IGFBP-3-expression in cultured human preadipocytes and adipocytes. Horm Metab Res 2000;32:555–9.
18. Chan S, Twigg S, Firth S, et al. Insulin-like growth factor binding protein 3 leads to insulin resistance in adipocytes. J Clin Endocrinol Metab 2005;90:6588–95.
19. Baxter RB, Twigg SM. Actions of IGF binding proteins and related proteins in adipose tissue. Trends Endocrinol Metab 2009;20:499–505.
20. Siddals KW, Westwood M, Gibson JM, et al. IGF-binding protein-1 inhibits IGF effects on adipocyte function: implications for insulin-like actions at the adipocyte. J Endocrinol 2002;174:289–97.
21. Rajkumar K, Modric T, Murphy LJ. Impaired adipogenesis in insulin-like growth factor binding protein-1 transgenic mice. J Endocrinol 1999;162:457–65.
22. Wheatcroft SB, Kearney MT, Shah AM, et al. IGF-binding protein-2 protects against the development of obesity and insulin resistance. Diabetes 2007;56:285–94.
23. Iida K, Takahashi Y, Kaji H, et al. Diverse regulation of full-length and truncated growth hormone receptor expression in 3T3-L1 adipocytes. Mol Cell Endocrinol 2003;210:21–9.
24. Bäck K, Arnqvist HJ. Changes in insulin and IGF-I receptor expression during differentiation of human preadipocytes. Growth Horm IGF Res 2009;19:101–11.
25. Gardan D, Mourot J, Louveau I. Decreased expression of the IGF-II gene during porcine adipose cell differentiation. Mol Cell Endocrinol 2008;292:63–8.
26. Rosenfeld RG, Hwa V. New molecular mechanisms of GH resistance. Eur J Endocrinol 2004;151:S11–5.
27. Clarkson RW, Chen CM, Harrison S, et al. Early responses of trans-activating factors to growth hormone in preadipocytes: differential regulation of CCAAT enhancer-binding protein-beta (C/EBP beta) and C/EBP delta. Mol Endocrinol 1995;9:108–20.
28. Kilgour E, Gout I, Anderson NG. Requirement for phosphoinositide 3-OH kinase in growth hormone signalling to the mitogen-activated protein kinase and p70s6k pathways. Biochem J 1996;315:517–22.

29. VanderKuur JA, Butch ER, Waters SB, et al. Signalling molecules involved in coupling growth hormone receptor to MAP kinase activation. Endocrinology 1997;138:4301–7.
30. Vesterlund M, Zadjali F, Persson T, et al. The SOCS2 ubiquitin ligase complex regulates growth hormone receptor levels. PLoS One 2011;6:e25358.
31. Picard F, Kurtev M, Chung N, et al. Sirt1 promotes fat mobilization in white adipocytes by repressing PPAR-gamma. Nature 2004;429:771–6.
32. Fischer-Posovszky P, Kukulus V, Tews D, et al. Resveratrol regulates human adipocyte number and function in a Sirt1-dependent manner. Am J Clin Nutr 2010;92:5–15.
33. Qin Y, Tian YP. Exploring the molecular mechanisms underlying the potentiation of exogenous growth hormone on alcohol-induced fatty liver diseases in mice. J Transl Med 2010;8:120.
34. Cuesta S, Kireev R, Forman K, et al. Growth hormone can improve insulin resistance and differentiation in pancreas of senescence accelerated prone male mice (SAMP8). Growth Horm IGF Res 2011;21:63–8.
35. Kralisch S, Klein J, Lossner U, et al. Hormonal regulation of the novel adipocytokine visfatin in 3T3-L1 adipocytes. J Endocrinol 2005;185(3):R1–8.
36. Soliman GA, Acosta-Jaquez HA, Fingar DC. mTORC1 inhibition via rapamycin promotes triacylglycerol lipolysis and release of free fatty acids in 3T3-L1 adipocytes. Lipids 2010;45:1089–100.
37. Hayashi AA, Proud CG. The rapid activation of protein synthesis by growth hormone requires signaling through mTOR. Am J Physiol Endocrinol Metab 2007; 292:E1647–55.
38. Thirone AC, Carvalho CR, Saad MJ. Growth hormone stimulates the tyrosine kinase activity of JAK2 and induces tyrosine phosphorylation of insulin receptor substrates and Shc in rat tissues. Endocrinology 1999;140:55–62.
39. Huang Y, Kim SO, Yang N, et al. Physical and functional interaction of growth hormone and insulin-like growth factor-I signaling elements. Mol Endocrinol 2004;18: 1471–85.
40. Laplante M, Sabatini DM. An emerging role of mTOR in lipid biosynthesis. Curr Biol 2009;19:R1046–52.
41. Sekimoto H, Boney CM. C-terminal Src kinase (CSK) modulates insulin-like growth factor-I signaling through Src in 3T3-L1 differentiation. Endocrinology 2003;144:2546–52.
42. Jiang ZY, Zhou QL, Holik J, et al. Identification of WNK1 as a substrate of Akt/protein kinase B and a negative regulator of insulin-stimulated mitogenesis in 3T3-L1 cells. J Biol Chem 2005;280(22):21622–8.
43. Sasaki-Suzuki N, Arai K, Ogata T, et al. Growth hormone inhibition of glucose uptake in adipocytes occurs without affecting GLUT4 translocation through an insulin receptor substrate-2-phosphatidylinositol 3-kinase-dependent pathway. J Biol Chem 2009;284:6061–70.
44. Fukuoka H, Iida K, Nishizawa H, et al. IGF-I stimulates reactive oxygen species (ROS) production and inhibits insulin-dependent glucose uptake via ROS in 3T3-L1 adipocytes. Growth Horm IGF Res 2010;20:212–9.
45. Chan SS, Schedlich LJ, Twigg SM, et al. Inhibition of adipocyte differentiation by insulin-like growth factor-binding protein-3. Am J Physiol Endocrinol Metab 2009; 296:E654–63.
46. Ricort JM, Binoux M. Insulin-like growth factor binding protein-3 stimulates phosphatidylinositol 3-kinase in MCF-7 breast carcinoma cells. Biochem Biophys Res Commun 2004;314:1044–9.

47. Morikawa M, Nixon T, Green H. Growth hormone and the adipose conversion of 3T3 cells. Cell 1982;29:783–9.
48. Fischer-Posovszky P, Tornqvist H, Debatin KM, et al. Inhibition of death-receptor mediated apoptosis in human adipocytes by the insulin-like growth factor I (IGF-I)/IGF-I receptor autocrine circuit. Endocrinology 2004;145:1849–59.
49. Scavo LM, Karas M, Murray M, et al. Insulin-like growth factor-I stimulates both cell growth and lipogenesis during differentiation of human mesenchymal stem cells into adipocytes. J Clin Endocrinol Metab 2004;89:3543–53.
50. Hauner H, Entenmann G, Wabitsch M, et al. Promoting effect of glucocorticoids on the differentiation of human adipocyte precursor cells cultured in a chemically defined medium. J Clin Invest 1989;84:1663–70.
51. Maison P, Griffin S, Nicoue-Beglah M, et al. Impact of growth hormone (GH) treatment on cardiovascular risk factors in GH-deficient adults: a metaanalysis of blinded, randomized, placebo-controlled trials. J Clin Endocrinol Metab 2004; 89:2192–9.
52. Ukropec J, Penesová A, Skopková M, et al. Adipokine protein expression pattern in growth hormone deficiency predisposes to the increased fat cell size and the whole body metabolic derangements. J Clin Endocrinol Metab 2008;93:2255–62.
53. Erman A, Veilleux A, Tchernof A, et al. Human growth hormone receptor (GHR) expression in obesity: I. GHR mRNA expression in omental and subcutaneous adipose tissues of obese women. Int J Obes (Lond) 2011;35:1511–9.
54. Kreitschmann-Andermahr I, Suarez P, Jennings R, et al. GH/IGF-I regulation in obesity—mechanisms and practical consequences in children and adults. Horm Res Paediatr 2010;73:153–60.
55. Thomas GA, Kraemer WJ, Kennett MJ, et al. Immunoreactive and bioactive growth hormone responses to resistance exercise in men who are lean or obese. J Appl Physiol 2011;111:465–72.
56. Kratzsch J, Dehmel B, Pulzer F, et al. Increased serum GHBP levels in obese pubertal children and adolescents: relationship to body composition, leptin and indicators of metabolic disturbances. Int J Obes Relat Metab Disord 1997;21:1130–6.
57. Cornford AS, Barkan AL, Horowitz JF. Rapid suppression of growth hormone concentration by overeating: potential mediation by hyperinsulinemia. J Clin Endocrinol Metab 2011;96:824–30.
58. Nam SY, Lee EJ, Kim KR, et al. Effect of obesity on total and free insulin-like growth factor (IGF)-1, and their relationship to IGF-binding protein (BP)-1, IGFBP-2, IGFBP-3, insulin, and growth hormone. Int J Obes Relat Metab Disord 1997;21:355–9.
59. Laron Z, Avitzur Y, Klinger B. Carbohydrate metabolism in primary growth hormone resistance (Laron syndrome) before and during insulin-like growth factor-I treatment. Metabolism 1995;44(Suppl 4):113–8.
60. Laron Z, Ginsberg S, Lilos P, et al. Body composition in untreated adult patients with Laron syndrome (primary GH insensitivity). Clin Endocrinol (Oxf) 2006;65:114–7.
61. Mauras N, Martinez V, Rini A, et al. Recombinant human insulin-like growth factor I has significant anabolic effects in adults with growth hormone receptor deficiency: studies on protein, glucose, and lipid metabolism. J Clin Endocrinol Metab 2000;85:3036–42.
62. Tchkonia T, Tchoukalova YD, Giorgadze N, et al. Abundance of two human preadipocyte subtypes with distinct capacities for replication, adipogenesis, and apoptosis varies among fat depots. Am J Physiol Endocrinol Metab 2005;288:E267–77.

63. McLaughlin T, Lamendola C, Liu A, et al. Preferential fat deposition in subcutaneous versus visceral depots is associated with insulin sensitivity. J Clin Endocrinol Metab 2011;96:E1756–60.
64. DiGirolamo M, Fine JB, Tagra K, et al. Qualitative regional differences in adipose tissue growth and cellularity in male Wistar rats fed ad libitum. Am J Physiol 1998; 274:R1460–7.
65. Villafuerte BC, Fine JB, Bai Y, et al. Expressions of leptin and insulin-like growth factor-I are highly correlated and region-specific in adipose tissue of growing rats. Obes Res 2000;8:646–55.
66. Cleveland-Donovan K, Maile LA, Tsiaras WG, et al. IGF-I activation of the AKT pathway is impaired in visceral but not subcutaneous preadipocytes from obese subjects. Endocrinology 2010;151:3752–63.
67. Bashan N, Dorfman K, Tarnovscki T, et al. Mitogen-activated protein kinases, inhibitory-kappaB kinase, and insulin signaling in human omental versus subcutaneous adipose tissue in obesity. Endocrinology 2007;148:2955–62.
68. Freda PU, Shen W, Heymsfield SB, et al. Lower visceral and subcutaneous but higher intermuscular adipose tissue depots in patients with growth hormone and insulin-like growth factor I excess due to acromegaly. J Clin Endocrinol Metab 2008;9:2334–43.
69. Shepherd PR, Gnudi L, Tozzo E, et al. Adipose tissue hyperplasia and enhanced glucose disposal in transgenic mice over-expressing GLUT 4 selectively in adipose tissue. J Biol Chem 1993;268:22243–6.
70. Ozanne SE, Jensen CB, Tingey JK, et al. Decreased protein levels of key insulin signaling molecules in adipose tissue from young men with a low birthweight— potential link to increased risk of diabetes? Diabetologia 2006;49:2993–9.
71. Iñiguez G, Ormazabal P, López T, et al. IGF-1R/ERK content and response to IGF-I and insulin in adipocytes from small for gestational age children. Growth Horm IGF Res 2009;19:256–61.
72. Yakar S, Setser J, Zhao H, et al. Inhibition of growth hormone action improves insulin sensitivity in liver IGF-1-deficient mice. J Clin Invest 2004;113:96–105.
73. Gravholt CH, Schmitz O, Simonsen L, et al. Effects of a physiological GH pulse on interstitial glycerol in abdominal and femoral adipose tissue. Am J Physiol 1999; 277:E848–54.
74. Wurzburger MI, Prelevic GM, Sonksen PH, et al. The effect of recombinant human growth hormone on regulation of growth hormone secretion and blood glucose in insulin-dependent diabetes. J Clin Endocrinol Metab 1993;77:267–72.
75. Varela-Nieto I, Hartl M, Gorospe I, et al. Anti-apoptotic actions of insulin-like growth factors: lessons from development and implications in neoplastic cell transformation. Curr Pharm Des 2007;13:687–703.
76. Paharkova-Vatchkova V, Lee KW. Nuclear export and mitochondrial and endoplasmic reticulum localization of IGF-binding protein 3 regulate its apoptotic properties. Endocr Relat Cancer 2010;17:293–302.

Probiotics, Prebiotics, Energy Balance, and Obesity

Mechanistic Insights and Therapeutic Implications

Federica Molinaro, MD[a,1], Elena Paschetta, MD[a,1],
Maurizio Cassader, PhD[a], Roberto Gambino, PhD[a],
Giovanni Musso, MD[b,*]

KEYWORDS

- Microbiota • Endotoxin • Obesity • Probiotics • Prebiotics

KEY POINTS

- Increased consumption of foods with high energy is involved in obesity development, which is a well-known risk factor for type 2 diabetes mellitus (T2DM) and cardiovascular disease.
- Several studies have demonstrated that gut microbiota can modulate host energy homeostasis and adiposity through different mechanisms: energy harvest from diet, fat storage and expenditure, incretins secretion, and systemic inflammation.
- Although experimental data suggest gut microbiota manipulation with probiotics and prebiotics can beneficially affect host adiposity and glucose metabolism, their effects are transient and diminish gradually after cessation.
- This review analyzes the potential gut microbiota-driven pathways that could represent novel target for treatment of obesity.

INTRODUCTION

Obesity-related disorders are related to energy homeostasis and inflammation; gut microbiota are involved in several host metabolic functions and may play an important role in this context through several mechanisms: increased energy harvest from the diet, regulation of host metabolism, and modulation of inflammation.

Human gut flora comprises at least 10^{14} bacteria belonging to 3 bacterial phyla: the gram-positive Firmicutes and Actinobacteria and the gram-negative Bacteroidetes.

This article originally appeared in Gastroenterology Clinics of North America, Volume 41, Issue 4, December 2012.
[a] Department of Medical Sciences, Corso AM Dogliotti 14 10124, University of Turin, Italy;
[b] Department of Emergency Medicine, Gradenigo Hospital, Gradenigo Hospital, Turin, Corso Regina Margherita 8, Turin 10132, Italy
[1] Equal first author.
* Corresponding author.
E-mail address: giovanni_musso@yahoo.it

2352-7986/14/$ – see front matter © 2014 Elsevier Inc. All rights reserved.

Firmicutes is the largest bacterial phylum and comprises more than 200 genera, including *Lactobacillus, Mycoplasma, Bacillus*, and *Clostridium* species.[1] Although each subject has a specific gut microbiota, a core human gut microbiome is shared among family members despite different environments[2]; nevertheless, the microbiome dynamically changes in response to some factors, including dietary nutrients, illness, and antibiotic use.

This review discusses the interaction of gut microbiota with host metabolism and the impact of manipulating microbiota composition on the pathogenesis and the treatment of obesity.

ASSOCIATION BETWEEN GUT MICROBIOTA AND OBESITY: PATHOPHYSIOLOGICAL MECHANISMS

Several data suggest that gut microflora play a role in the regulation of host energy homeostasis (Table 1).

Table I
Gut microbiota modulation of host energy homeostasis: mechanisms

Mechanisms	Mediators	Metabolic Effects
Reduced intestinal transit rate	Production of SCFA , that increase Gpr41-/Gpr43-mediated PYY secretion	Increased energy harvest from the diet
Polysaccharide degradation to monosaccharides	Microbial transport proteins and enzymes	Increased CHO absobtion and portal flow
Increased glucose absorption	Increased intestinal Glut1 expression	
Increased monosaccharides portal low	Increased capillaries density in intestinal villi	
Increased de novo lipogenesis	ChREBP and SREBP-1 mediated expression of lipogenic enzyme	Increased hepatic/adipose Tg contents
Increased adipociyte uptake of circulating FFA	Increased adipose LPL activity through reduction of intestinal Fiaf secretion	
Reduced FFA oxidation	Reduced Fiaf-induced (PGC)-1α and AMPK-induced expression of mitochondrial FFA oxidative enzymes	Reduced hepatic/muscle FFA oxidation
Regulation of GLP-2 secretion	Modulation of intestinal L-cell activity	Modulation of intestinal barrier function
LPS production	LPS-TLR4-mediated induction of hepatic/adipose/macrophagical pro-inflammatory cytokines SOCS-1, SOCS-3, IL-6, TNF-α, MCP-1	Modulation of systemic/hepatic/adipose inflammation
Modulation of gut barrier integrity	Stimulation of L-cell differentiation and GLP-2 secretion	
Regulation of hepatic/adipose fatty acid composition	Increased linoleic acid conversion to c9, t11 CLA , increased hepatic and adipose contents of DHA and EPA	Modulation of tissue composition of fatty acid

Animal models suggest obesity is associated with alteration of gut microbiota: germ-free mice have less total body fat than conventionally raised mice. The colonization of germ-free mice with a normal microbiota (composed mainly of *Bacteroides* and *Clostridium* genera) results in an increase in total body fat, hepatic triglycerides, fasting plasma glucose, and insulin resistance, despite a reduced food intake.[3] Similarly, conventionalization of germ-free mice with flora from obese donors induces a greater increase in total body fat than colonization with microbiota from lean mice.[4]

Moreover, germ-free mice are protected against the Western diet–induced insulin resistance and gained less body weight and fat mass than conventionalized mice.[5]

Genetically obese leptin-deficient ob/ob mice harbour a significantly higher percentage of Firmicutes and a 50% lower percentage of Bacteroidetes compared with their wild-type littermates fed the same polysaccharide-rich diet.[6] Consistently, in the high-fat/high-sugar Western diet mice, a model of dietary obesity, the development of obesity was associated with enrichment in Firmicutes at the expense of the Bacteriodetes compared with mice receiving a low-fat/high polysaccharide diet.[7] Metagenomic analysis of the obese microbiome showed a depletion of genes involved in motility and an enrichment in genes enabling the capacity of extract energy from the diet, including glycoside hydrolases, phosphotransferases, β-fructosidase and in other transport proteins and fermentation enzymes further processing breakdown products.

Although Bifidobacterium is not a predominating phylum in the gut, it seems to play an important role in host metabolism. In mice, a high-fat diet led to a reduction in Bifidobacterium, associated with increased fat mass, insulin resistance, and inflammatory activity.[8]

Gut microbiota is also connected to metabolic disorders through the modulation of the innate immune system. Mice genetically deficient in Toll-like receptor (TLR) 5, a component of innate immune system in the gut, developed hallmark features of metabolic syndrome, including hyperlipidemia, hypertension, insulin resistance, and increased adiposity, associated with changes in the composition of the gut microbiota. Transplantation of microbiota from TLR5-deficient mice to wild-type germ-free mice conferred many features of metabolic syndrome to the recipients.[9]

Increased Energy Harvest from the Diet

Nutrient absorption and gut motility can be modulated by short chain fatty acids (SCFAs), the major end products of bacterial fermentation. SCFAs (propionate, acetate, and butyrate) represent more than 60% of energy content of carbohydrates from the diet[10] and are ligands for Gpr41 and Gpr43, 2 G protein–coupled receptors that induce intestinal secretion of peptide YY (PYY) and leptin.

Gpr41 functional deletion was related with a reduction in PYY expression, a faster intestinal transit rate, and a reduction of energy uptake from the diet.[11] Consistently, Grp43-deficient mice showed lower total body fat and improved insulin sensitivity; moreover, GPR43 inhibition was associated with higher energy expenditure accompanied by higher core body temperature and increased food intake.[12]

Collectively, these findings disclose the pivotal role for Gpr41 and Gpr43 in mediating microbiota regulation of energy harvest from the diet.

Regulation of Host Energy Storage

In conventionalized mice, microbiota promotes absorption of monosaccharides from the gut lumen.[5] Increased carbohydrate availability promotes de novo lipogenesis in the liver and the adipose tissue by stimulating carbohydrate response element binding protein–mediated and sterol response element binding protein 1–mediated transcription of genes encoding 2 rate-limiting lipogenetic enzymes: acetyl-CoA carboxylase 1 and fatty acid synthase.[13] This mechanism leads to an accumulation of triglycerides in the liver and in adipose tissue.

Fasting-induced adipose factor (Fiaf), also called angiopoietin-like protein 4, is an inhibitor of adipose lipoprotein lipase produced by enterocytes, hepatocytes, skeletal myocytes, and adipocytes in response to fasting, peroxisome proliferator-activated receptor-γ activation, and inflammatory prostaglandins, PGD_2 and PGJ_2.[14] Fiaf also modulates fatty acid oxidation in skeletal muscle and in adipocytes, increasing the nuclear transcription factor peroxisomal proliferator-activated receptor coactivator 1α, a coactivator of genes encoding key enzymes involved in mitochondrial fatty acid oxidation.[15]

Gut microbiota affect storage of circulating triglycerides into adipocytes by regulating intestinal secretion of Fiaf: conventionalization of germ-free mice suppressed intestinal expression of Fiaf in differentiated villous epithelial cells in the ileum; consistently, germ-free Fiaf-KO mice fed a high-fat/high-carbohydrate diet were not protected against diet-induced obesity.[5] Specific microbiota has different effects on expression of Fiaf: mice fed a high-fat diet supplemented with *Lactobacillus paracasei* showed increased levels of Fiaf and displayed significantly less body fat and reduced triglyceride levels. In coculture experiments, Lactobacillus also induced Fiaf gene expression.[16] These data suggest that modulation of Fiaf through manipulating gut flora could be an important therapeutic target.

Microbiota may regulate the fatty acid metabolism also by affecting adenosine AMP–AMP (AMPK) activation. AMPK stimulates fatty acid oxidative pathways in the liver and the skeletal muscle through activation of mitochondrial enzymes, such as acetyl-CoA carboxylase and carnitine palmitoyltransferase I, and reduces hepatic glycogen-synthase activity and glycogen stores, improving hepatic and muscle insulin sensitivity.[17]

Gut flora may have an inhibitory effect on AMPK-regulated fatty acid oxidation, because germ-free mice present a persistent activation of hepatic and muscle AMPK, whereas AMPK activity and related metabolic pathways were suppressed in conventionalized mice.[5]

Regulation of Chronic Low-grade Endotoxinemia and Host Inflammatory Response

Chronic activation of the immune system is linked to the development of obesity and T2DM; TLR4-activated inflammatory pathway has been specifically connected with the low-grade chronic inflammation, which characterizes obesity-related disorders.

Gram-negative microbiota may affect host metabolism through lipopolysaccharide (LPS), which binds the complex of CD14 and TLR4 at the surface of innate immune cells, activating inflammatory pathways implicated in the pathogenesis of obesity, insulin-resistance, and T2DM.[18]

Beside LPS, free fatty acid and products from dying cell can bind TLR4 and stimulate inflammatory response in cell expressing TLR4 (gut immune cells, adipocytes, endothelial cells, tissue macrophages, hepatocytes, and hepatic Kupffer and stellate cells). The hepatic Kupffer cells may have an independent role in this contest: in mice, high-fat diet promotes the activation of Kupffer cells, resulting in insulin resistance and glucose intolerance, whereas selective depletion of these cells restores hepatic insulin sensitivity and improves whole-body and hepatic fat accumulation, without affecting adipose tissue macrophages.[19,20]

Metabolic endotoxiemia is also associated with nonalcoholic steatohepatitis, through hepatic inflammasome activation: a recent study reported, in a mouse model of nonalcoholic steatohepatitis, saturated fatty acids upregulation of the inflammasome that led to sensitization to LPS-induced inflammasome activation.[21] LPS administration modifies the gut microbiota composition (reduction of *Bifidobacteria* and *Eubacteria* spp) and determines metabolic effects, such as systemic insulin resistance, increased plasma and hepatic triglyceride content, and reduction of high-density lipoprotein levels[22,23]; mice fed a high-fat diet shown the same change in microbiota, associated with a low-grade elevation in circulating LPS levels (metabolic endotoxemia).[22] Consistently, LPS receptor deletion or changes of gut microbiota composition induced by antibiotic administration prevented the metabolic alteration of a high-fat diet.[22]

Modification in gut microbiota composition results in change of metabolic endotoxiemia level: prebiotic fermentable oligofructose (OFS) administration increased the intestinal proportion of *Lactobacilli* and *Bifidobacteria* in ob/ob mice, restored normal intestinal permeability through stimulation of epithelial tight-junction proteins, and reduced systemic endotoxiemia, in association with enhanced intestinal glucagon-like peptide (GLP)-2 levels.[24]

Gut microbiota modulates the gut-derived peptide secretion, promoting L-cell differentiation in the proximal colon of rats and increasing GLP-1 secretion in response to a meal in healthy humans[2]; deletion of GLP-1 abolished the beneficial effects of prebiotics on weight gain, glucose metabolism, and inflammatory pathway activation.[25] Furthermore, gut microbiota may modulate gut barrier integrity and endotoxinemia through GLP-2, a 33-amino acid peptide with known intestinotrophic properties, which is cosecreted with GLP-1 by enteroendocrine L cells.

Ob/ob mice treated with prebiotic plus carbohydrates diet presented an increased circulating GLP-1 and GLP-2, which were associated with an altered gut flora composition (increased proportion of *Lactobacilli* and *Bifidobacteria*), restored tight junction integrity and intestinal barrier function, and lowered endotoxinemia.[24] Administration of a GLP-2 antagonist prevented these effects, which were mimicked by the administration of a GLP-2 agonist, suggesting that GLP-2 could mediate the effects of prebiotics.[24]

Microbiota, such as *Bifidobacterium* and *Lactobacillus*, may exert an anti-inflammatory effect through the synthesis of bioactive isomers of conjugated linoleic acid, which shows antidiabetic, antiatherosclerotic, hypocholesterolemic, hypotriglyceridemic, and immunomodulatory activity.[26,27]

In different mammalian models, dietary supplementation of linoleic acid plus *Bifidobacterium breve* altered the profile of polyunsaturated fatty acid composition, resulting in higher intestinal, hepatic, and adipose tissue content of c9,t11 conjugated linoleic acid; the animals also present a higher adipose tissue concentrations of eicosapentaenoic acid and docosahexaenoic acid, 2 omega-3 polynsatured fatty acids with anti-inflammatory and lipid-lowering properties.[28] These changes were associated with a reduced expression of proinflammatory cytokines, such as tumor necrosis factor α, interleukin-6, interleukin-1β, and interleukin-8, accompanied with a higher anti-inflammatory interleukin-10 secretion.

Finally, SCFAs elevation also could result in a reduction of the inflammation and an improvement of insulin sensitivity. Butyrate shows anti-inflammatory properties that could improve epithelial permeability.[29] Acetate raised plasma PYY and GLP-1 and suppressed proinflammatory cytokines.[30]

Collectively, these data suggest that endotoxinemia is involved in the pathogenesis of obesity-related diseases, is affected by dietary nutrient composition, and may be modulated by manipulation of gut microbiota composition.

The Role of Vitamin D

Vitamin D deficiency has been associated with allergic diseases development and increased body mass index.[31]

Vitamin D plays a role in immunomodulation and a decreased vitamin D uptake has been correlated with a change in fecal microbiota composition in one study,[32] although this association needs to be confirmed in larger cohorts.

Mice lacking the vitamin D receptor present chronic, low-grade inflammation in the gastrointestinal tract[33] and the absence of the vitamin D receptor results in enhanced inflammation in response to normally nonpathogenic bacterial flora.[34] Moreover, intestinal vitamin D receptor has also been shown to negatively regulate bacterial-induced intestinal nuclear factor κB activation and to attenuate response to infection, suggesting that the vitamin D may affect the impact of intestinal flora on inflammatory disorders.[35]

THE ROLE OF GUT MICROBIOTA IN HUMAN OBESITY

Obese humans show an increase in Firmicutes/Bacteroidetes ratio; dietary-induced or surgically induced weight loss results in a reduction in this ratio, with a proportion of Bacteroidetes and Firmicutes similar to that found in lean humans, irrespective of the type of diet (fat or carbohydrate restricted).[36–40]

A metagenomic analysis of 154 individuals, including monozygotic and dizygotic twins concordant for leanness or obesity, and their mothers also showed that obesity was associated with a relative depletion of Bacteroidetes and a higher proportion of Actinobacteria compared with leanness.[2] Consistently, one prospective study found that children with lower proportion of Bifidobacterium and higher levels of *Staphylococus aureus* in their infancy gained significantly more weight at 7 years.[41]

The aforementioned changes in gut microbiota composition in human obesity were not uniformly found by different investigators. Some investigators reported no differences or even lower ratios of Firmicutes to Bacteroidetes in obese human adults compared with lean controls; however, significant diet dependent reductions in a group of butyrate-producing Firmicutes were found.[38,42] Arumugam and colleagues[40] investigated the phylogenetic composition of 39 fecal samples from individuals representing 6 nationalities. They characterized 3 clusters of individual microbiotal composition, referred to as enterotypes, that were not nation specific or continent specific. They identified 3 marker molecules that correlate strongly with the host's body mass index, 2 of which are ATPase complexes, supporting the link found between energy harvest and obesity in the host and suggesting the importance of metagenomic-derived functional biomarkers over phylogenetic ones.

Changes in energy harvesting from diet is also associated with the uptake of SCFAs, end products of bacterial fermentation: in obese humans, the amount of SCFAs in fecal samples was greater than in lean subjects,[42] although the diets rich in nondigestible fibers decrease body weight and severity of diabetes[44]; these contradictory findings could be explained by the anti-inflammatory effects of butyrate.

Furthermore, another pathway has been better studied in humans: the linkage between microbiota and systemic inflammation. LPS administration induces acute inflammation and systemic insulin resistance, stimulating the systemic and adipose tissue expression of proinflammatory and insulin resistance-inducing cytokines.[45]

Consistently in healthy human subjects, total energy intake and high-fat/high-carbohydrate meals, but not fruit/fiber meals, can acutely increased plasma LPS levels, coupled with enhanced TLR4 expression.[22,46]

In summary, the different pathophysiologic factors that explain the association of microbiota with metabolic disturbances have not been studied in depth in human in comparison with animal models, although growing evidences link gut microbiota with endotoxemia and energy harvest from diet.

THERAPEUTIC TARGETS

The mechanisms connecting gut microbiota to obesity could have relevant implications for treatment.

Probiotics

Probiotics are food supplements that contain living bacteria, such as *Bifidobacteria, Lactobacilli, Streptococci*, and nonpathogenic strains of *Escherichia coli*. When administered, they confer beneficial effects to the host because of changes in the gut microbiota that are transient and diminish gradually with time after cessation.[47] Different studies suggest that probiotics influence the intestinal lumen rather than the gut-epithelium, possibly explaining the transient effect of probiotics.[48,49] This thesis was tested by Goossens and colleagues[48]: they compared the effects of consuming *Lactobacillus plantarum* on the microbial colonization of feces and biopsies from the ascending colon and rectum. Within fecal samples, the amount of *Lactobacilli* was significantly increased. The biopsies did not, however, confirm a growth of *Lactobacilli*. Recently, van Baarlen and colleagues[50] described changes in the expression of up to thousands of genes in duodenal biopsies after administration of 3 types of *Lactobacilli*. Alterations in the gut microbiota as a result of probiotics are commonly observed but evidence showing that probiotica administration directly affects inflammatory state has only recently been demonstrated in humans.[51,52] In contrast, studies on the effects of probiotics on characteristics of T2DM are mostly performed in animal models, reporting beneficial effects by various strains of *Lactobacilli* on characteristics of T2DM.[47] Both antidiabetic and anti-inflammatory effects of *Lactobacillus casei* in diet-induced obese mice were recently described.[53] In addition, diet-induced obese mice showed a reduction in body weight gain after they were supplemented with *Lactobacillus rhamnosus PL60* plus an adequate diet.[54] In the same way, Kang and colleagues[55] studied the effects of *Lactobacillus gasseri* BNR17 on diet-induced overweight rats; they found that the percent increase in body weight and fat pad mass was significantly lower in the BNR17 group. Although these animal findings are interesting, the relevance of lactobacilli supplementation for the control of adiposity is a matter of debate. To clarify the effect of Lactobacillus-containing probiotics on weight, Million and colleagues[56] performed a meta-analysis of clinical studies and experimental models. They included 17 RCTs in humans, 51 studies on farm animals, and 14 experimental models and they concluded that different Lactobacillus species are associated different effects on weight change that are host-specific. In particular, *Lactobacillus fermentum* and *Lactobacillus ingluviei* were associated with weight gain in animals; *Lactobacillus plantarum* was associated with weight loss in animals and *Lactobacillus gasseri* was associated with weight loss both in obese humans and in animals.

Prebiotics

Prebiotics (mostly oligosaccharides) are nondigestible but fermentable food ingredients that selectively stimulate the growth or activity of one or multiple gut microbes that are beneficial to their human hosts.[47] The beneficial metabolic effects of prebiotics are in part mediated by a reduction in metabolic endotoxiemia. In physiologic situations, *Bifidobacteria* are capable of lowering LPS levels.[57,58] The number of *Bifidobacteria* was inversely correlated with the development of fat mass, glucose intolerance, and LPS level.[57] High-fat diets promote the growth of LPS-producing gut microbiota and subsequently restrict the amount of *Bifidobacteria*. *Bifidobacterium* spp and *Lactobacillus* spp are sensitive to the administration of certain prebiotics.[59] Prebiotics containing OFS specifically stimulate the growth of these intestinal bacteria.[60,61] OFS administration completely restored *Bifidobacteria* spp and normalized plasma endotoxin levels, leading to improved glucose tolerance, increased satiety, and weight loss in human subjects.[8,62,63] Besides modulating endotoxemia, OFS can alter metabolism in various other manners. Cani and colleagues[64] showed that effects of OFS were mediated via a GLP1-dependent pathway. High-fat–fed diabetic mice on OFS treatment demonstrated improved glucose tolerance, diminished body weight, and decreased endogenous glucose production. Either adding the GLP-1 receptor antagonist exendin 9–39 or using GLP-1 knockout mice resulted in a complete lack of the OFS-mediated beneficial effects, thus showing the causal role of GLP-1 in this pathway in animals. Attempts to translate these findings to human subjects are ambiguous, showing that OFS tends to dose dependently decrease energy intake and increase PYY plasma concentrations,[63,65] but reported effects on satiety are conflicting.[44] Everard and colleagues[66] found that in ob/ob mice, prebiotic feeding decreased Firmicutes and increased Bacteroidetes phyla, improved glucose tolerance, increased L-cell number and associated parameters (intestinal proglucagon mRNA expression and plasma GLP-1 levels), and reduced fat-mass development, oxidative stress, and low-grade inflammation. In high-fat–fed mice, prebiotic treatment improved leptin sensitivity as well as metabolic parameters. Furthermore, OFS fermentation directly affects SFCA butyrate synthesis from extracellular acetate and lactate, implicating the therapeutic potential of prebiotics.[67] In addition, insulin-type fructance decreased the activity of the endocannabinoid system (by reducing the expression of cannabinoid receptor 1, restoring the expression of anandamide-degrading enzyme, and decreasing anandamide levels in the intestinal and adipose tissues), a phenomenon that contributes to an improvement barrier function of the gut and adipogenesis.[68] Finally, insulin-type fructan prebiotics counteract the overespression of GPR43 in the adipose tissue, which is related to a decrease rate of differentiation and a reduce adipocyte size.[69] Thus, available evidence supports the hypothesis that prebiotics can influence metabolic disturbances. The beneficial effect on clinical endpoints in metabolic disturbances remains to be demonstrated in large prospective randomized controlled trials.

SUMMARY

Increased consumption of foods with high energy is involved obesity development, which is a well-known risk factor for T2DM and cardiovascular disease.

Several studies demonstrate gut microbiota can modulate host energy homeostasis and adiposity through different mechanisms: energy harvest from diet, fat storage and expenditure, incretins secretion, and systemic inflammation.

Although experimental data suggest gut microbiota manipulation with probiotics and prebiotics can beneficially affect host adiposity and glucose metabolism, their effects are transient and diminish gradually after cessation. This review analyzes the potential gut microbiota-driven pathways that could represent novel target for treatment of obesity.

REFERENCES

1. Zoetendal EG, Vaughan EE, de Vos WM. A microbial world within us. Mol Microbiol 2006;59:1639–50.
2. Turnbaugh PJ, Hamady M, Yatsunenko T, et al. A core gut microbiome in obese and lean twins. Nature 2009;457:480–4.
3. Backhed F, Ding H, Wang T, et al. The gut microbiota as an environmental factor that regulates fat storage. Proc Natl Acad Sci U S A 2004;101:15718–23.

4. Turnbaugh PJ, Ley RE, Mahowald MA, et al. An obesity-associated gut microbiome with increased capacity for energy harvest. Nature 2006;444:1027–31.
5. Backhed F, Manchester JK, Semenkovich CF, et al. Mechanisms underlying the resistance to diet-induced obesity in germ-free mice. Proc Natl Acad Sci U S A 2007;104:979–84.
6. Ley RE, Bäckhed F, Turnbaugh P, et al. Obesity alters gut microbial ecology. Proc Natl Acad Sci U S A 2005;102:11070–5.
7. Turnbaugh PJ, Bäckhed F, Fulton L, et al. Diet-induced obesity is linked to marked but reversible alterations in the mouse distal gut microbiome. Cell Host Microbe 2008;3:213–23.
8. Cani PD, Amar J, Iglesias MA, et al. Metabolic endotoxemia initiates obesity and insulin resistance. Diabetes 2007;56:1761–72.
9. Vijay-Kumar M, Aitken JD, Carvalho FA, et al. Metabolic syndrome and altered gut microbiota in mice lacking Toll-like receptor 5. Science 2010;328:228–31.
10. Louis P, Flint HJ. Diversity, metabolism and microbial ecology of butyrate producing bacteria from the human large intestine. FEMS Microbiol Lett 2009;294:1–8.
11. Samuel BS, Shaito A, Motoike T, et al. Effects of the gut microbiota on host adiposity are modulated by the short-chain fatty acid binding G proteincoupled receptor, Gpr41. Proc Natl Acad Sci U S A 2008;105:16767–72.
12. Bjursell M, Admyre T, Göransson M, et al. Improved glucose control and reduced body fat mass in free fatty acid receptor 2-deficient mice fed a highfat diet. Am J Physiol Endocrinol Metab 2011;300:211–20.
13. Musso G, Gambino R, Cassader M. Recent insights into hepatic lipid metabolism in non-alcoholic fatty liver disease (NAFLD). Prog Lipid Res 2009;48:1–26.
14. Dutton S, Trayhurn P. Regulation of angiopoietin-like protein 4/fasting-induced adipose factor (Angptl4/FIAF) expression in mouse white adipose tissue and 3T3-L1 adipocytes. Br J Nutr 2008;100:18–26.
15. Musso G, Gambino R, Cassander M. Interactions between gut microbiota and host metabolism predisposing to obesity and diabetes. Annu Rev Med 2011;62:361–80.
16. Aronsson L, Huang Y, Parini P, et al. Decreased fat storage by Lactobacillus paracasei is associated with increased levels of angiopoietin-like 4 protein (ANGPTL4). PLoS One 2010;5:13087.
17. Musso G, Gambino R, Cassader M. Emerging molecular targets for the treatment of nonalcoholic fatty liver disease. Annu Rev Med 2010;61:375–92.
18. Seki E, Brenner DA. TLR and adaptor molecules in liver disease: update. Hepatology 2008;48:322–35.
19. Neyrinck AM, Cani PD, Dewulf EM, et al. Critical role of Kupffer cells in the management of diet-induced diabetes and obesity. Biochem Biophys Res Commun 2009;385:351–6.
20. Huang W, Metlakunta A, Dedousis N, et al. Depletion of liver Kupffer cells prevents the development of diet-induced hepatic steatosis and insulin resistance. Diabetes 2010;59:347–57.
21. Csak T, Ganz M, Pespisa J, et al. Fatty acid and endotoxin activate inflammasomes in mouse hepatocytes that release danger signals to stimulate immune cells. Hepatology 2011;54(1):133–44.
22. Cani PD, Bibiloni R, Knauf C, et al. Changes in gut microbiota control metabolic endotoxemia-induced inflammation in high-fat diet–induced obesity and diabetes in mice. Diabetes 2008;57:1470–81.
23. Osto M, Zini E, Franchini M, et al. Subacute endotoxemia induces adipose inflammation and changes in lipid and lipoprotein metabolism in cats. Endocrinology 2011;152:804–15.

24. Cani PD, Possemiers S, Van de Wiele T, et al. Changes in gut microbiota control inflammation in obese mice through a mechanism involving GLP-2-driven improvement of gut permeability. Gut 2009;58:1091–103.
25. Zhou J, Martin RJ, Tulley RT, et al. Dietary resistant starch upregulates total GLP-1 and PYY in a sustained day-long manner through fermentation in rodents. Am J Physiol Endocrinol Metab 2008;295:E1160–6.
26. Gorissen L, Raes K, Weckx S, et al. Production of conjugated linoleic acid and conjugated linolenic acid isomers by Bifidobacterium species. Appl Microbiol Biotechnol 2010;87:2257–66.
27. Devillard E, McIntosh FM, Paillard D, et al. Differences between human subjects in the composition of the faecal bacterial community and faecal metabolism of linoleic acid. Microbiology 2009;155(Pt 2):513–20.
28. Wall R, Ross RP, Shanahan F, et al. Metabolic activity of the enteric microbiota influences the fatty acid composition of murine and porcine liver and adipose tissues. Am J Clin Nutr 2009;89:1393–401.
29. Lewis K, Lutgendorff F, Phan V, et al. Enhanced translocation of bacteria across metabolically stressed epithelia is reduced by butyrate. Inflamm Bowel Dis 2010; 16:1138–48.
30. Freeland KR, Wolever TM. Acute effects of intravenous and rectal acetate on glucagon-like peptide-1, peptide YY, ghrelin, adiponectin and tumour necrosis factor-alpha. Br J Nutr 2010;103:460–6.
31. Parikh SJ, Edelman M, Uwaifo GI, et al. The relationship between obesity and serum 1,25-dihydroxy vitamin D concentrations in healthy adults. J Clin Endocrinol Metab 2004;89:1196–9.
32. Mai V, McCrary QM, Sinha R, et al. Associations between dietary habits and body mass index with gut microbiota composition and fecal water genotoxicity: an observational study in African American and Caucasian American volunteers. Nutr J 2009;8:49.
33. Adorini L, Penna G. Dendritic cell tolerogenicity: a key mechanism in immunomodulation by vitamin D receptor agonists. Hum Immunol 2009;70:345–52.
34. Yu S, Bruce D, Froicu M, et al. Failure of T cell homing, reduced CD4/CD8alphaalpha intraepithelial lymphocytes, and inflammation in the gut of vitamin D receptor KO mice. Proc Natl Acad Sci U S A 2008;105:20834–9.
35. Wu S, Liao AP, Xia Y, et al. Vitamin D receptor negatively regulates bacterial-stimulated NF-kappaB activity in intestine. Am J Pathol 2010;177:686–97.
36. Ley RE, Turnbaugh PJ, Klein S, et al. Microbial ecology: human gut microbes associated with obesity. Nature 2006;444:1022–3.
37. Zhang H, DiBaise JK, Zuccolo A, et al. Human gut microbiota in obesity and after gastric bypass. Proc Natl Acad Sci U S A 2009;106:2365–70.
38. Duncan SH, Lobley GE, Holtrop G, et al. Human colonic microbiota associated with diet, obesity and weight loss. Int J Obes 2008;32:1720–4.
39. Santacruz A, Marcos A, Wärnberg J, et al. Interplay between weight loss and gut microbiota composition in overweight adolescents. Obesity (Silver Spring) 2009; 17:1906–15.
40. Nadal I, Santacruz A, Marcos A, et al. Shifts in clostridia, bacteroides and immunoglobulin-coating fecal bacteria associated with weight loss in obese adolescents. Int J Obes 2009;33:758–67.
41. Kalliomaki M, Collado MC, Salminen S, et al. Early differences in fecal microbiota composition in children may predict overweight. Am J Clin Nutr 2008;87:534–8.
42. Schwiertz A, Taras D, Schäfer K, et al. Microbiota and SCFA in lean and overweight healthy subjects. Obesity (Silver Spring) 2010;18(1):190–5.

43. Arumugam M, Raes J, Pelletier E, et al. Enterotypes of the human gut micro-biome. Nature 2011;473(7346):174–80 [Erratum appears in Nature 2011;474(7353):666].

44. Cani PD, Joly E, Horsmans Y, et al. Oligofructose promotes satiety in healthy human: a pilot study. Eur J Clin Nutr 2006;60:567–72.

45. Mehta N, McGillicuddy FC, Anderson PD, et al. Experimental endotoxemia in-duces adipose inflammation and insulin resistance in humans. Diabetes 2010; 59:172–81.

46. Ghanim H, Abuaysheh S, Sia CL, et al. Increase in plasma endotoxin concentra-tions and the expression of Toll-like receptors and suppressor of cytokine signaling-3 in mononuclear cells after a high-fat, high-carbohydrate meal: impli-cations for insulin resistance. Diabetes Care 2009;32:2281–7.

47. Kootte RS, Vrieze A, Holleman F, et al. The therapeutic potential of manipulating gut microbiota in obesity and type 2 diabetes mellitus. Diabetes Obes Metab 2012;14(2):112–20.

48. Goossens DA, Jonkers DM, Russel MG, et al. The effect of a probiotic drink with Lactobacillus plantarum 299v on the bacterial composition in faeces and mucosal biopsies of rectum and ascending colon. Aliment Pharmacol Ther 2006;23(2):255–63.

49. Martin FP, Wang Y, Sprenger N, et al. Probiotic modulation of symbiotic gut microbial-host metabolic interactions in a humanized microbiome mouse model. Mol Syst Biol 2008;4:157.

50. van Baarlen P, Troost F, van der Meer C, et al. Human mucosal in vivo transcrip-tome responses to three lactobacilli indicate how probiotics may modulate human cellular pathways. Proc Natl Acad Sci U S A 2011;108(Suppl 1):4562–9.

51. Konstantinov SR, Smidt H, de Vos WM, et al. S layer protein A of Lactobacillus acidophilus NCFM regulates immature dendritic cell and T cell functions. Proc Natl Acad Sci U S A 2008;105:19474–9.

52. van Baarlen P, Troost FJ, van HS, et al. Differential NF-kappaB pathways induc-tion by Lactobacillus plantarum in the duodenum of healthy humans correlating with immune tolerance. Proc Natl Acad Sci U S A 2009;106:2371–6.

53. Naito E, Yoshida Y, Makino K, et al. Beneficial effect of oral administration of Lactobacillus casei strain Shirota on insulin resistance in diet-induced obesity mice. J Appl Microbiol 2011;110:650–7.

54. Lee HY, Park JH, Seok SH, et al. Human originated bacteria, Lactobacillus rham-nosus PL60, produce conjugated linoleic acid and show anti-obesity effects in diet-induced obese mice. Biochim Biophys Acta 2006;1761:736–44.

55. Kang JH, Yun SI, Park HO. Effects of Lactobacillus gasseri BNR17 on body weight and adipose tissue mass in diet-induced overweight rats. J Microbiol 2010;48:712–4.

56. Million M, Angelakis E, Paul M, et al. Comparative meta-analysis of the effect of Lactobacillus species on weight gain in humans and animals. Microb Pathog 2012;53(2):100–8.

57. Cani PD, Neyrinck AM, Fava F, et al. Selective increases of bifidobacteria in gut microflora improve high-fat-diet-induced diabetes in mice through a mechanism associated with endotoxaemia. Diabetologia 2007;50:2374–83.

58. Griffiths EA, Duffy LC, Schanbacher FL, et al. In vivo effects of bifidobacteria and lactoferrin on gut endotoxin concentration and mucosal immunity in Balb/c mice. Dig Dis Sci 2004;49:579–89.

59. Meyer D, Stasse-Wolthuis M. The bifidogenic effect of inulin and oligofructose and its consequences for gut health. Eur J Clin Nutr 2009;63(11):1277–89.

60. Silk DB, Davis A, Vulevic J, et al. Clinical trial: the effects of a trans-galactooligosaccharide prebiotic on faecal microbiota and symptoms in irritable bowel syndrome. Aliment Pharmacol Ther 2009;29(5):508–18.
61. Tuohy KM, Rouzaud GC, Bruck WM, et al. Modulation of the human gut microflora towards improved health using prebiotics—assessment of efficacy. Curr Pharm Des 2005;11(1):75–90.
62. Cani PD, Lecourt E, Dewulf EM, et al. Gut microbiota fermentation of prebiotics increases satietogenic and incretin gut peptide production with consequences for appetite sensation and glucose response after a meal. Am J Clin Nutr 2009;90(5):1236–43.
63. Parnell JA, Reimer RA. Weight loss during oligofructose supplementation is associated with decreased ghrelin and increased peptide YY in overweight and obese adults. Am J Clin Nutr 2009;89(6):1751–9.
64. Cani PD, Knauf C, Iglesias MA, et al. Improvement of glucose tolerance and hepatic insulin sensitivity by oligofructose requires a functional glucagon-like peptide 1 receptor. Diabetes 2006;55:1484–90.
65. Verhoef SP, Meyer D, Westerterp KR. Effects of oligofructose on appetite profile, glucagon-like peptide 1 and peptide YY3-36 concentrations and energy intake. Br J Nutr 2011;106:1757–62.
66. Everard A, Lazarevic V, Derrien M, et al. Responses of gut microbiota and glucose and lipid metabolism to prebiotics in genetic obese and diet-induced leptin-resistant mice. Diabetes 2011;60(11):2775–86.
67. Morrison DJ, Mackay WG, Edwards CA, et al. Butyrate production from oligofructose fermentation by the human faecal flora: what is the contribution of extracellular acetate and lactate? Br J Nutr 2006;96(3):570.
68. Muccioli GG, Naslain D, Backhed F, et al. The endocannabinoid system links gut microbiota to adipogenesis. Mol Syst Biol 2010;6:392.
69. Dewulf EM, Cani PD, Nevrinck AM, et al. Inulin-type fructans with prebiotic properties counteract GPR43 overexpression and PPARγ-related adipogenesis in the white adipose tissue of high-fat diet-fed mice. J Nutr Biochem 2011;22(8): 712–22.

Surgical Management of Adolescent Obesity

Sean J. Barnett, MD, MS

KEYWORDS

• Morbid obesity • Adolescents • Bariatric surgery • Comorbidities • Weight loss

KEY POINTS

- Morbid obesity continues to see a rapid increase in pediatric and adolescent populations. Morbidly obese adolescents develop significant comorbidities that continue on into adulthood. Although medical management in the overweight population of children can be helpful, morbidly obese adolescents do not show significant long-term weight reduction with lifestyle modification.
- Bariatric surgery is a safe and long-term solution in selected morbidly obese adolescents who are physically and psychosocially mature.
- Adolescent bariatric surgical patients require lifelong dietary modification and follow-up to ensure adequate nutritional supplementation. Roux-en-Y gastric bypass (RYGB) remains the gold standard operation but sleeve gastrectomy (SG) continues to gain rapid prominence, given its simplicity and reduced postoperative complication rates.
- The adjustable gastric band (AGB) in the adolescent population can be efficacious compared with medical therapy but has demonstrated significantly higher complication and reoperation rates compared with its use in adults. More long-term, longitudinal studies are necessary to firmly establish guidelines for patient selection and optimal procedure choice.

INTRODUCTION

It has been estimated that approximately 18% of all children and adolescents meet the criteria of being overweight or obese in the United States, a rate that has almost tripled over the past 30 years [1]. Of these overweight children, 50% to 77% will continue to be obese into adulthood, carrying with them all the associated comorbidities [2–4]. More alarming, however, are the approximately 4% to 7% of all children and adolescents (more than 2 million) considered morbidly obese (body mass index [BMI] >99th percentile) in this country [2,5,6]. These data parallel recent National Health and Nutrition Examination Survey (NHANES) data demonstrating that approximately two-thirds

---

This article originally appeared in Advances in Pediatrics, Volume 60, 2013.
Disclosures: The author has no relevant financial relationships to disclose.
Division of Pediatric General & Thoracic Surgery, Cincinnati Children's Hospital Medical Center, 3333 Burnet Avenue, Cincinnati, OH 45215, USA
E-mail address: sean.barnett@cchmc.org

Clinics Collections 3 (2014) 233–246
http://dx.doi.org/10.1016/j.ccol.2014.09.043
2352-7986/14/$ – see front matter © 2014 Elsevier Inc. All rights reserved.

of US adults are considered overweight and more than one-third considered obese [7]. The importance of these data cannot be overlooked given the long-term health, psychosocial, and economic ramifications of childhood obesity.

Although behavioral weight management programs have been shown to have lasting effects in some children, these approaches are ineffective in those patients who are morbidly obese [8]. Of those morbidly obese children undergoing behavioral weight loss, one-third to one-half cannot even complete a program. Those who complete a program lose, on average, 5 pounds (3% weight loss), which is not maintained 7 months later [8]. These findings lend toward performing bariatric surgery on morbidly obese adolescents to provide longer-lasting overall weight loss and comorbidity reduction. This article discusses the definition of pediatric obesity and the comorbidities of morbid obesity in children and adolescents, provides guidelines for performing bariatric surgery in adolescents, discusses the procedures and their outcomes in this patient population, and provides a framework for postoperative care.

DEFINITION

The prevailing standard for measurement of obesity in the adult population is body mass index (BMI kg/m^2). This is a simple way to define obesity in those who have attained their full adult height. By definition, adults are considered overweight with a BMI greater than 25 kg/m^2 and considered obese with a BMI greater than or equal to 30 kg/m^2. These numbers can be extrapolated over different ethnic groups and populations to allow for easy formation of guidelines for treatment.

In children and adolescents, the use of BMI becomes more complicated due to the physiologic changes in adiposity with height and weight changes during normal growth. Therefore, growth charts are used for most children and adolescents that are both age specific and gender specific to better define obesity throughout childhood [9]. General guidelines throughout the literature define pediatric obesity as a BMI greater than the 95th percentile for age and gender, with those greater than the 99th percentile considered severely obese (BMI >35 kg/m^2, consistent with the definition for adults) [10]. These definitions present unique problems in defining those individuals at the extreme categories of obesity, given the relative paucity of population-based data to calculate these percentile boundaries. This definition is compounded by the small number of children and adolescents with a BMI greater than 40 kg/m^2 represented in the data sets used to formulate pediatric growth charts, namely NHANES. Because most adolescents with a BMI greater than 35 kg/m^2 are greater than the 99th BMI percentile for current growth charts [2], it is appropriate to use adult selection criterion for the use of bariatric surgery in this patient population. Thresholds should be considered general guidelines and those with significant comorbidities should also be considered for bariatric surgery despite regard for BMI.

COMORBIDITIES ASSOCIATED WITH MORBID OBESITY IN ADOLESCENTS

Given the relative explosion in the prevalence of pediatric obesity over the past 30 years, there has been a parallel increase in the frequency and severity of obesity-related comorbidities in morbidly obese adolescents. These disease states are frequently seen at a much younger age than previously encountered, encompass a wide range of organ systems, and carry subsequent increased risks into adulthood [11–14].

Glucose intolerance

Although a frequent manifestation of adult obesity, it has been demonstrated that there has been a significant (more than 10-fold) increase in the prevalence of type 2 diabetes mellitus in adolescents over the past decade [15]. Even more striking is the finding that up to 25% of all obese children and adolescents have some form of impaired glucose intolerance [16]. Insulin resistance has been clearly linked with childhood obesity [17], and studies suggest that type 2 diabetes mellitus developing in childhood or in adolescence can progress more rapidly than in adults [18]. Type 2 diabetes mellitus in adolescents is considered a chronic and progressive disease associated with many other comorbidities, including dyslipidemia, hypertension, cardiac disease, and nonalcoholic liver disease [19,20]. In a recent study published by the Centers for Disease Control and Prevention, epidemiologists predict that type 2 diabetes mellitus is expected to develop in 33% to 50% of all Americans born in the year 2000 [21].

Cardiovascular disease

Risk factors for atherosclerosis and coronary artery disease are common in obese adolescents [22–24], with approximately 60% of obese children in the Bogalusa Heart Study having 1 of these factors and 20% having 2 or more of these factors [25]. Hypertension occurs at a 9-fold increased rate in obese children [26] and is a well-known risk factor for the development of cardiac disease in adults. Furthermore, there has been a linear increase in the development of cardiovascular risk factors in relation to increased BMI in children [27]. The incidence of left ventricular hypertrophy has also been shown significantly increased in young adults as a direct consequence of comorbidities related to adolescent obesity, namely obstructive sleep apnea [28].

Obstructive sleep apnea

Up to 20% of school-aged children with obesity are reported to have either moderate or severe sleep apnea [29]. Data associates poor school performance with sleep deprivation and disordered sleep patterns [30,31], both of which are common in obese children and adolescents,as well as placing them at increased risk for hyperactivity and learning difficulties throughout life [32]. Adolescents with sleep apnea also exhibit significant left ventricular hypertrophy [28] and abnormal ventricular dimensions [33], which have not been found improved with medical weight loss alone [34].

Nonalcoholic fatty liver disease and nonalcoholic steatohepatitis

Approximately 38% of obese adolescents have steatosis and 9% have nonalcoholic steatohepatitis (NASH) compared with 5% and 1%, respectively, in their lean counterparts [35]. Of those undergoing bariatric surgery at Cincinnati Children's Hospital, 83% have evidence of fatty liver disease, with 20% formally demonstrating NASH [36]. The most serious consequence of liver damage associated with obesity is fibrosis coupled with accelerated cirrhosis, ultimately leading to end-stage liver disease.

Pseudotumor cerebri

Pseudotumor cerebri is a rare progressive childhood disorder associated with increased intracranial pressure that often leads to papilledema and blindness. The relationship between obesity and symptom onset is unclear. As many as 50% of children with pseudotumor cerebri are obese [37] and, with extensive weight loss after bariatric surgery, it can improve in both adults [38] and in adolescents [39].

Psychological aspects

A significant number of adolescents seeking treatment of their obesity present with differing stages of clinical depression [40]. Many obese adolescents have been found to have low self-esteem and can engage in high-risk behaviors [41], and obesity has been found to have a significant negative effect on their quality of life [42]. Obese adolescents also demonstrate significantly lower quality-of-life scores than lean children with scores and are comparable with pediatric cancer patients [43]. Women who were overweight as adolescents are also less likely to marry and have completed fewer years of school compared with their lean counterparts [44]. A recent longitudinal study demonstrated a significant improvement in depressive symptoms and quality of life over the first postoperative period after bariatric surgery in adolescents [45].

Summary

The large mounting body of literature demonstrating the significant number of comorbidities associated with obesity coupled with their relative lack of resolution by medical weight loss means in the morbidly obese has led to a large body of evidence in support of the use of modern weight loss operations for selected, morbidly obese adolescents. Bariatric surgery has been shown to completely resolve type 2 diabetes mellitus in adolescents who have undergone gastric bypass [46]. It has also shown a dramatic reduction in the severity of obstructive sleep apnea symptoms in all patients, with complete resolution of symptoms in 90% [47]. A decrease in the degree of steatosis and regression of hepatic fibrosis has been found in some patients after bariatric surgery [48]. These data, coupled with the improvements in pseudotumor cerebri and psychosocial behaviors (discussed previously), support the early use of bariatric surgical procedures in the adolescent population.

GUIDELINES FOR SURGERY

Best practice guidelines by the American Society for Metabolic and Bariatric Surgery have been recently updated and published [49]. As discussed previously, most adolescents with a BMI greater than 35 kg/m^2 are greater than the 99th percentile; therefore, adult criteria for selection are considered appropriate for adolescents. Current recommendations have not changed significantly since the last best practice guidelines were set in 2009 (**Table 1**) [50]. In summary, these include those individuals with a BMI greater than or equal to 35 kg/m^2 with significant major comorbidities, which include type 2 diabetes mellitus, pseudotumor cerebri, severe NASH, and moderate to severe obstructive sleep apnea (apnea-hypopnea index >15). Those individuals with a BMI greater than or equal to 40 kg/m^2 with less severe comorbid disease, including glucose intolerance, hypertension, dyslipidemia, mild to moderate obstructive sleep apnea (apnea-hypopnea index >5), and impaired quality of life, are also thought to meet criteria for bariatric surgery [49]. Given that these are merely guidelines for treatment, exceptions can be made in extenuating circumstances if the potential long-term health risks outweigh the risks of bariatric surgery.

Because adolescence represents an extensive period of growth, the timing for surgical treatment remains controversial and depends on the compelling needs of patients. For those adolescents who have attained the majority of linear growth

Table 1	
Patient selection criteria for adolescent weight loss surgery	
BMI (kg/m^2)	**Comorbidities**
>35	Type 2 diabetes mellitus, moderate of severe obstructive sleep apnea, pseudotumor cerebri, severe NASH
>40	Mild obstructive sleep apnea, hypertension, insulin resistance, glucose intolerance, dyslipidemia, impaired quality of life

Data from Michalsky M, Reichard K, Inge T, et al. ASMBS pediatric committee best practice guidelines. Surg Obes Relat Dis 2012;8:1–7.

(>95%), there is little reason to believe that bariatric surgery will impair growth. Physiologic maturation is generally complete by sexual maturation (Tanner stage 4) [51]. Skeletal maturation (adult stature) is normally attained by the age 13 to 14 in girls and age 15 to 16 in boys [52]. The onset of menarche is also a sign of physiologic maturity in girls, with growth usually complete within 2 years after menarche. For those patients for whom physical maturation is uncertain, bone age can be assessed by plain radiography of the hand or wrist and estimated by a radiologist via nomograms.

Coupled with physiologic factors of maturation in adolescents is the determination of a patient's psychosocial maturity level. Patients should not only be able to demonstrate a general understanding of the risks and benefits of surgery but also the long-term ramifications after bariatric surgical procedures and ability to comply with vitamin and nutritional recommendations. Although the majority of patients cannot consent for themselves, it is expected that patients provide assent for the procedure. It is paramount that a patient's parents are readily involved in the entire process in order to assess support mechanisms, determine and ensure the likelihood of postoperative compliance, and provide adequate consent for the procedure.

Specific recommendations regarding team member qualifications have been made to maximize the multidisciplinary approach required for bariatric surgery in adolescents [49]. These include, but are not limited to, the following:

- Surgeon: The surgeon performing adolescent bariatric surgery should meet the general certification requirements of the American Board of Surgery and have appropriate training and experience in performing bariatric procedures. The individual should be credentialed by the institution to perform such procedures, but it is not necessary to be boarded specifically in pediatric surgery. As an example, Cincinnati Children's Hospital has 4 board-certified surgeons (adult and pediatric) who have extensive knowledge and training in the various bariatric surgical procedures performed.

- Medical specialist: Includes at least one physician with specialty training in endocrinology, gastroenterology, nutrition, or adolescent medicine. The main responsibilities of this team member are the screening and management of a patient's comorbid conditions with the team and the patient's primary care physician. My program uses a board-certified pediatric gastroenterologist as its medical director (which comes in handy for those patients who require preoperative and postoperative endoscopy) and a board-certified adolescent medicine physician who assists with the care of the majority of female patients who experience menstrual dysfunction.

- Registered dietitian: Arguably the most important part of the overall program, the dietitian should have extensive experience in treating adolescents and their families with obesity. The dietician sets the tone during the preoperative phase of the program and helps manage patient questions and concerns throughout the postoperative phase.

- Mental health specialist: Includes a psychologist, psychiatrist, or other independently licensed metal health provider with specific training in pediatric, adolescent, and family treatment. The individual should also have experience in treating those patients with obesity and eating disorders. My psychologist plays a pivotal role during the initial assessment to ensure that patients are psychologically ready to begin the program and to help garner the necessary resources required to move past the preoperative phase.

- Program coordinator: Includes a registered nurse, social worker, or business specialist whose main responsibility is the coordinating of care to help facilitate compliance and follow-up. My coordinator also works with patients' insurance companies to ensure coverage for treatment and procedures.

- Exercise physiologist or specialist: This specialist provides safe physical activity education for morbidly obese patients.
- Social worker: A dedicated social worker is not required but is highly recommended. In my program, she monitors patients' psychosocial health as well as communicates with patient therapists on a regular basis. She also manages the support group, access to resources, and various functions throughout the year.
- Nurse practioner: This position is not required but is an integral part of the team at Cincinnati Children's Hospital. She has an ongoing dialogue with all my patients and literally has her hands on the pulse of the program. She also helps manage many of the medical problems of the patients within the program on a daily basis.

With the various team members comes a significant commitment of the institution to provide safe and quality care for these difficult patients. A recent article, published in *Pediatrics* in 2011, sought to develop certain criteria for pediatric/adolescent bariatric surgery programs [53]. Michalsky and colleagues [53] propose 10 criteria for proposed specialty programs, including (1) institutional commitment, (2) a defined medical home for patients, (3) routine experience in laparoscopic bariatric procedures, (4) program staffing (discussed previously), (5) multidisciplinary review for each patient, (6) specialized equipment (hospital beds, patient transfer systems, operating room tables, and adequate radiologic facilities), (7) standardized care using clinical pathways, (8) follow-up care, (9) support groups, and (10) transition of care as patients move into adulthood. The ability to meet these criteria help to ensure a well-rounded program that is able to meet all the needs of morbidly obese adolescents.

PROCEDURES AND OUTCOMES

The experience of several small series suggests that gastric bypass, AGB, and SG can be performed routinely, safely, and effectively in adolescents [54,55–65]. To date, however, adolescent bariatric surgery has not been evaluated in a longitudinal or prospective manner. To address these shortcomings in outcomes for adolescent bariatric surgery, a consortium of 5 pediatric institutions is currently involved in a National Institutes of Health–funded study, designed to collect standardized prospective preoperative and postoperative clinical data longitudinally (Teen–Longitudinal Assessment of Bariatric Surgery [Teen-Labs]). Accrual of patients for the study is complete and the initial data are being analyzed with initial results set to be published by the end of this year.

There have been many bariatric operations performed in adolescents in the past but the remainder of this section focuses on the 3 most commonly performed operations to date. These include the AGB, RYGB, and SG (**Fig. 1**). All the operations are performed laparoscopically. Minimally invasive bariatric surgery has significant advantages over open surgery, namely the reduction of complications, length of stay, and pain postoperatively, but is one of the most technically difficult procedures performed [66].

ADJUSTABLE GASTRIC BAND

The Food and Drug Administration approved the use of Lap-Band (Allergan, Irvine, California) for use in adults in the United States in 2001 and the Realize Band (Ethicon, Cincinnati, Ohio) shortly thereafter. Prior to its introduction into the United States, the AGB procedure was the most commonly performed procedure in Europe, Latin America, and Australia. It is not currently approved for patients under age 18 by the Food

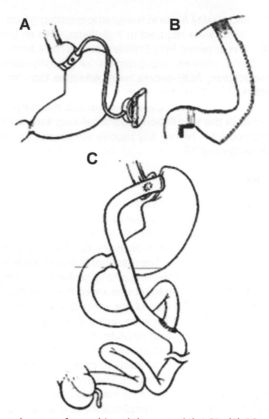

Fig. 1. Bariatric procedures performed in adolescents: (A) AGB, (B) SG, and (C) RYGB.

and Drug Administration, with results of an ongoing national study awaiting publication. Given its current restrictions, studies in adolescents are generally found to originate from outside the United States.

The laparoscopically placed gastric band creates a small pouch in the upper portion of the stomach, acting solely as a restrictive procedure. A balloon on the inside of the band is connected to a port placed in the subcutaneous tissues of the upper abdomen (see **Fig. 1A**). The port can be accessed by a small-gauge needle to perform periodic adjustments by placing or removing sterile water into the system. This in turn changes the size of the balloon around the stomach, thus changing the size of the functional stoma that it creates. These periodic adjustments are critical for the overall success of the band and require as many as 10 visits over the course of the first postoperative year. The procedure generally requires 45 to 60 minutes to complete, patients are discharged on the same day or next day, and there is no cutting or stapling of the stomach or intestine. Complications include gastric prolapse, stomal obstruction, band erosion, and, most commonly, access port or tubing problems. These seem similar when comparing adolescent AGBs with their adult counterparts.

A recent study from Australia followed patients with a BMI greater than 35 for 2 years randomized to either supervised lifestyle intervention or gastric banding [57]. The main outcomes were weight loss and adverse outcomes; 24 of the 25 gastric banding patients and 18 of 25 lifestyle modification patients completed the study. A mean excess weight loss of 78.8% was seen in the banding group and 13.2% in the lifestyle modification group. The study also noted significant improvement in features of the metabolic syndrome and quality of life in the gastric banding group. Alarmingly, however, 8 reoperations (33%) were required in 7 patients, with an overall complication rate of 48% over the 2-year period [57]. Smaller studies have achieved similar results with many experiencing marked improvement of obesity-related comorbidities [63,64]. Given these studies, AGB seems more effective than lifestyle modification alone and can result in a significant reduction in comorbidities. Given the much higher complication rate in adolescents compared with adults, the surgeon must be careful when considering AGB in this population. Additional long-term data are forthcoming from industry-sponsored trials before any recommendation can be made regarding their use in patients under age 18.

SLEEVE GASTRECTOMY

The SG is rapidly gaining acceptance as a primary operation in both adult and adolescent populations. Once considered only part of the larger duodenal switch operation, it has been shown to offer significant weight loss with fewer complications than gastric bypass [67]. This restrictive procedure involves the longitudinal resection of the stomach along a narrow 34-French bougie. The resection extends approximately 6 cm from the pylorus to the angle of His, thus creating a long gastric tube along the lesser curve of the stomach. The fundus and greater curvature of the stomach are removed (see **Fig. 1B**). The mechanism of weight loss is not yet understood but may be the result of both restriction and alteration of appetite and satiety signals from the gut to the brain, including changes in ghrelin and peptide YY levels [68]. Literature regarding its effectiveness in the pediatric population is growing [62,67–72] but continues to be sparse. The largest single institutional study to date reported outcomes of 108 adolescents undergoing SG in Saudi Arabia [62]. The investigators reported a significant reduction in BMI of 37% at 1 year, similar to previously reported studies in this country after gastric bypass [73], with no major complications or deaths. Significant reductions in type 2 diabetes mellitus, sleep apnea, hypertension, and dyslipidemia were also noted.

Given these promising findings, and with the help of additional longitudinal prospective studies like the current Teen-Labs study, SG seems a viable option for bariatric surgery in adolescents.

ROUX-EN-Y GASTRIC BYPASS

RYGB is both a restrictive and malabsorptive procedure and is considered the gold standard for bariatric surgical procedures in the United States. The restrictive component is a small gastric pouch (approximately 15–20 mL in size) coupled with a small gastric outlet (2–3 cm in diameter) that results in early and sustained satiety. The malabsorptive component involves re-establishing intestinal continuity with a gastric bypass segment of varying lengths between 100 cm and 150 cm (see **Fig. 1C**).

Currently, there have been no procedure-related deaths reported in adolescents undergoing RYGB. Early complications include pulmonary embolism, wound infections, stomal stenosis, and marginal ulcers. Late complications have included small bowel obstruction, incisional hernias, symptomatic cholelithiasis, protein calorie and micronutrient deficiencies, and late weight regain (10%–15% incidence) [53,65,73]. These complications parallel their adult counterparts and stress the requirement of lifelong follow-up. The majority of weight can be expected to be lost within the first 18 to 24 months after surgery.

Two recent studies in adolescents have demonstrated similar postoperative outcomes compared with adults. A recent meta-analysis of 6 studies involving adolescent

RYGB demonstrated a significant reduction in excess body weight with improvement in associated comorbidities [74]. A recent report from Cincinnati Children's Hospital demonstrated a significant reduction in BMI (35%–37%) within the first year after RYGB in adolescents [73]. One finding from that article showed an equal percentage of weight reduction despite the preoperative BMI. Unfortunately, those patients who started out heavier (BMI >60), despite losing a significant amount of weight, remained morbidly obese at 1 year. This demonstrates the need for earlier referral to ensure adequate weight loss to maximize comorbidity reduction. Several studies (cited previously in this review) demonstrate the resolution of numerous comorbid states in adolescents, including hypertension [74], sleep apnea [75], and type 2 diabetes mellitus [46], and psychosocial improvements [45]. Given these findings, the current literature supports the use of RYGB as a safe and efficacious means for significant weight loss and comorbidity reduction. As discussed previously, the Teen-Labs study should help strengthen the literature once outcomes are reported.

POSTOPERATIVE MANAGEMENT

It is of the utmost importance for a bariatric patient's primary care physician to become familiar with the physiologic changes that occur after bariatric surgery. This allows for effective partnership between the bariatric team and the primary physician for the care of the patient after the operation.

Patients generally spend between 2 and 3 nights after their operation in the hospital and are discharged home on clear liquids. They are advanced fairly quickly to a high-protein liquid diet, which is usually maintained for at least 1 month after surgery. The postoperative diet is methodically advanced by introducing new food choices toward the goal of a well-balanced, small-portion (approximately 1 cup) diet, ensuring a daily intake of 1 g of protein per kilogram of ideal body weight. Patients are encouraged to eat proteins first during every meal to ensure their adequate intake. Nonsteroidal anti-inflammatory medications are generally avoided to reduce the risk of ulcer formation. Postoperative nausea is common after SG and most patients are discharged home on antinausea medications. The nausea tends to resolve within the first week after surgery. Reflux is also common after SG with approximately half of my patients requiring proton pump inhibitors for at least the first 6 postoperative months. Routine postoperative vitamin supplementation is the key for all operations, given the significant reduction in nutrients (AGB and SG) and combined malabsorption (RYGB). The typical regimen consists of 2 pediatric chewable multivitamins, a calcium supplement, and an iron supplement for menstruating women. B-complex vitamins are also supplemented beyond the typical multivitamin primarily to augment thiamine and folate supplementation (**Table 2**) [76]. Severe complications can arise with their deficiency, specifically in those who undergo RYGB [77].

There are 5 basic rules that are routinely emphasized with patients and family at each visit: (1) eat protein first; (2) drink 64 oz to 96 oz of water or sugar-free liquids daily; (3) no snacking between meals; (4) exercise at least 30 minutes per day; and (5) always remember vitamins and minerals.

All bariatric surgeries, to varying degrees, result in surgically enforced, low-calorie, low-carbohydrate intake, which, in turn, requires intensive attention to ensure adequate intake of important macronutrients and micronutrients. Postoperative follow-up consists of an initial visit 2 weeks after surgery. After this initial visit, patients are seen during regular intervals within my program (6 weeks, and then generally every 3 months for the first 18 months postoperatively). Patients are then generally seen on an annual basis. Serum chemistries, complete blood cell count, urine specific gravity,

Table 2	
Recommended nutritional supplementation after weight loss surgery	
Supplement	**Recommendation**
Multivitamin (with folic acid)	1 to 2 Daily
Calcium citrate with vitamin D	1500–1800 mg/d
Vitamin D	1000 IU/d (if deficiency found preoperatiavely)
Vitamin B$_{12}$	500 μg/d Oral or 1000 μg/mo intramuscular
Elemental iron	65 mg Elemental iron for menstruating women
Vitamin B$_1$	Consider 50 mg daily in first 6 mo
Vitamins A and K	Treat if symptomatic

Laboratory results are checked at 6 months postoperatively and then yearly unless symptoms arise.
Data from Xanthakos SA. Nutritional deficiencies in obesity and after bariatric surgery. Pediatr Clin North Am 2009;56(5):1105–21.

prothrombin time (evidence of vitamin K adequacy), and representative B-complex vitamin levels (eg, B$_1$, B$_{12}$, and folate) are obtained at regular intervals. Upper gastro-intestinal series are usually obtained yearly in our SG patients and on an as-needed basis otherwise.

SUMMARY

Morbid obesity continues to see a rapid increase in pediatric and adolescent populations. These patients develop significant comorbidities that continue into adulthood. Although medical management in the overweight population of children can be helpful, the morbidly obese adolescents do not show significant long-term weight reduction with lifestyle modification. Bariatric surgery is a safe and long-term solution in selected morbidly obese adolescents who are physically and psychosocially mature. Adolescent bariatric surgical patients require lifelong dietary modification and follow-up to ensure adequate nutritional supplementation. RYGB remains the gold standard operation but SG continues to gain rapid prominence, given its simplicity and reduced postoperative complication rates. AGB in the adolescent population can be efficacious compared with medical therapy but has demonstrated significantly higher complication and reoperation rates compared with its use in adults. It remains to be approved by the Food and Drug Administration only for those 18 years of age and older. More long-term, longitudinal studies are necessary to firmly establish guidelines for patient selection and optimal procedure choice.

REFERENCES

[1]. Ogden CL, Carroll MD, Curtin LR, et al. Prevalence of overweight and obesity in the United States, 1999-2004. JAMA 2006;295(13):1549–55.
[2]. Freedman DS, Mei Z, Srinivasan SR, et al. Cardiovascular risk factors and excess adiposity among overweight children and adolescents: the Bogalusa Heart Study. J Pediatr 2007;150:12–7.
[3]. Strauss RS, Pollack HA. Epidemic increase in childhood overweight. 1986-1998. JAMA 2001;286:2845–8.
[4]. Parsons TJ, Powers C, Logan S, et al. Childhood predictors of adult obesity: a systematic review. Int J Obes Relat Metab Disord 1999;23(Suppl 8):S1–107.
[5]. Skelton JA, Cook SR, Auinger P, et al. Prevalence and trends of severe obesity among US children and adolescents. Acad Pediatr 2009;9:322–9.

[6]. Koebnick C, Smith N, Coleman KJ, et al. Prevalence of extreme obesity in a multiethnic cohort of children and adolescents. J Pediatr 2010;157:26–31.e2.

[7]. Flegal KM, Carroll MD, Kit BK, et al. Prevalence of obesity and Trends in the distribution of body mass index amoung US adults, 1999-2010. JAMA 2012;307: 491–7.

[8]. Levine MD, Ringham RM, Kalarchian MA, et al. Is family-based behavioral weight control appropriate for severe pediatric obesity? Int J Eat Disord 2001; 30(3):318–28.

[9]. Michels KB. Early life predictors of chronic disease. J Womens Health (Larchmt) 2003;12(2):157–61.

[10]. Wahlqvist ML. Chronic disease prevention: a life-cycle approach which takes account of the environmental impact and opportunities of food, nutrition and public health policies—the rationale for an eco-nutritional disease nomenclature. Asia Pac J Clin Nutr 2002;11(Suppl 9):S759–62.

[11]. Pi-Sunyer FX. The obesity epidemic: pathophysiology and consequences of obesity. Obes Res 2002;10(Suppl 2):97S–104S.

[12]. Whitaker RC. Understanding the complex journey to obesity in early adulthood. Ann Intern Med 2002;136(12):923–5.

[13]. Must A, Jacques PF, Dallal GE, et al. Long-term morbidity and mortality of overweight adolescents; A follow-up of the Harvard Growth Study of 1922-1935. N Engl J Med 1992;327:1350–5.

[14]. Dietz WH. Health consequences of obesity in youth: childhood predictors of adult disease. Pediatrics 1998;101(3 pt 2):518–25.

[15]. Pinhas-Hamiel O, Dolan LM, Daniels SR, et al. Increased incidence of non-insulin dependent diabetes mellitus among adolescents. J Pediatr 1996;128: 608–15.

[16]. Sinha R, Fisch G, Teague B, et al. Prevalence of impaired glucose tolerance among children and adolescents with marked obesity. N Engl J Med 2002; 346(11):802–10.

[17]. Caprio S. Insulin resistance in childhood obesity. J Pediatr Endocrinol Metab 2002;15(Suppl 1):487–92.

[18]. Type 2 diabetes in children and adolescents. American Diabetes Association. Pediatrics 2000;105:671–80.

[19]. Scott A, Toomath R, Boucher D, et al. First national audit of the outcomes of care in young people with diabetes in New Zealand: high prevalence of nephropathy in Maori and Pacific Oslanders. N Z Med J 2006;119:U2015.

[20]. Scott A, Whitcombe S, Bouchier D, et al. Diabetes in children and young adults in Waikato Province, New Zealand: outcomes of care. N Z Med J 2004;117: U1219.

[21]. Narayan K, Boyle J, Thompson T, et al. Lifetime risk for diabetes mellitus in the United States. JAMA 2003;290(14):1884–90.

[22]. Daniels SR. Cardiovascular disease risk factors and atherosclerosis in children and adolescents. Curr Atheroscler Rep 2001;3:479–85.

[23]. Freedman DS, Srinivasan SR, Harsha DW, et al. Relation of body fat patterning to lipid and lipoprotein concentrations in children and adolescents: the Bogalusa Heart Study. Am J Clin Nutr 1989;50:930–9.

[24]. May AL, Kuklina EV, Yoon PW. Prevalence of cardiovascular disease risk factors among US adolescents, 1999-2008. Pediatrics 2012;129:1035–41.

[25]. Freedman DS, Khan LK, Dietz WH, et al. Relationship of childhood obesity to coronary heart disease risk factors in adulthood: the Bogalusa Heart Study. Pediatrics 2001;108:712–8.

[26]. Rosner B, Prineas R, Daniels SR, et al. Blood pressure difference between blacks and whites in relation to body size and among US children and adolescents. Am J Epidemiol 2000;151:1007–19.

[27]. Katsuren K, Nakamura K, Ohta T. Effect of body mass index-z score on adverse levels of cardiovascular disease risk factors. Pediatr Int 2012;54:200–4.

[28]. Li AM, Nelson EA, Wing YK. Obstructive sleep apnea and obesity. Hong Kong Med J 2004;10:144.

[29]. Verhulst SL, Schrauwen N, Haentjens D, et al. Sleep-disordered breathing in overweight and obese children and adolescents: prevalence, characteristics, and the role of fat distribution. Arch Dis Child 2007;92:205–8.

[30]. Gozal D. Sleep-disordered breathing and school performance in children. Pediatrics 1998;102:616–20.

[31]. Gozal D, Wang M, Pope DW. Objective sleepiness measures in pediatric obstructive sleep apnea. Pediatrics 2001;108:693–7.

[32]. Chervin RD, Dillon JE, Archbold KH, et al. Conduct problems and symptoms of sleep disorders in children. J Am Acad Child Adolesc Psychiatry 2003;42: 201–8.

[33]. Amin RS, Kimball TR, Bean JA, et al. Left ventricular hypertrophy and abnormal ventricular geometry in children and adolescents with obstructive sleep apnea. Am J Respir Crit Care Med 2002;165:1395–9.

[34]. Ippisch HM, Inge TH, Daniels SR, et al. Reversibility of cardiac abnormalities in morbidly obese adolescents. J AM Coll Cardiol 2008;51(14):1342–8.

[35]. Schwimmer JB, Deutsch R, Kahen T, et al. Prevalence of fatty liver in children and adolescents. Pediatrics 2006;118:1388–93.

[36]. Xanthakos S, Miles L, Bucuvalas J, et al. Histologic Spectrum of NASH in Morbidly Obese Adolescents Differs from Adults. Clin Gastroenterol Hepatol 2006;4(2):226–32.

[37]. Weisberg LA, Chutorian AM. Pseudotumor cerebri of childhood. Am J Dis Child 1977;131:1243–8.

[38]. Sugarman HJ, Felton WL III, Sismanis A, et al. Gastric surgery for pseudotumor cerebri associated with severe obesity. Ann Surg 1999;229:634–42.

[39]. Chandra V, Dutta S, Albanese CT, et al. Clinical resolution of severely symptomatic pseudotumor cerebri after gastric bypass in an adolescent. Surg Obes Relat Dis 2007;3:198–200.

[40]. Zeller MH, Modi AC. Predictors of health-related quality of life in obese youth. Obesity (Silver Spring) 2006;14:122–30.

[41]. Strauss RS. Childhood obesity and self-esteem. Pediatrics 2000;105:e15.

[42]. Ball K, Crawford D, Kenardy J. Longitudinal relationships among overweight, life satisfaction, and aspirations in young women. Obes Res 2004;12:1019–30.

[43]. Schwimmer JB, Burwinkle TM, Varni JW. Health-related quality of life of severely obese children and adolescents. JAMA 2003;289:1813–9.

[44]. Gortmaker SL, Must A, Perrin JM, et al. Social and economic consequences of overweight in adolescence and young adulthood. N Engl J Med 1993;329: 1008–12.

[45]. Zeller MH, Modi AC, Noll JG, et al. Psychosocial functioning improves following adolescent bariatric surgery. Obesity (Silver Spring) 2009;17:985–90.

[46]. Inge TH, Miyano G, Bean J, et al. Reversal of type 2 diabetes mellitus and improvements in cardiovascular risk factors after surgical weight loss in adolescents. Pediatrics 2009;123(1):214–22.

[47]. Kaira M, Inge T. Effect of bariatric surgery on obstructive sleep apnea in adolescents. Paediatr Respir Rev 2006;7(4):260–7.

[48]. Kral JG, Thung SN, Biron S, et al. Effects of surigcal treatment of the metabolic syndrome on liver fibrosis and cirrhosis. Surgery 2004;135:48–58.

[49]. Michalsky M, Reichard K, Inge T, et al. ASMBS pediatric committee best practice guidelines. Surg Obes Relat Dis 2012;8:1–7.

[50]. Pratt JS, Lenders CM, Dionne EA, et al. Best practice updates for pediatric/adolescent weight loss surgery. Obesity (Silver Spring) 2009;17:901–10.

[51]. Tanner JM. Growth at adolescence. 2nd edition. Oxford (United Kingdom): Blackwell Scientific Publications; 1962.

[52]. Tanner JM, Davies PS. Clinical longitudinal standards for height and weight velocity for North American children. J Pediatr 1985;107:317–29.

[53]. Michalsky M, Kramer RE, Fullmer MA, et al. Developing criteria for pediatric/adolescent bariatric surgery programs. Pediatrics 2001;128(2):S65.

[54]. Sugerman HJ, Sugerman EL, DeMaria EJ, et al. Bariatric surgery for severely obese adolescents. J Gastrointest Surg 2003;7:102–8.

[55]. Rand CS, MacGregor AM. Adolescents having obesity surgery: a 6 year follow-up. South Med J 1999;87:1208–13.

[56]. Barnett SJ, Stanley C, Hanlon M, et al. Long-term follow-up and the role of surgery in adolescents with morbid obesity. Surg Obes Relat Dis 2005;1:394–8.

[57]. O'Brien PE, Sawyer SM, Laurie S, et al. Laparoscopic adjustable gastric banding in severeley obese adolescents; a randomized trial. JAMA 2010;303:519–26.

[58]. Alqahtani AR, Antonisamy B, Alamri H, et al. Laparoscopic sleeve gastrectomy in 108 obese children and adolescents aged 5 to 21 years. Ann Surg 2012;256(2):266–73.

[59]. Jen HC, Rickard DG, Shew SB, et al. Trends and outcomes of adolescent bariatric surgery in California, 2005-2007. Pediatrics 2010;126:e746–53.

[60]. Zitsman JL, Fennoy I, Witt MA, et al. Laparoscopic adjustable gastric banding in adolescents: short-term results. J Pediatr Surg 2011;46:157–62.

[61]. Lawson ML, Kirk S, Mitchell T, et al. One year outcomes of Roux-en-Y gastric bypass for morbidly obese adolescents: a multicenter study from the Pediatric Bariatric Study Group. J Pediatr Surg 2006;41:137–43.

[62]. Al-Qahtani AR. Laparoscopic adjustable gastric banding in adolescents: safety and efficacy. J Pediatr Surg 2007;42:894–7.

[63]. Dolan K, Creighton L, Hopkins G, et al. Laparoscopic gastic banding in morbidly obese adolescents. Obes Surg 2003;13:101–5.

[64]. Angrisani L, Favretti F, Furbetta F, et al. Obese teenagers treated by Lap-Band System: the Italian experience. Surgery 2005;138:877–81.

[65]. Strauss RS, Bradley LJ, Brolin RE. Gastric bypass in adolescents with morbid obesity. J Pediatr 2001;138:499–504.

[66]. Schauer PR, Ikramuddin S. Laparoscopic surgery for morbid obesity. Surg Clin North Am 2001;81:1145–79.

[67]. Rosenthal RJ. International sleeve gastrectomy expert panel consensus statement: best practice guidleines based on experience of > 12,000 cases. Surg Obes Relat Dis 2012;8:8–19.

[68]. Langer FB, Reza Hoda MA, Bohdjalian A, et al. Sleeve gastrectomy and gastric banding: effects on plasma ghrelin levels. Obes Surg 2005;15:1024–9.

[69]. Lee CM, Cirangle PT, Jossart GH. Vertical gastrectomy for morbid obesity in 216 patients: resport of two year results. Surg Endosc 2007;21:1810–6.

[70]. Till H, Bluher S, Hirsch W, et al. Efficacy of laparoscopic sleeve gastrectomy (LGS) as a stand-alone techniwque for children with morbid obesity. Obes Surg 2008;18:1047–9.

[71]. Till H, Muenstere O, Keller A, et al. Laparoscopic sleeve gastrectomy acheives substantial weight loss ni an adolescnet girl with morbid obesity. Eur J Pediatr 2008;1:47–9.

[72]. Boza C, Viscido G, Salina J, et al. Laparscopic sleeve gastrectomy I obese adolescents: results in 51 patients. Surg Obes Relat Dis 2012;8:133–9.

[73]. Inge TH, Jnekins TM, Zeller M, et al. Baseline BMI is a strong predictor of nadir BMI after adolescent gastric bypass. J Pediatr 2010;156:103–8.

[74]. Treadwell JR, Sun F, Schoelles K. Systematic review and meta-analysis of bariatric surgery for pediatric obesity. Ann Surg 2008;248(5):763–76.

[75]. Ippisch HM, Inge TH, Daniels SR, et al. Reversibility of cardiac abnormalities in morbidly obese adolescents. J Am Coll Cardiol 2008;51:1342–8.

[76]. Xanthakos SA. Nutritional deficiencies in obesity and after bariatric surgery. Pediatr Clin North Am 2009;56(5):1105–21.

[77]. Towbin A, Inge TH, Garcia VF, et al. Beriberi after gastric bypass surgery in adolescence. J Pediatr 2004;145(2):263–7.

Morbidity and Effectiveness of Laparoscopic Sleeve Gastrectomy, Adjustable Gastric Band, and Gastric Bypass for Morbid Obesity

Timothy D. Jackson, MD, MPH[a,b], Matthew M. Hutter, MD, MPH[a,c],*

KEYWORDS

- Morbid obesity • Bariatric surgery • Sleeve gastrectomy • Adjustable gastric band
- Gastric bypass • Outcomes • Comparative effectiveness

KEY POINTS

- Laparoscopic sleeve gastrectomy (LSG), laparoscopic adjustable gastric band (LAGB) and laparoscopic Roux-en-Y gastric bypass are all considered acceptable contemporary surgical options for the treatment of morbid obesity.
- Recent quality improvement efforts have significantly reduced the morbidity and mortality associated with modern bariatric surgical procedures.
- LRYGB appears to be most effective although is associated with more risk when compared to both LAGB and LSG.
- LSG is positioned between the LRYGB and LABG in associated morbidity and effectiveness although long-term outcome data is lacking.

OBESITY AS A SURGICAL DISEASE

Obesity continues to be a leading public health concern [1]. Current data indicate that 34.4% of the United States population has class I obesity (body mass index [BMI] >30 kg/m^2) and 6% has class III obesity (BMI >40 kg/m^2) [2]. Obesity is associated with many comorbidities that significantly decrease life expectancy [3]. Estimates suggest that obesity accounts for up to 15% of all deaths annually in the United States and will soon emerge as the single leading cause of preventable death in the developed world [4].

This article originally appeared in Advances in Surgery, Volume 46, September 2012.

[a] The Codman Center for Clinical Effectiveness in Surgery, Massachusetts General Hospital, Boston, MA, USA; [b] Department of Surgery, University of Toronto, University Health Network, 399 Bathurst Street, 8MP-322, Toronto, Ontario, Canada M5T 2S8; [c] Division of General and Gastrointestinal Surgery, Department of Surgery, Massachusetts General Hospital, 15 Parkman Street WACC 460, Boston, MA 02114, USA

* Corresponding author. Division of General and Gastrointestinal Surgery, Department of Surgery, Massachusetts General Hospital, 15 Parkman Street WACC 460, Boston, MA 02114.
E-mail address: mhutter@partners.org

Clinics Collections 3 (2014) 247–259
http://dx.doi.org/10.1016/j.ccol.2014.09.044
2352-7986/14/$ – see front matter © 2014 Elsevier Inc. All rights reserved.

Surgery remains the only effective treatment modality for morbid obesity, resulting in long-term weight loss and sustained improvement in weight-related comorbidities [5]. At present, there are limited pharmacologic therapies, and medically supervised diets have yielded only modest results [6,7]. Results from the Swedish Obesity Subjects (SOS) study, a large prospective cohort study with more than 10 years of follow-up, showed bariatric surgery to be associated with long-term weight loss and decreased overall mortality [8]. There have been significant improvements in the safety of bariatric procedures in recent years [9], and bariatric surgery has repeatedly been shown to be a cost-effective intervention [10–12]. Eligibility for bariatric procedures continues to be determined by the National Institutes of Health (NIH) criteria [13] from 1991 in which surgery is indicated for patients with a BMI of 40 kg/m^2 or greater, or a BMI of 35 kg/m^2 or greater with significant weight-related comorbidities.

Examination of current trends in bariatric surgery shows 3 options emerging as the surgical procedures of choice: the laparoscopic sleeve gastrectomy (LSG), laparoscopic adjustable gastric band (LAGB), and laparoscopic Roux-en-Y gastric bypass (LRYGB) [14]. This article provides a current summary of recent available outcomes data on the LSG, LAGB, and LRYGB.

CONTEMPORARY SURGICAL OPTIONS

Contemporary surgical options for morbid obesity include the LSG, LAGB, and LRYGB. At present, greater than 90% of bariatric surgical procedures are performed via a laparoscopic approach [14], and this is thought to be an important factor in recent improved outcomes [15].

LSG

The LSG involves excision of the lateral aspect of the stomach to create a lesser curve–based gastric tube (**Fig. 1**). This procedure was initially performed as part of the biliopancreatic diversion with duodenal switch [16] and later as the first step in staged procedures for the superobese [17–19]. Since its description laparoscopically [20], sleeve gastrectomy has been gaining popularity as a stand-alone procedure despite the lack of long-term outcomes data [21,22]. It is currently being performed for 7.8% of primary bariatric operations, according to the American College of Surgeons (ACS) Bariatric Surgery Center Network (BSCN) data [23]. At present, the LSG is not a reimbursable procedure by the Centers for Medicare and Medicaid Services (CMS) but is covered by several insurers [24].

LAGB

The LAGB was initially described in 1993 but was not approved for use in the United States until 2001 [25]. This procedure involves placement of an adjustable gastric band around the cardia of the stomach via the pars flaccida connected with tubing to a subcutaneous port implanted on the rectus fascia (**Fig. 2**). The degree of restriction is titrated with fills through the subcutaneous port. The LAGB is potentially a fairly noninvasive surgical option and its popularity in North America has been increasing [26]. It is currently being performed for 46% of primary bariatric operations, according to ACS-BSCN data [23]. In Europe and Australia, where there is longer clinical experience with this procedure, the number of LAGB procedures is declining [14].

LRYGB

The modern gastric bypass reported by Mason and colleagues [27] was first described via a laparoscopic approach in 1994 [28] and had overtaken the open procedures by

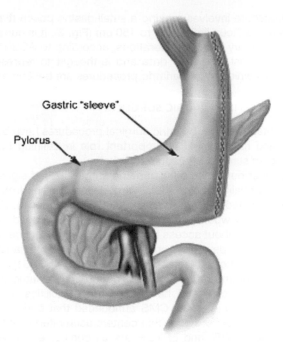

Fig. 1. Sleeve gastrectomy. (*From* Jones DB, Maithel SK, Schneider BE. Atlas of minimally invasive surgery. Woodbury, CT: Cine-Med, 2006. Copyright © Ciné-Med Inc; with permission.)

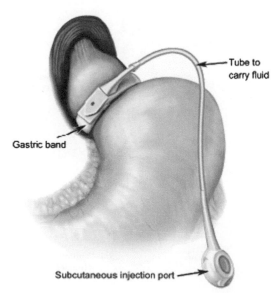

Fig. 2. Laparoscopic adjustable gastric band. (*From* Jones DB, Maithel SK, Schneider BE. Atlas of minimally invasive surgery. Woodbury, CT: Cine-Med, 2006. Copyright © Ciné-Med Inc; with permission.)

2004 [29]. This procedure involves making a small gastric pouch (typically 30 cm^3), which is connected to a Roux limb of 75 to 150 cm (**Fig. 3**). It is currently being performed for 44% of primary bariatric operations, according to ACS-BSCN data [23]. The LRYGB has the most long-term data and is thought to represent the current gold standard against which other bariatric procedures are benchmarked.

QUALITY IMPROVEMENT IN BARIATRIC SURGERY

Improvements in outcomes after bariatric surgical procedures have been achieved in the past decade and have played an important role in defining LSG, LAGB, and LRYGB as the modern surgical procedures of choice.

Early reports of poor outcomes after bariatric surgery raised significant concerns about the safety and quality of care [30]. Thirty-day mortalities from administrative claims data were estimated to be as high as 2% [30]. In response, CMS announced in November 2005 that it would no longer cover bariatric procedures. To address these and other concerns about access to safe surgical care, 2 large national surgical associations independently developed accreditation programs in bariatric surgery: the American Society of Bariatric and Metabolic Surgeons (ASMBS) [31] and the ACS [32]. Both accreditation programs require centers performing bariatric surgery to meet established standards of care and have appropriate facilities, organization, and trained personnel. In February 2006, CMS announced that bariatric surgery would be reimbursed only when performed within centers accredited by either the ASMBS or the ACS [24]. LSG, LAGB, and LRYGB are all considered acceptable surgical options for the purposes of accreditation.

Reporting of outcomes data is a mandatory requirement for accreditation as a center for bariatric surgery. The ACS has established the BSCN [33] Data Collection Program and the ASMBS has developed the Bariatric Outcomes Longitudinal Database

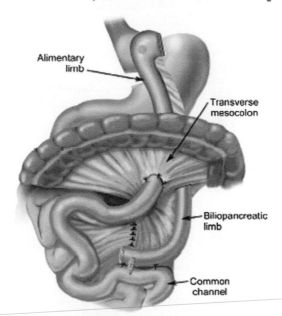

Fig. 3. Laparoscopic Roux-en-Y gastric bypass. (*From* Jones DB, Maithel SK, Schneider BE. Atlas of minimally invasive surgery. Woodbury, CT: Cine-Med, 2006. Copyright © Ciné-Med Inc; with permission.)

(BOLD) [34]. The ACS-BSCN database was built on the success and methodological rigor of the National Surgical Quality Improvement Program (NSQIP). Information from both prospective databases is playing an important role in ensuring quality of bariatric surgical care delivery and is helping to better define the real-world outcomes for LSG, LAGB, and LRYGB.

In addition to the introduction of accreditation in bariatric surgery, the widespread adoption of laparoscopic techniques, the increased clinical experience, and the development of fellowship training programs have also contributed to the reduced mortality and morbidity associated with these procedures.

MORTALITY

With recent quality improvement successes in bariatric surgery, the mortality associated with LSG, LAGB, and LRYGB has decreased significantly. Current mortalities for all patients are 15 to 20 times lower than the previously widely reported 2% mortality found in high-risk populations (see later discussion). The highest mortality has been associated with the LRYGB. In the first Longitudinal Assessment of Bariatric Surgery (LABS-1) study [35], a large NIH-funded multi-institutional prospective cohort study with 10 centers and 4776 patients, the 30-day mortality for Roux-en-Y gastric bypass (RYGB) was 0.2% compared with 0% in the LAGB group. The open RYGB (ORYGB) group had a 10-fold higher 30-day mortality at 2.1%. A subsequent analysis of all early mortalities within the LABS study cohort revealed that the recognized complications of anastomotic leak, cardiac events, and pulmonary complications accounted for most of the deaths [36].

Data from multiple large prospective cohorts of patients having bariatric surgery has allowed for an estimate of mortality outside of the study setting. An initial report from the NSQIP data showed a similar 30-day mortality for patients undergoing LAGB and LRYGB (0.09% vs 0.14%) in a sample of 4756 patients between 2005 and 2006 [37]. The baseline data from ASMBS-BOLD reports 30-day mortality of 0.09% and 90-day mortality of 0.11%, although the data were not stratified by procedure type [34].

Recent data from the Michigan Bariatric Surgery Collaborative (MBSC), which consists of 29 hospitals and 25,469 patients throughout Michigan, reported early mortality after LSG, LAGB, and LRYGB as 0.1%, 0.04%, and 0.1% respectively [38]. Data from the ACS-BSCN reports 0.11%, 0.05%, and 0.14% for 30-day mortality after LSG, LAGB, and LRYGB with data from 28,616 patients at 109 centers from across the United States (Table 1). Within the same cohort, 1-year mortality was reported at 0.21%, 0.08%, and 0.34% for LSG, LAGB, and LRYGB respectively. Considering

Table 1
Morbidity and mortality associated with LRYGB, LSG, and LAGB from the ACS-BSCN dataset

	LRYGB	LSG	LAGB
30-d mortality (%)	0.14	0.11	0.05
1-y mortality (%)	0.34	0.21	0.08
30-d morbidity (%)	5.91	5.61	1.44
30-d readmission (%)	6.47	5.40	1.71
30-d reoperation/intervention(%)	5.02	2.97	0.92

Data from Hutter MM, Schirmer BD, Jones DB, et al. First report from the American College of Surgeons Bariatric Surgery Center Network: laparoscopic sleeve gastrectomy has morbidity and effectiveness positioned between the band and the bypass. Ann Surg 2011;254(3):410–20 [discussion: 420–2].

these recent data, mortality is consistently low among all 3 procedures, with the LSG and LRYGB having higher rates than LAGB.

MORBIDITY

With mortality low across all procedure types, and because LSG, LAGB, and LRYGB are all considered to be safe options for the treatment of morbid obesity, increasing emphasis is being placed on their associated morbidity. Each procedure has unique risk profiles that continue to be better defined as more data become available.

The LSG has a 30-day morbidity of 5.61% reported in the first results from the ACS-BSCN; lower than LRYGB at 5.91% but significantly higher than LAGB at 1.44% (see **Table 1**) [23]. Readmission rates within 30 days after surgery followed a similar trend (LSG 5.40%, LAGB 1.71%, LRYGB 6.47%), as did the need for reoperation/intervention (LSG 2.97%, LAGB 0.92%, LRYGB 5.02%) [23]. Initial data from the MBSC also shows that the LSG is positioned between the LRYGB and LAGB in rates of postoperative complications. The number of patients experiencing more than 1 serious complication was 2.3% in LSG, 0.9% in LAGB, and 3.3% in LRYGB [38]. Similar findings are emerging from the ASMBS-BOLD data: the percentage of patients experiencing 1 or more complication was 10.84% in LSG, 4.62% in LAGB, and 14.87% in RYGB [34].

Although LSG was excluded from the analysis, in the LABS-1 study, the investigators also showed higher morbidity associated with LRYGB compared with LAGB. The LABS-1 composite end point (death, deep vein thrombosis [DVT]/PE, reintervention/reoperation, and failure to be discharged from hospital within 30 days) was 1.0% in the patients having LAGB compared with 4.8% in the LRYGB group [30].

Conversion to open rate was lowest in LSG at 0.1%, LAGB was 0.25%, and highest in LRYGB at 1.43% in the ACS-BSCN data [23].

Evaluation of anastomotic or staple line leaks reveals similar low rates in both LSG and LRYGB. This complication does not occur in the LAGB because there are no anastomoses or staple lines to dehisce. The MBSC reported a higher leak rate associated with LSG at 1% compared with 0.8% with LRYGB [38]. A similar low leak rate was found in the ACS-BSCN dataset: 0.74% for LSG and 0.78% for LRYGB. These recent leak rates are lower than typically reported in previous literature. In a meta-analysis of LSG with 36 studies and data from 2570 patients, the leak rate was determined to be 2.7% in patients undergoing LSG as a primary procedure [21]. Similarly, leaks after LRYGB have been reported at 1.5% [39] and 2.1% [40] in recent large case series. Although the leak rates of LSG and LRYGB are similar, managing leaks after LSG may represent a more challenging clinical problem [41,42].

Bleeding is a rare early complication that can occur after any bariatric procedure. Major bleeding, as defined by transfusion of more than 4 units of blood, occurred in 0.3% of patients having LSG, 0.04% in LAGB, and 0.7% in LRYGB in the MBSC data [38]. Minor bleeding was reported at 0.7%, 0.1%, and 2.0% for LSG, LAGB, and LRYGB respectively [38]. In the ACS-BSCN cohort, bleeding events occurred in 0.64% after LSG, 0.05% after LAGB, and 1.11% after LRYGB [23]. LSG is between LAGB and LRYGB in bleeding risk.

Medical complications can be an important source of morbidity during the postoperative period. The rates of venous thromboembolic (VTE) events seem to be similar in LSG and LRYGB and lower in LAGB. In the MBSC, VTE rates were 0.4% for both LSG and LRYGB and 0.1% for LAGB [38]. Rates of DVT were 0.11% for LSG, 0.03% for LAGB, and 0.14% for LRYGB from ACS-BSCN data [23]. Incidence of pulmonary embolism was also low and followed a similar trend in that study. Slightly higher rates of VTE were reported for LAGB (0.3%) and LRYGB (0.4%) in the LABS-1 study [35]. Cardiac events are typically rare after bariatric procedures. LRYGB seems to have the greatest associated cardiac risk, with cardiac events occurring in 0.1% [38] and 0.09% [23] of patients in the MBSC and ACS-BSCN databases respectively. In LAGB and LSG, cardiac events were rarer. Pulmonary complications such as pneumonia also occur with more frequency in LRYGB compared with LSG and are lowest in LAGB.

Later complications such as stricture, marginal ulcers, bowel obstructions, and nutritional deficiencies tend to occur more frequently after LRYGB compared with LSG and are infrequent after LAGB. In the ACS-BSCN cohort, strictures occurred in 1.42% of patients having LRYGB, 0.42% in LSG, and 0.13% LAGB [23]. Similarly, in the MBSC data, strictures developed in 1.8% of patients after LRYGB, 0.7% after LSG, and no strictures were reported in patients having LAGB [38]. Marginal ulcers occur with variable frequency after LRYGB, with reported incidences ranging from 0.6% to 16% in previous studies [43], depending on how and when they were identified. The 30-day marginal ulcer rate in the ACS-BSCN database was 0.47% [23]. Although most marginal ulcers respond well to medical therapy, some patients require surgical revision; 9% in a recent case series [43]. Another complication unique to LRYGB is the risk of developing internal hernias. Estimates of the incidence of internal hernias range from 0.5% to 9% in the literature [44]. Lack of long-term follow-up data after LRYGB makes lifetime risk difficult to estimate. If not recognized and treated early, the consequences of internal hernias can be devastating. Although any patient can develop nutritional deficiencies after a bariatric procedure, the risk is more pronounced in patients who have had LRYGB given its malabsorptive and restrictive mechanism of action. If patients are not monitored and do not take appropriate supplementation, they can develop micronutrient deficiencies associated with significant morbidity [45]. The potential for patients to develop strictures, marginal ulcers, internal hernias, and micronutrient deficiencies after LRGYB adds to the longer-term morbidity associated with this procedure.

Although early complications are rare with the LAGB, there exists considerable controversy about rates of long-term complications and failure. Within the ACS-BSCN data, 0.11% of patients having LAGB experienced early complications [23]. Similar findings were present in the MBSC, which showed that only 0.4% of patients having LAGB developed an early band complication requiring reoperation such as slippage, obstruction, gastric or esophageal perforation, and port site infection [38]. This low early morbidity associated with the LAGB has established this procedure as the lowest-risk surgical option, although longer-term data are calling this notion into question. A recent case series from Belgium with 12 years of follow-up showed that 39% of patients experienced major complications, 28% developed band erosion, 17% were converted to LRGYB, and only 51% of patients had their band in place at the end of the follow-up period [46]. Although the findings were dramatic, the study had significant limitations because it consisted of only 151 patients, was from a single surgeon, and had only 54.3% follow-up. Another recent small case series from Chile supports these findings, reporting a surgical failure rate greater than 40% and 24.1% reoperation rate in patients having LAGB after 5 years of follow-up [47]. A recent meta-analysis of 19 studies reports lower surgical failure rates, with rates of erosion and slippage of 1.03% and 4.93% after an average follow-up of more than 6 years [48]. Data from the University Health System Consortium Clinical Database with 10,151 patients undergoing LAGB showed even more favorable results, with a 0.76% band revision rate and 0.87% band explantation rate over the 3-year study period [49]. Changes in surgical technique, band devices, increased clinical experience, and process of care between early LAGB procedures and current LAGB procedures are being put forward to reconcile the large discrepancies in morbidity associated with LAGB in the current literature [50]. Longer-term data will continue to better define the morbidity associated with LAGB and allow a more complete estimate of risk.

At present, there is a paucity of medium-term to long-term data on the morbidity associated with the LSG. Studies with follow-up beyond 5 years are scarce, and needed to better define the risks of LSG compared with LRYGB and LAGB.

COMPARATIVE EFFECTIVENESS

LSG, LAGB, and LRYGB have variable results in achieving sustained weight loss and resolution of weight-related comorbidities. Short-term studies suggest that the sleeve lies between the bypass, which has greater weight loss and reduction in weight-related comorbidities, and the band, which seems to have a lesser impact.

Reduction in weight

LRYGB has consistently been shown to be the more effective procedure in achieving and sustaining reduction in weight compared with the LSG and LAGB. As highlighted in the first report form the ACS-BSCN data, the LRYGB resulted in average reduction in BMI of 15.34 kg/m^2 at 12 months compared with 11.87 kg/m^2 in the LSG group and 7.05 kg/m^2 in the LAGB group (**Table 2**) [23]. The follow-up at 12 months in this study was approximately 70%. Beyond 1 year, it seems that all procedures can result in sustained weight loss. A recent meta-analysis reported sustained weight loss in patients having both LAGB and LRYGB up to 3 years [51]. In patients having LAGB, mean percent excess body weight loss (%EBWL) was 42.6% at 1 year (data from 15 studies), 50.3% at 2 years (12 studies), and 55.2% at 3 years (9 studies). For patients having LRYGB, %EBWL was 61.5% at 1 year (10 studies), 69.7% at 2 years (5 studies), and 71.2% at 3 years (2 studies). In an updated meta-analysis, Buchwald and colleagues [52] also showed sustained weight in patients having both LAGB and LRYGB. LRYGB was found to result in a BMI reduction of 16 kg/m^2 (22 studies, 2757 patients) and %EBWL of 63.3%, whereas LAGB resulted in a reduction in BMI of 9.63 kg/m^2 (66 studies, 6128 patients) and %EBWL of 43.9% beyond 2 years. There is a paucity of data beyond 5 years with appropriate follow-up. A recent case series of 242 patients undergoing LRYGB with 19% follow-up at 10 years showed a mean %EBWL of 57% [53]. A case series of 151 patients having LAGB with 54.3% follow-up at 12 years reported a mean %EBWL of 42.8% [46]. Fewer data are available on the longer-term weight loss outcomes in LSG, although a cross-sectional review of patients undergoing LSG showed a sustained reduction in BMI of 11.1 kg/m^2 at 5 years [22].

Table 2
Effectiveness of LRYGB, LSG, and LRYGB at 1 year from the ACS-BSCN [23]. Reduction in BMI and percentage with improvement or resolution of select weighted related comorbidities. Estimates are limited by small numbers at time of follow-up

	LRYGB	LSG	LAGB
Reduction in BMI (kg/m^2)	15.34	11.87	7.05
Diabetes (%)	83	55	44
Hypertension (%)	79	68	44
Hyperlipidemia (%)	66	35	33
Obstructive sleep apnea (%)	66	62	38
Gastroesophageal reflux disease (%)	70	50	64

To summarize the available data, the LRGYB results in the most weight loss in the short term, followed by the LSG, whereas the LAGB seems to be the least effective option. Medium-term data suggest that the LSG, LAGB, and LRYGB all seem to provide sustained weight loss, although overall data are limited (and almost absent for the LSG). Long-term weight loss outcomes are still needed, and the percentage of patients followed up remains a challenge for most cohort studies.

Reduction in weight-related comorbidities

LSG, LAGB, and LRYGB all result in significant improvement in the comorbidities associated with obesity. These comorbidities include diabetes, hypertension, hyperlipidemia, obstructive sleep apnea (OSA), and gastroesophageal reflux disease (GERD). The extent to which these comorbidities improve is correlated with weight loss; the LRYGB tends to perform better than the LAGB and LSG, with the LSG being more effective that the LAGB.

Multiple studies have shown the effectiveness of these procedures in the treatment of diabetes. An analysis of 19 studies with 11,175 patients, follow-up greater than 2 years reporting diabetes-specific end points after bariatric surgery showed that diabetes resolved in 78% of patients and improved in 87% [52]. In these studies, LRYGB was more effective than LAGB with 70.9% resolution beyond 2 years compared with 58.3% in the patients having LAGB. This trend was shown in the ASC-BSCN data and placed the LSG between the LRYGB and LAGB: at 1 year, 83% of patients who underwent LRYGB had resolution or improvement in their diabetes compared with 55% of patients having LSG and 44% of patients having LAGB (see **Table 2**) [23]. The enhanced ability for LRYGB to improve diabetes compared with LSG and LAGB may be related to additional metabolic effects induced by intestinal bypass independently of weight loss alone [54].

Hypertension, hyperlipidemia, GERD, and OSA also all reliably improve after bariatric surgery, with LRYGB having the greatest treatment effect. In the ASC-BSCN data, the LSG consistently performed better than the LAGB but not as well as the LRYGB (see **Table 2**). The 1 exception was GERD, which improved or resolved in 50% who received the LSG, compared with 70% in patients having LRYGB and 64% in the LAGB group [23]. From the available literature, it seems that LRYGB results in both the most weight loss and resolution of weight-related comorbidities. LSG is positioned between the LAGB and the LRYGB, although long-term data are lacking.

TOWARD OPTIMIZING OUTCOMES

Remarkable progress has been made in recent years in improving patient safety and quality of care in bariatric surgery. The introduction of accreditation and mandatory reporting of outcomes has created a wealth of clinically rich data to better inform clinicians of the real-world morbidity and effectiveness associated with different surgical options. The LSG, LAGB, and LRYGB have emerged as the contemporary procedures of choice for the treatment of morbid obesity. Although there are ample data supporting the short-term safety of these procedures, the lack of long-term data limits the ability of clinicians to fully understand their effectiveness. Obesity is a chronic disease that requires lifelong treatment and monitoring. Efforts to improve follow-up after bariatric procedures are needed to ensure that potential late morbidity is reduced. Subsequent data from sources such as the ACS-BSCN, ASMBS-BOLD, MBSC, and the LABS consortium will better define long-term effectiveness and risks associated with these procedures. Furthermore, these data may inform future policy decisions on issues such as coverage determinations and the expansion of current surgical indications.

An improved understanding of the risk/benefit profile associated with each procedure type has the potential to improve the matching of patient to procedure type. The development of risk/benefit assessment tools derived from current outcomes data may better inform the procedure selection process for both patients and providers. Additional data collection evaluating more patient-centered outcomes and quality of life will help to better define the overall impact of these procedures in the treatment of morbid obesity.

SUMMARY

LSG, LAGB, and LRYGB are all safe and effective modern surgical options for the treatment of morbid obesity. Recent quality improvement successes in bariatric surgical care delivery have resulted in low mortality and morbidity after these procedures. All seem to result in sustained weight loss and improvement in weight-related comorbidities, although appropriate long-term outcomes data for all procedure types are needed. The LRYGB seems to be associated with the most risk but offers the most benefit, whereas the LAGB seems to have the lowest risk and to be least effective. The LSG seems to be positioned between the LRYGB and LAGB in associated morbidity and effectiveness in short-term and medium-term studies. Because the LSG has only recently been performed, there are currently no data about its long-term effectiveness. A better understanding of the unique risk/benefit profile associated with each procedure type will better inform patient selection and has the potential to further optimize outcomes.

REFERENCES

[1]. WHO. Obesity: preventing and managing the global epidemic. World Health Organ Tech Rep Ser 2000;894:1–253.

[2]. Shields M, Carroll M, Odgen C. Adult obesity prevalence in Canada and the United States. NCHS Data Brief 2011;56:1–8 [in French].

[3]. Fontaine KR, Redden DT, Wang C, et al. Years of life lost due to obesity. JAMA 2003;289(2):187–93.

[4]. Stewart ST, Cutler DM, Rosen AB. Forecasting the effects of obesity and smoking on U.S. life expectancy. N Engl J Med 2009;361(23):2252–60.

[5]. Buchwald H, Avidor Y, Braunwald E, et al. Bariatric surgery: a systematic review and meta-analysis. JAMA 2004;292(14):1724–37.

[6]. Appel LJ, Clark JM, Yeh HC, et al. Comparative effectiveness of weight-loss interventions in clinical practice. N Engl J Med 2011;365(21):1959–68.

[7]. Wadden TA, Volger S, Sarwer DB, et al. A two-year randomized trial of obesity treatment in primary care practice. N Engl J Med 2011;365(21):1969–79.

[8]. Sjostrom L, Narbro K, Sjostrom CD, et al. Effects of bariatric surgery on mortality in Swedish obese subjects. N Engl J Med 2007;357(8):741–52.

[9]. Encinosa WE, Bernard DM, Du D, et al. Recent improvements in bariatric surgery outcomes. Med Care 2009;47(5):531–5.

[10]. Picot J, Jones J, Colquitt JL, et al. The clinical effectiveness and cost-effectiveness of bariatric (weight loss) surgery for obesity: a systematic review and economic evaluation. Health Technol Assess 2009;13(41):1–190, 215–357, iii–iv.

[11]. Cremieux PY, Ghosh A, Yang HE, et al. Return on investment for bariatric surgery. Am J Manag Care 2008;14(11):e5–6.

[12]. Sampalis JS, Liberman M, Auger S, et al. The impact of weight reduction surgery on health-care costs in morbidly obese patients. Obes Surg 2004;14(7):939–47.

[13]. NIH. Gastrointestinal surgery for severe obesity. 1991. Available at: http://consensus.nih.gov/1991/1991gisurgeryobesity084html.htm. Accessed November 27, 2011.

[14]. Buchwald H, Oien DM. Metabolic/bariatric surgery worldwide 2008. Obes Surg 2009;19(12):1605–11.

[15]. Reoch J, Mottillo S, Shimony A, et al. Safety of laparoscopic vs open bariatric surgery: a systematic review and meta-analysis. Arch Surg 2011;146(11):1314–22.

[16]. Hess DS, Hess DW. Biliopancreatic diversion with a duodenal switch. Obes Surg 1998;8(3):267–82.

[17]. Almogy G, Crookes PF, Anthone GJ. Longitudinal gastrectomy as a treatment for the high-risk super-obese patient. Obes Surg 2004;14(4):492–7.

[18]. Hamoui N, Anthone GJ, Kaufman HS, et al. Sleeve gastrectomy in the high-risk patient. Obes Surg 2006;16(11):1445–9.

[19]. Cottam D, Qureshi FG, Mattar SG, et al. Laparoscopic sleeve gastrectomy as an initial weight-loss procedure for high-risk patients with morbid obesity. Surg Endosc 2006;20(6):859–63.

[20]. Ren CJ, Patterson E, Gagner M. Early results of laparoscopic biliopancreatic diversion with duodenal switch: a case series of 40 consecutive patients. Obes Surg 2000;10(6):514–23 [discussion: 524].

[21]. Brethauer SA, Hammel JP, Schauer PR. Systematic review of sleeve gastrectomy as staging and primary bariatric procedure. Surg Obes Relat Dis 2009; 5(4):469–75.

[22]. Strain GW, Saif T, Gagner M, et al. Cross-sectional review of effects of laparoscopic sleeve gastrectomy at 1, 3, and 5 years. Surg Obes Relat Dis 2011; 7(6):714–9.

[23]. Hutter MM, Schirmer BD, Jones DB, et al. First report from the American College of Surgeons Bariatric Surgery Center Network: laparoscopic sleeve gastrectomy has morbidity and effectiveness positioned between the band and the bypass. Ann Surg 2011;254(3):410–20 [discussion: 420–2].

[24]. CMS. Decision memo for bariatric surgery for the treatment of morbid obesity. Available at: http://www.cms.gov/medicare-coverage-database/details/ncd-details.aspx?NCDId=57&ncdver=3&bc=AgAAgAAAAAAA&. Accessed November 27, 2011.

[25]. Belachew M, Zimmermann JM. Evolution of a paradigm for laparoscopic adjustable gastric banding. Am J Surg 2002;184(6B):21S–5S.

[26]. Hinojosa MW, Varela JE, Parikh D, et al. National trends in use and outcome of laparoscopic adjustable gastric banding. Surg Obes Relat Dis 2009;5(2):150–5.

[27]. Mason EE, Printen KJ, Blommers TJ, et al. Gastric bypass in morbid obesity. Am J Clin Nutr 1980;33(Suppl 2):395–405.

[28]. Wittgrove AC, Clark GW, Tremblay LJ. Laparoscopic gastric bypass, Roux-en-Y: preliminary report of five cases. Obes Surg 1994;4(4):353–7.

[29]. Nguyen NT, Root J, Zainabadi K, et al. Accelerated growth of bariatric surgery with the introduction of minimally invasive surgery. Arch Surg 2005;140(12): 1198–202 [discussion: 1203].

[30]. Flum DR, Salem L, Elrod JA, et al. Early mortality among Medicare beneficiaries undergoing bariatric surgical procedures. JAMA 2005;294(15):1903–8.

[31]. ASMBS-BSCOE. The American Society of Metabolic and Bariatric Surgery - Bariatric Surgery Center of Excellence. 2011. Available at: http://www.surgicalreview.org/. Accessed November 27, 2011.

[32]. ACS-BSCN. American College of Surgeons Bariatric Surgery Center Network. 2011. Available at: http://www.acsbscn.org. Accessed November 27, 2011.

[33]. Schirmer B, Jones DB. The American College Of Surgeons Bariatric Surgery Center Network: establishing standards. Bull Am Coll Surg 2007;92(8):21–7.

[34]. DeMaria EJ, Pate V, Warthen M, et al. Baseline data from American Society for Metabolic and Bariatric Surgery-designated Bariatric Surgery Centers of Excellence using the Bariatric Outcomes Longitudinal Database. Surg Obes Relat Dis 2010;6(4):347–55.

[35]. Flum DR, Belle SH, King WC, et al. Perioperative safety in the longitudinal assessment of bariatric surgery. N Engl J Med 2009;361(5):445–54.

[36]. Smith MD, Patterson E, Wahed AS, et al. Thirty-day mortality after bariatric surgery: independently adjudicated causes of death in the longitudinal assessment of bariatric surgery. Obes Surg 2011;21(11):1687–92.

[37]. Lancaster RT, Hutter MM. Bands and bypasses: 30-day morbidity and mortality of bariatric surgical procedures as assessed by prospective, multi-center, risk-adjusted ACS-NSQIP data. Surg Endosc 2008;22(12):2554–63.

[38]. Finks JF, Kole KL, Yenumula PR, et al. Predicting risk for serious complications with bariatric surgery: results from the Michigan Bariatric Surgery Collaborative. Ann Surg 2011;254(4):633–40.

[39]. Durak E, Inabnet WB, Schrope B, et al. Incidence and management of enteric leaks after gastric bypass for morbid obesity during a 10-year period. Surg Obes Relat Dis 2008;4(3):389–93.

[40]. Gonzalez R, Sarr MG, Smith CD, et al. Diagnosis and contemporary management of anastomotic leaks after gastric bypass for obesity. J Am Coll Surg 2007;204(1):47–55.

[41]. Tan JT, Kariyawasam S, Wijeratne T, et al. Diagnosis and management of gastric leaks after laparoscopic sleeve gastrectomy for morbid obesity. Obes Surg 2010;20(4):403–9.

[42]. Csendes A, Braghetto I, Leon P, et al. Management of leaks after laparoscopic sleeve gastrectomy in patients with obesity. J Gastrointest Surg 2010;14(9):1343–8.

[43]. Azagury DE, Abu Dayyeh BK, Greenwalt IT, et al. Marginal ulceration after Roux-en-Y gastric bypass surgery: characteristics, risk factors, treatment, and outcomes. Endoscopy 2011;43(11):950–4.

[44]. O'Rourke RW. Management strategies for internal hernia after gastric bypass. J Gastrointest Surg 2011;15(6):1049–54.

[45]. Kaplan LM. Gastrointestinal management of the bariatric surgery patient. Gastroenterol Clin North Am 2005;34(1):105–25.

[46]. Himpens J, Cadiere GB, Bazi M, et al. Long-term outcomes of laparoscopic adjustable gastric banding. Arch Surg 2011;146(7):802–7.

[47]. Boza C, Gamboa C, Perez G, et al. Laparoscopic adjustable gastric banding (LAGB): surgical results and 5-year follow-up. Surg Endosc 2011;25(1):292–7.

[48]. Singhal R, Bryant C, Kitchen M, et al. Band slippage and erosion after laparoscopic gastric banding: a meta-analysis. Surg Endosc 2010;24(12):2980–6.

[49]. Nguyen NT, Hohmann S, Nguyen XM, et al. Outcome of laparoscopic adjustable gastric banding and prevalence of band revision and explantation at academic centers: 2007-2009. Surg Obes Relat Dis 2011. [Epub ahead of print].

[50]. O'Brien P. Comment on: outcome of laparoscopic adjustable gastric banding and the prevalence of band revision and explantation at academic centers: 2007-2009. Surg Obes Relat Dis 2011. [Epub ahead of print].

[51]. Garb J, Welch G, Zagarins S, et al. Bariatric surgery for the treatment of morbid obesity: a meta-analysis of weight loss outcomes for laparoscopic adjustable

gastric banding and laparoscopic gastric bypass. Obes Surg 2009;19(10): 1447–55.

[52]. Buchwald H, Estok R, Fahrbach K, et al. Weight and type 2 diabetes after bariatric surgery: systematic review and meta-analysis. Am J Med 2009;122(3): 248–56 e245.

[53]. Higa K, Ho T, Tercero F, et al. Laparoscopic Roux-en-Y gastric bypass: 10-year follow-up. Surg Obes Relat Dis 2011;7(4):516–25.

[54]. Ikramuddin S, Buchwald H. How bariatric and metabolic operations control metabolic syndrome. Br J Surg 2011;98(10):1339–41.

The Potential Role of Sports Psychology in the Obesity Epidemic

Vincent Morelli, MD[a],*, Carolyn Davis, PhD[b]

KEYWORDS

• Sports psychology • Childhood obesity • Psychological disorders in athletes

KEY POINTS

• Sports psychologists play an important role in enhancing performance among athletes.
• Sports psychologists can also lend their expertise to assist with injury prevention and recovery, as well as compliance issues.
• Sports psychology also has a role in helping to reverse the growing obesity epidemic among school-aged children.
• These professionals, working with coaches, can increase children's levels of physical activity.
• Cognitive-behavioral techniques (eg, confidence building, anger management) could lead to enhanced enjoyment, increased participation, improved school performance, and a reduction in obesity.

DEFINING SPORTS PSYCHOLOGY

In psychology, there are many subfields with unique practices and specific areas of focus. Sport psychology is 1 such subfield, requiring the practicing professional to be appropriately educated, trained, and focused in this area of expertise. The definition from the American Psychological Association's (Exercise and Sport Psychology) Web site states: "Exercise and sport psychology is the scientific study of the psychological factors that are associated with participation and performance in sport, exercise, and other types of physical activity. It is important to note that although overlap exists, 'doing therapy' with a person who happens to be an athlete is *not* considered sport psychology."[1]

This article originally appeared in Primary Care: Clinics in Office Practice, Volume 40, Issue 2, June 2013.

[a] Department of Family and Community Medicine, Meharry Medical College, 1005 Dr D. B. Todd Boulevard, Nashville, TN 37208, USA; [b] Department of Counseling Psychology, Walden University, 100 Washington Avenue, Suite 900, Minneapolis, MN 55401, USA
* Corresponding author.
E-mail address: morellivincent@yahoo.com

Clinics Collections 3 (2014) 261–277
http://dx.doi.org/10.1016/j.ccol.2014.09.045
2352-7986/14/$ – see front matter © 2014 Elsevier Inc. All rights reserved.

THE ROLE OF THE SPORTS PSYCHOLOGIST

Interest and involvement in sport psychology have grown tremendously in the last 15 to 20 years.[2] This change is, in part, a result of the increased awareness of how psychological and physiologic factors interact to enhance performance and how a balanced integration of these 2 facets can provide athletes with a winning edge.[3]

Although performance enhancement has heightened the awareness and popularity of sports psychology, there is still much about the role of the sports psychologist that needs to be emphasized to involved team physicians. Research has also shown that sports psychology can play an important role in injury prevention and healing (discussed later), in improving the athlete's self-care, improving mood, improving quality of life, and increasing the athlete's sense of internal control.[4] Physiologic advantages such as improvement in immune response, decreased postoperative pain and anxiety, shortened hospital stays, and decreased use of pain medications have also been proved to be enhanced by proper sports psychology intervention in athletes.[5]

Another area that is vital for team physicians to heed is recognition and management of psychological disorders in athletes (discussed later). Most current texts in sports psychology contain an abundance of information on cognitive-behavioral techniques, goal setting, imagery, and visualization for performance enhancement, but contain only limited discussions of the presence of psychological maladies in athletes and little examination of the dynamics at play inside the athlete's mind. There may be discussions between patients and team physicians about anxiety disorders or disordered eating, but mood or other personality disorders may be overlooked. It is possible that such disorders are more common in this population than is suspected.

For example, many of the behaviors associated with advanced or exceptional performance can be closely aligned with disordered personality diagnoses such as obsessive compulsive behavior patterns and perfectionist tendencies. Some individuals may even show characteristics of borderline personality and narcissistic personality disorders as a function of participation in their particular sport. Sports physicians and team psychologists need to be particularly aware of this potential for psychopathology in athletes to optimally manage such issues.

An area that may benefit the team physician is an awareness of the sports psychologist's role in recognizing the athletic identity: the degree with which an individual identifies with an athlete role.[6] This is an important self-concept that influences an individual's experiences, relationships with others, and pursuit of sport activity.[7] Strong athletic identification has been correlated with a firm sense of self-identity, more social interactions, increased confidence, and more positive athletic experiences.[8]

On the other hand, athletes who place too much emphasis on this identity may be at risk for psychological problems, particularly during sport transition periods such as adaptation to injury or retirement. The recognition of this overidentification by the sports psychologist or team physician may allow intervention to prevent transitional hardships for the athlete.[9]

SPORTS PSYCHOLOGIST AND SPORTS PHYSICIAN PARTNERSHIP

As discussed earlier, there are several areas in which a team physician and sports psychologist may work together to more effectively serve the athletes under their care. Such interaction may be used to address health issues such as stress, anxiety, depression, risky behavior, and unhealthy habits. Interactions with the sports psychologist and the team physician may also help athletes better deal with injury, maintain psychological well-being, and improve the athlete's performance to better prepare them for future life transitions. The following sections describe 5 specific areas of potential partnership.

Psychiatric Disorders in Athletes

Overall, the prevalence of psychiatric disorders in the athletic population is no different from that found in the general nonathletic population.[10–12] For example, the incidence of depression in college athletes (a significant 21%) is the same as that found in nonathletic college students.[13] Other maladies such as anxiety, obsessive compulsive disorder, and exercise addiction are much discussed in the sports psychology literature, but the incidence and prevalence of these disorders in athletics have been minimally studied. One caveat here is that there are increased incidences of certain disorders in certain types of athletics. For example, in aesthetic sports (eg, ballet, figure skating), 15% of athletes have been reported to suffer from anorexia or bulimia[14] compared with 1.2% to 2.3% in the general population.[15–18] In bulk/strength athletic endeavors, 23% of male athletes and up to 56% of female athletes taking anabolic steroids have reported major symptoms of mood disorders.[19,20]

With these points in mind, it is important for the team physician to be aware of the frequency of mood disorders, eating disorders, and other psychiatric conditions in the athletic population. A partnership between team physician and sports psychologist may heighten awareness, better educate coaching staff, and more effectively provide prompt therapeutic intervention when needed.

Overtraining

Overtraining syndrome is an ill-defined malady characterized by an increased perception of effort during sport, lack of energy, muscle soreness, sleep disturbances, loss of appetite, weight loss, mood disturbances, decreased self-confidence, inability to concentrate, and frequent upper respiratory tract infections.[21–23] These symptoms often overlap or are described as indistinguishable from depression/major mood disorders.[24]

Overtraining increases the incidence of injury and may also predispose some athletes to an increased incidence of long-term illness, such as diabetes in athletes who are continuingly bulking up; continued eating disorders in ballet dancers, skaters, gymnasts, and wrestlers; and long-term arthritis and other maladies in contact sports.

In addition to physical risks, overtrained athletes (especially elite athletes) may be more susceptible to a narrowed sense of identity[25] which has been linked with psychological stress and depression, especially when challenged by injury, failure, aging, or retirement.[26] In younger elite athletes, overtraining may lead to the development of a one-dimensional identity, unrealistic expectations, perceptions of conditional love, and perfectionistic traits.[27]

Elite athletes have a reported seasonal incidence of overtraining syndrome of 7% to 20%,[21] and younger elite athletes may be even more at risk with an incidence reported at 20% to 30%.[27] Still higher rates have been reported in basketball players during training camp (33%), professional soccer players during the season (50%), and in elite runners, with career prevalence rates of up to 60%.[28,29]

It is well for the sports physician to be aware of the frequency of overtraining syndrome, of groups that may be at particularly high risk, and of the signs and symptoms shown by affected athletes. Such awareness allows the team physician and sports psychologist to promptly address any physical or psychological issues, educate coaches, and prevent potential injury.

Injury Prevention

The American College of Sports Medicine Consensus Statement on psychological issues related to injuries in athletes notes that although there is no clear injury-prone personality type, (eg, perfectionist, introvert, extrovert), psychological factors can predispose athletes to injury and also play an important role in the rehabilitation and recovery from injury.[30,31] In particular, stress and stressful life events (eg, divorce, death, financial crisis) are clearly associated with increased injury rates, and a team physician should be aware of this, make coaches aware, and monitor athletes (as much as possible) for the occurrence of such events. When encountered by the team physician, stress reduction techniques and psychological support with a sports psychologist or mental health worker have proved effective.

Injury Rehabilitation

Psychological factors also play a role in the rehabilitation of athletes because during this time they can experience, medical, social, financial, sport-related, or personal stressors (eg, loss of identity, fear of reinjury, loss of confidence, mood swings, obsession with return-to-play issues).[32,33] All such emotional responses during rehabilitation can adversely affect recovery and future athletic participation. Just as patient mood and attitude have been proved to prolong surgical recovery times,[34] such factors should also be taken into consideration when setting goals and predicting recovery times for athletes in postinjury rehabilitation.

Team physicians should be mindful of the potential effect of psychological factors on injury and recovery and should be aware of the need for both physical and psychological rehabilitation.[30] The integration of a sports psychologist or other mental health provider into team dynamics can help with such issues of injury recovery.

Athletic Performance Enhancement

Although performance enhancement is an important and exciting area of sports psychology, such concerns usually lie outside the team physician's purview. Issues such as overcoming performance anxiety, building confidence, enhancing motivation, using imagery, decision making, anger management, resiliency, self-talk, team-building strategies, goal setting, peak performance, coach-athlete relationships, and so forth are more in the domain of coaches and sports psychologists rather than in the team physician's realm of overall health and wellness. Still, the team physician may wish to be aware of these programs and methods, both from general interest and as a method of relationship building with coaches and athletes.

Summary of Sports Psychologist and Sports Physician Partnership

With the increasing acceptance and widening use of sports psychology in professional and university settings,[35] team physicians need to be aware of the role that sports psychologists play in performance enhancement, injury prevention and recovery,[30,36] compliance, and the overall psychological and physical health of the athlete. The team physician must be aware of the role that life stressors play in increasing the risk of injury[37] and must help to recognize and address such issues when they arise. In addition, the team physician may play a role in helping to recognize pathologic personality disorders, risk-taking behavior, and unhealthy choices. In these instances, the team physician may aid in facilitating proper referral and treatment.

A partnership between the sports physician and the sports psychologist is vital if athletes and teams are to perform well, prevent and recover from injuries, promote overall health, maximize human potential, and contribute optimally to society.

NEW AND EMERGING TRENDS IN SPORTS PSYCHOLOGY

Although there is much ongoing and exciting research in performance enhancement and virtually every other area of sports psychology, we would like to propose 1 new area in which sports psychology could potentially be applied, an area that is important to the health of the nation.

A Potential Role for Sports Psychology in Affecting the Obesity Epidemic

Exercise effects on physical and mental health

In the United States, more than 250,000 deaths per year (12% of the total deaths/y) are attributable to a lack of regular physical activity.[38,39] It is well established that regular physical activity is protective against diabetes,[40] heart disease,[41] obesity, hypertension, and breast, prostate, and colon cancer, and results in a lower all-cause mortality.[42] Observational studies have also shown exercise to be protective against dementia and cognitive decline in elderly people.[43,44] In addition, exercise can benefit those with established heart disease, diabetes, hypertension, peripheral artery disease, heart failure, osteoarthritis, depression, anxiety, and several other chronic medical conditions.[45–48]

Studies also report that physical activity is associated with improvements in self-esteem,[49] well-being, satisfaction with appearance,[50] and symptoms of anxiety and depression.[51–53] It may protect against the development of depression as well.[45,54] Physical activity is believed to lessen depression and anxiety by both physiologic (increasing neurotransmitting amines and endorphins)[55,56] and psychological mechanisms (distracting patients from unpleasant situations, increasing social interaction, and increasing feelings of self-competence).[57,58]

It is clear that physical activity is vital to a healthy existence.

THE PROBLEM OF OBESITY

In the United States, roughly 60% of adults are overweight and 24% are obese.[59] Finkelstein and colleagues[60] estimated the total annual costs related to weight issues in the United States to be more than 78 billion dollars, accounting for 9.1% of total medical expenditures in 1998. Projections estimate that if these obesity trends continue, by 2030 costs will reach nearly 100 billion dollars and account for nearly 16% of total health care expenditures.

International studies indicate that obesity and obesity-related costs are global issues. Australia's adult overweight/obesity prevalence is 40%,[61] with an estimated annual cost of 21 billion dollars (2005),[62] and Canada's overweight/obesity prevalence is nearly 60%,[63] with direct costs estimated at 6 billion dollars. In Europe, an estimated 50% of adults are overweight or obese.[64] Global estimates in 2005 found that 23.2% of the world's adults were overweight (937 million people) and 9.8% were obese (396 million people).[65]

As stated earlier, the health and mental health effects of this epidemic are devastating both on an individual and societal level.

THE PROBLEM OF OBESITY IN CHILDREN

It is estimated that one-third of children and adolescents in the United States are overweight or obese[66] and, if trends continue, more than 40% will be obese by 2036.[67] Approximately 50% of obese 6-year-olds will remain so as adults,[68,69] whereas only 9% of normal-weight children will become obese as adults.[70] One long-term international study noted that more than 80% of obese children remained obese into adulthood when evaluated 23 years later.[71] There is also strong evidence that once obesity is established, it is difficult to reverse through interventions.[72]

As with adults, the health problems associated with childhood obesity are well known. However, it is important to keep in mind that childhood health risks associated with obesity are carried forward into adulthood, with a higher incidence of both childhood disease and adult medical conditions manifesting in these overweight and obese patients (eg, asthma, sleep apnea, hypertension, hyperlipidemia, coronary artery disease, diabetes, cancers).[73,74]

In addition to medical risks, overweight children can also experience psychological stressors, including discrimination from their peers, lowered self-esteem, depression, sadness, loneliness, nervousness, and other psychological maladies and psychosocial problems, which may persist into adulthood.[75,76]

If overweight or obese children normalize their body mass index (BMI) by adulthood, a marked reduction in these conditions is proved to occur. This is the goal of all intervention programs.[74]

Habits Started in Childhood

Childhood is a critical time for effective health promotion because children are more amenable to changing their habits, and because healthy habits acquired in childhood are more likely to persist into adulthood.[77–79] The transition from childhood to adolescence is a particularly crucial period when children are at increased risk for unnecessary weight gain.[80,81] During this time (age 10–12 years), children are afforded more dietary decision-making power (often choosing poorly) and more freedom as to how they spend their leisure time. They may also initiate unhealthy behaviors such as skipping breakfast, dropping out of organized sports, or increasing screen time/computer use.[82]

The Benefits of Physical Activity in Children

It is well established that physical activity aids in disease prevention, promotes mental health and well-being,[83] and enhances social skills.[84]

A report in 2010 from the Centers for Disease Control[85] concludes "there is substantial evidence that physical activity can help improve academic achievement, including grades and standardized test scores." These findings are corroborated by the most recent 2012 review,[86] which concludes, "physical activity is positively related to academic performance in children."

Physical activity in childhood and adolescence also predicts higher educational achievement[87,88] and greater socioeconomic success in adulthood.[89,90] These benefits are seen regardless of a child's socioeconomic background.

Recent Cuts in Physical Education Programs

Informed by these findings, the recent political trend to cut physical education (PE) programs and budgets[91] is misguided if long-term health and productivity are judged to be important by society. Currently, only 5 states (Illinois, Iowa, Massachusetts, New Mexico, and Vermont) require PE every year from kindergarten to 12th grade, and no federal law requires it be offered. However, in light of the current obesity epidemic, Congress may soon be forced to address the issue on a national level.[92]

Numbers of Children Participating in Physical Activity

Although the exact numbers and percentages of children engaging in school-based and after-school physical activity are not well documented, it is likely that these numbers have declined recently as obesity rates have increased. Childhood habits, carried forward into adulthood, likely contribute to the fact that only 37% of men and 24% of women in the United Kingdom engage in 30 minutes of exercise per day[93] and that only 50% of US adults do so.[94]

Reasons Why Children Participate

A 2006 review of reasons why children and adolescents participate in sports[95] examined 24 high-quality studies and concluded that among adolescents, weight management, social interaction, and enjoyment were common reasons for participation in sport and physical activity. More importantly, from our perspective, were the motivating factors and barriers to exercise in the younger age groups. These children were motivated by a love of experimentation, an interest in engaging in unusual activities, and parenteral involvement and support. Barriers included involvement in competitive sports or highly structured activity.

A Review of Obesity Prevention Programs: Models that Promote Behavioral Change

Weight gain, overweight, and obesity are a result of an imbalance between food intake, physical activity,[64] and a variety of genetic, behavioral, cultural, environmental, and economic factors.[96] In addition, in the United States and other developed countries, there is a significant tie between obesity and lower socioeconomic status, as well as a racial bias. In the United States, blacks and Hispanic children have a rate of obesity twice that of white/non-Hispanic children.[97]

Various multidisciplinary approaches to the problem of obesity and physical inactivity have been undertaken in the recent past, with varying results. For example, 1 program[98] was instituted in grammar schools in 2007 to 2008 in which professional educators taught kindergarteners to second-graders about health-related topics, including nutrition, physical activity, bullying, and germ prevention. Their interventions proved to significantly increase the knowledge of taught topics but failed to report significant effects on BMI. An extension of this pilot program called *Wholesome Routines* taught similar topics to third-graders to fifth-graders and included teachers, families, and food service providers to approach the issue from multiple angles. Results of the program interventions over the course of 1 year (2007–2008) revealed that 8.3% of students reduced BMI by 5% to 10%, and 39% of students reported increasing their physical activity by an hour per week. Although this result represents some progress, it is certainly not enough to recommend widespread program adaptation or to engender much enthusiasm.

Several other obesity prevention programs are currently in use (or are being investigated) in the United States and other developed countries. Whereas some programs report effectiveness, modest weight loss, (eg, CATCH [Coordinated Approach To Child Health],[99] HOP'N [Healthy Opportunities for Physical Activity and Nutrition][100]), increased physical activity, or decreased screen time, others do not.[101] Overall, only 50% of obesity intervention programs reviewed in 2006 were found to be effective.[102–104]

In reviewing the literature, a 2011 Cochrane meta-analysis of obesity prevention programs[105] evaluated 37 programs with 27,946 participating children (most between ages 6 and 12 years). The analysis concluded that overall, the programs, were "effective at reducing adiposity" and that children in the intervention groups experienced a mean difference in adiposity of 0.15 kg/m^2 or about a 180-g (0.4-pound) weight loss for an average 6-year-old or a 230-g (half-pound) weight loss for an average 12-year-old. Again, this result was not nearly significant enough to engender enthusiasm, especially because several of the interventions took place over several years.

The review noted that in assessing programs, common elements that contributed to effectiveness were: (1) a school-based curriculum that included healthy eating, physical activity, and body image; (2) increased sessions for physical activity and the development of movement skills; (3) improvements in the nutritional quality of foods supplied in schools; (4) environments and cultural practices that support children eating healthier foods and being active throughout each day; (5) support for teachers and other staff to implement health promotion strategies; and (6) parental support so that they may encourage these behaviors at home.

The Cochrane review's conclusion notes that, although positive, the results may be biased by the omission of smaller studies with negative outcomes. It also states that the data do not identify which components of which programs were most effective, and that the duration of the beneficial effects could not be shown over the long-term. This conclusion, along with the minimal amount of weight loss discussed earlier, is again hardly a ringing endorsement of current intervention programs.

The latest 2012 review of obesity prevention programs focused on children aged 4 to 6 years[106] and concluded that parental knowledge (eg, via informational handouts, newsletters) alone is insufficient in obesity prevention. Successful programs instead require parental engagement, including physical activity modeling, especially for male caregivers. It states that this strategy is vital and that parents/caregivers should be a major target of intervention programs.[107] The review recommends that physical and dietary behaviors be targeted together and that activity programs should encourage at least 120 minutes/d of physical activity (only 60 minutes/d is recommended by the US Centers for Disease Control [CDC]) and that dietary interventions should include child education, parental education and an examination of barriers to healthy food choices. Optimal programs should also limit leisure screen time to 1 hour per day and offer a variety of physical activities,[79] so that all children are encouraged to participate. The review also notes that forced competition can be counterproductive.

The Cochrane review, this review, and others[108–111] emphasize the importance of clear and simple messages. These messages must be grounded in scholarship, be designed to effect positive behavioral change, and be effectively communicated with all teachers, leaders, and parents involved in the programs.

The American Association of Pediatrics recommends that in treating and preventing obesity, physicians can help induce behavioral change by tracking weight and BMI, promoting a healthy diet, and encouraging increased activity.[112] However, despite these recommendations, many primary care physicians report that they believe that they lack skills to appropriately address the problem.[113] Therefore, current thinking holds that obesity is best approached in a multidisciplinary fashion, with physicians, allied health personnel, and behaviorists all involved and playing significant roles.

The literature supports family lifestyle intervention programs that emphasize education, parent and family involvement, goal formation, and monitoring. Such programs have been shown to be more effective than education-only programs.[114–116] Several studies have emphasized that parents must be included if interventions are to be successful, both because they can help offer children healthy alternatives and because of the importance of modeling.[117] A recent study found that parental confidence (in the ability of a program to effect change) was the strongest predictor of the success of a program.[118] Parents are also vital in discussions of barriers to weight loss and in identifying social networks (eg, peers, neighbors, family members) that could help or hinder weight loss efforts.[119] In addition to the important role that parents play, family intervention can also often assess factors that predict poor response to weight loss, such as depression, loneliness, teasing, and other social issues that the child may experience. Such intervention may also help identify appetite patterns such as poor satiety response, binge eating, or night eating syndrome.[120]

The most successful obesity interventions offer a socioenvironmental approach, one that recognizes the important inclusion of parents, family, the home environment, peers, and the community.[121–123] This model, rather than placing the responsibility for behavioral change solely on the individual and individual willpower, recognizes the role that the environment plays in both the problem and the solution. The socioenvironmental model requires parental involvement for the purpose of providing modeling, rule setting, and environmental interventions. Such environmental interventions include removing unhealthy choices (eg, excessive screen time, high-fat/high-sugar food choices) and making activity and healthful choices more accessible. In addition, this model incorporates positive peer influence and community resources whenever possible. This approach also requires that interventions be repetitive and intense enough to engrain new habits and patterns of behavior. Recent evidence supports this approach for sustainable weight loss.[121,122,124] As part of this approach, health care providers should schedule follow-up sessions with families and patients every 3 months to track weight and overall health, assess patient adaptation, compliance and attitudes, and to reinforce teachings and inculcate healthful habits.[125]

Many of the reviews discussed recommend that programs should have a common framework, but with enough flexibility built in to provide teachers/leaders with the opportunity to modify the program to account for cultural differences, community differences, and individual differences among participants.

A ROLE FOR SPORTS PSYCHOLOGY IN OBESITY PREVENTION

The shortcomings in obesity prevention programs beg for an innovative approach to the problem. One such innovative approach is to educate school coaches and PE teachers in sports psychology. Although many of the reviewed programs do have behavioral components, to the best of our knowledge, no programs to date have instituted sports psychology training in an attempt to increase participation, increase activity, and prevent obesity. We believe that this oversight demands to be addressed. Naturally, such a sports psychology component would be used in conjunction with successful components of established programs, as noted earlier. We believe that our novel sports psychology in obesity prevention program fits well into the socioenvironmental model and offers both a way to further positively affect the child's environment and a practical way to continue to teach and inculcate healthful values.

In addition, research has shown that athletes evaluate psychosocially trained coaches more positively than nontrained coaches[126,127] and that such coaches have been proved to increases athletes' self-esteem to a greater degree than nontrained coaches.[128,129] This situation, in turn, can lead to greater enjoyment and increased participation. Barnett and colleagues[129] found that 95% of youth who played for psychologically trained coaches returned to participate the following year, whereas only 74% of those who played for nontrained coaches returned.

An innovative advancement might be to incorporate a sports psychology component into an already proven prevention program, for the following reasons:

- Because physical inactivity has been reported as the most prevalent chronic disease risk factor, costing developed countries billions of dollars each year[130]
- Because sport is a major platform for encouraging the general population to become more physically active, and a key element of obesity reduction and health promotion strategies in developed countries[131]
- Because childhood habits are carried forward into adulthood[77–79]

- Because physical activity and childhood participation in activity are so vital to long-term health, school performance, and socioeconomic gain[89,90]
- Because decreased PE time in schools, insufficient safe areas for after-school play, and competing sedentary behaviors such as computers, TV and video games are making it more challenging to meet physical activity goals[132]
- Because coaches trained in sports psychology have been proved to increase children's participation in sport and increase participant enjoyment of physical activity[129]
- Because, as summarized earlier, existing obesity prevention programs have limited effectiveness on weight and physical activity in children
- Because to date, no obesity prevention programs have included educating elementary school coaches and PE teachers in sports psychology

This strategy could positively affect the outcomes of enhanced enjoyment, increased participation, improved school performance, and a reduction of overweight and obesity. It is certainly a question worth exploring.

REFERENCES

1. Aoyagi MW, Portenga ST. The role of positive ethics and virtues in the context of sport and performance psychology service delivery. Prof Psychol Res Pr 2010; 41(3):253–9.
2. Costa C. The status and future of sport management: a Delphi study. J Sport Manag 2005;19(2):117–42.
3. Buckworth J, Dishman RK. Determinants of exercise and physical activity. In: Buckworth J, Dishman RK, editors. Exercise psychology. Champaign (IL): Human Kinetics; 2002. p. 3–15.
4. Armatas V, Chondrou E, Yiannakos A. Psychological aspects of rehabilitation following serious athletic injuries with special reference to goal setting: a review study. Physical Training. 2007. Available at: http://ejmas.com/pt/ptframe.htm. Accessed October 14, 2012.
5. Dworsky D, Krane V. Using the mind to health body. Association for Applied Sport Psychology. Available at: http://www.appliedsportpsych.org/resource-center/injury-&-rehabilitation/articles/imagery. Accessed September 12, 2012.
6. Brewer BW, Cornelius AE. Self-protective changes in athletic identity following anterior cruciate ligament reconstruction. Psychol Sport Exerc 2010;11(1): 1–5.
7. Cornelius A. The relationship between athletic identity, peer and faculty socialization, and college student development. J Coll Stud Dev 1995;36(6):560–73.
8. Griffith KA, Johnson KA. Athletic identity and life role of Division-I and Division-III collegiate athletes. 2002. Available at: http://murphylibrary.uwlax.edu/digital/jur/2002/griffith-johnson.pdf. Accessed September 12, 2012.
9. Brewer BW, Van Raalte JL, Linder DE. Athletic identity: Hercules' muscles or Achilles heel? Int J Sport Psychol 1993;24:237–54.
10. Markser VZ. Sport psychiatry and psychotherapy. Mental strains and disorders in professional sports. Challenge and answer to societal changes. Eur Arch Psychiatry Clin Neurosci 2011;261(Suppl 2):S182–5.
11. Yang J, Peek-Asa C, Corlette JD, et al. Prevalence of and risk factors associated with symptoms of depression in competitive collegiate students athletes. Clin J Sport Med 2007;17(6):481–7.
12. Donohue B, Covassin T, Lancer K, et al. Examination of psychiatric symptoms in student athletes. J Genet Psychol 2004;131:29–36.

13. Kelly WE, Kelly KE, Brown FC, et al. Gender differences in depression among college students: a multi-cultural perspective. Coll Student J 1999;33:72–6. Available at: http://www.freepatentsonline.com/article/College-Student-Journal/62894055.html. Accessed October 15, 2012.

14. Byrne S, McLean N. Elite athletes: effects of the pressure to be thin. J Sci Med Sport 2002;5:80–94.

15. Bulik CM, Sullivan PF, Tozzi F, et al. Prevalence, heritability, and prospective risk factors for anorexia nervosa. Arch Gen Psychiatry 2006;63:305–12.

16. Keski-Rahkonen A, Sihvola E, Raevuori A, et al. Reliability of self-reported eating disorders: optimizing population screening. Int J Eat Disord 2006; 39(8):754–62.

17. Hudson JI, Hiripi E, Pope HG Jr, et al. The prevalence and correlates of eating disorders in the National Comorbidity Survey Replication. Biol Psychiatry 2007; 61(3):348–58.

18. Keski-Rahkonen A, Hoek HW, Linna MS, et al. Incidence and outcomes of bulimia nervosa: a nationwide population-based study. Psychol Med 2009;39: 823–31.

19. Pope HG Jr, Katz DL. Psychiatric and medical effects of anabolic-androgenic steroid use. A controlled study of 160 athletes. Arch Gen Psychiatry 1994; 51(5):375–82.

20. Gruber AJ, Pope HG Jr. Psychiatric and medical effects of anabolic-androgenic steroid use in women. Psychother Psychosom 2000;69(1):19–26.

21. Morgan WP, Brown DR, Raglin JS, et al. Psychological monitoring of overtraining and staleness. Br J Sports Med 1987;21(3):107–14.

22. Hawley CJ, Schoene RB. Overtraining syndrome: why training too hard, too long, doesn't work. Phys Sportsmed 2003;31(6):47–8.

23. Budgett R, Newsholme E, Lehmann M, et al. Redefining the overtraining syndrome as the unexplained underperformance syndrome. Br J Sports Med 2000;34(1):67–8.

24. Schwenk TL. The stigmatization and denial of mental illness in athletes. Br J Sports Med 2000;34(1):4–5.

25. Cresswell SL, Eklund RC. Athlete burnout: a longitudinal qualitative investigation. Sport Psychol 2007;21:1–20.

26. Reardon CL, Factor RM. Sport psychiatry: a systematic review of diagnosis and medical treatment of mental illness in athletes. Sports Med 2010;40:61–80.

27. Winsley R, Matos N. Overtraining and elite young athletes. Med Sport Sci 2011; 56:97–105.

28. Morgan WP, O'Connor PJ, Sparling PB, et al. Psychologic characterization of the elite female distance runner. Int J Sports Med 1987;8(Suppl 2):124–31.

29. Morgan WP, O'Connor PJO, Ellickson KA, et al. Personality structure, mood states, and performance in elite male distance runners. Int J Sport Psychol 1988;19:247–63.

30. American College of Sports Medicine, American Academy of Family Physicians, American Academy of Orthopaedic Surgeons, et al. Psychological issues related to injury in athletes and the team physician: a consensus statement. Med Sci Sports Exerc 2006;38(11):2030–4.

31. Wiese-Bjornstal DM. Psychology and socioculture affect injury risk, response, and recovery in high-intensity athletes: a consensus statement. Scand J Med Sci Sports 2010;20(Suppl 2):103–11.

32. Evans L, Wadey R, Hanton S, et al. Stressors experienced by injured athletes. J Sports Sci 2012;30(9):917–27.

33. Podlog L, Dimmock J, Miller J. A review of return to sport concerns following injury rehabilitation: practitioner strategies for enhancing recovery outcomes. Phys Ther Sport 2011;12(1):36–42.
34. Rosenberger PH, Jokl P, Ickovics J, et al. Psychosocial factors and surgical outcomes: an evidence-based literature review. J Am Acad Orthop Surg 2006; 14(7):397–405.
35. Williams JM. Sport psychology: past, present, future. In: Williams JM, editor. Applied sports psychology. 6th edition. Philadelphia: McGraw Hill Higher Education; 2009. p. 7–13.
36. Ahern DK, Lohr BA. Psychosocial factors in sports injury rehabilitation. Clin Sports Med 1997;16(4):755–68.
37. Williams JM, Andersen MB. Psychological antecedents of sport and injury: review and critique of the stress and injury model. J Appl Sport Psychol 1998;10:5–25.
38. Hahn RA, Teutsch SM, Rothenberg RB, et al. Excess deaths from nine chronic diseases in the United States. JAMA 1990;264:2654–9.
39. McGinnis JM, Foege WH. Actual causes of death in the United States. JAMA 1993;270:2207–12.
40. Helmrich SP, Ragland DR, Leung RW, et al. Physical activity and reduced occurrence of non-insulin-dependent diabetes mellitus. N Engl J Med 1991;325: 147–52.
41. Kodama S, Saito K, Tanaka S, et al. Cardiorespiratory fitness as a quantitative predictor of all-cause mortality and cardiovascular events in healthy men and women: a meta-analysis. JAMA 2009;301:2024.
42. Paffenbarger RS Jr, Hyde RT, Wing AL, et al. The association of changes in physical-activity level and other lifestyle characteristics with mortality among men. N Engl J Med 1993;328:538.
43. Simonsick EM. Fitness and cognition: encouraging findings and methodological considerations for future work. J Am Geriatr Soc 2003;51:570.
44. Coyle JT. Use it or lose it–do effortful mental activities protect against dementia? N Engl J Med 2003;348:2489.
45. Pate RR, Pratt M, Blair SN, et al. Physical activity and public health. A recommendation from the Centers for Disease Control and Prevention and the American College of Sports Medicine. JAMA 1995;273(5):402–7.
46. Martinsen EW. Physical activity and depression: clinical experience. Acta Psychiatr Scand 1994;377(Suppl):23–7.
47. Dimeo F, Bauer M, Varahram I, et al. Benefits from aerobic exercise in patients with major depression: a pilot study. Br J Sports Med 2001;35(2):114–7.
48. Dunn AL, Trivedi MH, O'Neal HA. Physical activity dose-response effects on outcomes of depression and anxiety. Med Sci Sports Exerc 2001;33(Suppl 6): 587–97.
49. Martinsen EW, Hoffart A, Solberg O. Aerobic and non-aerobic forms of exercise in the treatment of anxiety disorders. Stress Med 1989;5:115–20.
50. Paluska SA, Schwenk TL. Physical activity and mental health: current concepts. Sports Med 2000;29(3):167–80.
51. Mead GE, Morley W, Campbell P, et al. Exercise for depression. Cochrane Database Syst Rev 2009;(3):CD004366.
52. Krogh J, Nordentoft M, Sterne JA, et al. The effect of exercise in clinically depressed adults: systematic review and meta-analysis of randomized controlled trials. J Clin Psychiatry 2011;72(4):529–38.
53. Conn VS. Depressive symptom outcomes of physical activity interventions: meta-analysis findings. Ann Behav Med 2010;39(2):128–38.

54. Raglin JS. Exercise and mental health. Beneficial and detrimental effects. Sports Med 1990;9(6):323–9.
55. Ransford CP. A role for amines in the antidepressant effect of exercise: a review. Med Sci Sports Exerc 1982;4(1):1–10.
56. Morgan WP. Affective beneficence of vigorous physical activity. Med Sci Sports Exerc 1985;17:94–100.
57. North TC, McCullagh P, Tran ZV. Effect of exercise on depression. Exerc Sport Sci Rev 1990;18:379–415.
58. Peluso MA, Guerra de Andrade LH. Physical activity and mental health: the association between exercise and mood. Clinics (Sao Paulo) 2005;60(1):61–70.
59. Centers for Disease Control and Prevention (CDC). State-specific prevalence of obesity among adults–United States, 2005. MMWR Morb Mortal Wkly Rep 2006; 55(36):985–8.
60. Finkelstein E, Fiebelkorn I, Wang G. National medical expenditures attributable to overweight and obesity: how much and who's paying? Health Aff (Millwood) 2003;(Suppl Web Exclusives):W3-219-26.
61. Dunstan DR, Zimmet P, Welborn T, et al. Diabesity & associated disorders in Australia–2000: the accelerating epidemic. The Australian Diabetes, Obesity and Lifestyle Study (AusDiab). Melbourne (Victoria): International Diabetes Institute; 2001.
62. Colagiuri S, Lee CM, Colagiuri R, et al. The cost of overweight and obesity in Australia. Med J Aust 2010;192(5):260–4.
63. Anis AH, Zhang W, Bansback N, et al. Obesity and overweight in Canada: an updated cost-of-illness study. Obes Rev 2010;11(1):31–40.
64. Brug J, Lien N, Klepp KI, et al. Exploring overweight, obesity and their behavioural correlates among children and adolescents: results from the Health-promotion through Obesity Prevention across Europe project. Public Health Nutr 2010;13(10A):1676–9.
65. Kelly T, Yang W, Chen CS, et al. Global burden of obesity in 2005 and projections to 2030. Int J Obes (Lond) 2008;32(9):1431–7.
66. Ogden CL, Carroll MD, Kit BK, et al. Prevalence of obesity and trends in body mass index among US children and adolescents, 1999-2010. JAMA 2012;307:483.
67. Kopelman PG. Obesity as a medical problem. Nature 2000;404:635–43.
68. Whitaker RC, Wright JA, Pepe MS, et al. Predicting obesity in young adulthood from childhood and parental obesity. N Engl J Med 1997;337:869.
69. Singh AS, Chin A, Paw MJ, et al. Dutch obesity intervention in teenagers: effectiveness of a schoolbased program on body composition and behavior. Arch Pediatr Adolesc Med 2009;163(4):309–17.
70. Freedman DS, Khan LK, Serdula MK, et al. Racial differences in the tracking of childhood BMI to adulthood. Obes Res 2005;13(5):928–35.
71. Herman KM, Craig CL, Gauvin L, et al. Tracking of obesity and physical activity from childhood to adulthood: the Physical Activity Longitudinal Study. Int J Pediatr Obes 2009;4:281.
72. Oude Luttikhuis H, Baur L, Jansen H, et al. Interventions for treating obesity in children. Cochrane Database Syst Rev 2009;(1):CD001872.
73. Daniels SR. The consequences of childhood overweight and obesity. Future Child 2006;16(1):47–67.
74. Juonala M, Magnussen CG, Berenson GS, et al. Childhood adiposity, adult adiposity, and cardiovascular risk factors. N Engl J Med 2011;365:1876.
75. Strauss R. Childhood obesity and self-esteem. Pediatrics 2000;105:e15.

76. Dietz WH. Health consequences of obesity in youth: childhood predictors of adult disease. Pediatrics 1998;101(3 Pt 2):518–25.
77. Tripodi A, Severi S, Midili S, et al. "Community projects" in Modena (Italy): promote regular physical activity and healthy nutrition habits since childhood. Int J Pediatr Obes 2011;6(Suppl 2):54–6.
78. te Velde SJ, Twisk JW, Brug J. Tracking of fruit and vegetable consumption from adolescence into adulthood and its longitudinal association with overweight. Br J Nutr 2007;98(2):431–8.
79. Cleland V, Dwyer T, Venn A. Which domains of childhood physical activity predict physical activity in adulthood? A 20-year prospective tracking study. Br J Sports Med 2012;46(8):595–602.
80. Demory-Luce D, Morales M, Nicklas T, et al. Changes in food group consumption patterns from childhood to young adulthood: the Bogalusa Heart Study. J Am Diet Assoc 2004;104:1684–91.
81. Kimm SY, Glynn NW, Obarzanek E, et al. Relation between the changes in physical activity and body-mass index during adolescence: a multicentre longitudinal study. Lancet 2005;366:301–7.
82. Windle M, Grunbaum JA, Elliott M, et al. Healthy passages–a multilevel, multimethod longitudinal study of adolescent health. Am J Prev Med 2004;27: 164–72.
83. Biddle SJH, Fox KR. The way forward for physical activity and the promotion of psychological well-being. In: Biddle SJH, Fox KR, Boutcher SH, editors. Physical activity and psychological well-being. London: Routledge; 2000. p. 154–68.
84. Mahoney L, Carns B, Farmer T. Promoting interpersonal competence and educational success through extracurricular activity participation. J Educ Psychol 2003;95:409–18.
85. Rasberry CN, Lee SM, Robin L, et al. The association between school-based physical activity, including physical education, and academic performance: a systematic review of the literature. Prev Med 2011;52(Suppl 1):S10–20.
86. Singh A, Uijtdewilligen L, Twisk JW, et al. Physical activity and performance at school: a systematic review of the literature including a methodological quality assessment. Arch Pediatr Adolesc Med 2012;166(1):49–55.
87. Taras H. Physical activity and student performance at school. J Sch Health 2005;75:214–8.
88. Dwyer T, Sallis JF, Blizzard L. Relation of academic performance to physical activity and fitness in children. Pediatr Exerc Sci 2001;13:225–37.
89. Koivusilta LK, Nupponen H, Rimpelä AH. Adolescent physical activity predicts high education and socio-economic position in adulthood. Eur J Public Health 2012;22(2):203–9.
90. Aarnio M, Winter T, Kujala U, et al. Associations of health related behaviour, social relationships, and health status with persistent physical activity and inactivity: a study of Finnish adolescent twins. Br J Sports Med 2002;36: 360–4.
91. Roslow Research Group. Physical education trends in our nation's schools a survey of practicing K-12 physical education teachers. National Association for Sport and Physical Education (NASPE); 2009. Available at: http://www.aahperd.org/naspe/about/announcements/upload/PE-Trends-Report.pdf. Accessed November 2, 2012.
92. Perna FM, Oh A, Chriqui JF, et al. The association of state law to physical education time allocation in US public schools. Am J Public Health 2012;102(8): 1594–9.

93. Joint Health Surveys Unit. Health survey for England 1998. London: HMSO; 1999.
94. Haskell WL, Lee IM, Pate RR, et al. Physical activity and public health updated recommendation for adults from the American College of Sports Medicine and the American Heart Association. Med Sci Sports Exerc 2007;39(8):1423–34.
95. Allender S, Cowburn G, Foster C. Understanding participation in sport and physical activity among children and adults: a review of qualitative studies. Health Educ Res 2006;21(6):826–35.
96. Lobstein T, Bauer L, Uauy R. Obesity in children and young people: a crisis in public health. Obes Rev 2004;5(Suppl 1):1–104.
97. Ogden CL, Flegal KM, Carroll MD, et al. Prevalence and trends in overweight among US children and adolescents, 1999–2000. JAMA 2002;288:1728–32.
98. Vinsel D. Shedding old habits to create a new future. Interactive program targets childhood obesity by teaching healthy lifestyle choices. Healthc Exec 2010; 25(3):70, 72.
99. Hoelscher DM, Springer AE, Ranjit N, et al. Reductions in child obesity among disadvantaged school children with community involvement: the Travis County CATCH Trial. Obesity (Silver Spring) 2010;18(Suppl 1):S36–44.
100. Dzewaltowski DA, Rosenkranz RR, Geller KS, et al. HOP'N after-school project: an obesity prevention randomized controlled trial. Int J Behav Nutr Phys Act 2010;7:90.
101. Croker H, Viner RM, Nicholls D, et al. Family-based behavioural treatment of childhood obesity in a UK National Health Service setting: randomized controlled trial. Int J Obes (Lond) 2012;36(1):16–26.
102. Doak CM, Visscher TL, Renders CM, et al. The prevention of overweight and obesity in children and adolescents: a review of interventions and programmes. Obes Rev 2006;7:111–36.
103. Campbell K, Waters E, O'Meara S, et al. Interventions for preventing obesity in childhood. A systematic review. Obes Rev 2001;2:149–57.
104. Hardeman W, Griffin S, Johnston M, et al. Interventions to prevent weight gain: a systematic review of psychological models and behaviour change methods. Int J Obes Relat Metab Disord 2000;24:131–43.
105. Waters E, de Silva-Sanigorski A, Hall BJ, et al. Interventions for preventing obesity in children. Cochrane Database Syst Rev 2011;(12):CD001871.
106. Summerbell CD, Moore HJ, Vögele C, et al. Evidence-based recommendations for the development of obesity prevention programs targeted at preschool children. ToyBox-study group. Obes Rev 2012;13(Suppl 1):129–32.
107. Doak C, Heitmann B, Summerbell C, et al. Prevention of childhood obesity–what type of evidence should we consider relevant? Obes Rev 2009;10:350–6.
108. Haerens L, Vereecken C, Maes L, et al. Relationship of physical activity and dietary habits with body mass index in the transition from childhood to adolescence: a 4-year longitudinal study. Public Health Nutr 2010;13(10A):1722–8.
109. Robinson TN. Television viewing and childhood obesity. Pediatr Clin North Am 2001;48:1017–25.
110. Gortmaker SL, Cheung LW, Peterson KE, et al. Impact of a school-based interdisciplinary intervention on diet and physical activity among urban primary school children: eat well and keep moving. Arch Pediatr Adolesc Med 1999; 153:975–83.
111. James J, Thomas P, Cavan D, et al. Preventing childhood obesity by reducing consumption of carbonated drinks: cluster randomized controlled trial. BMJ 2004;328:1237.

112. Krebs NF, Jacobson MS. Prevention of pediatric overweight and obesity. Pediatrics 2003;112(2):424–30.
113. Holt N, Schetzina KE, Dalton WT 3rd, et al. Primary care practice addressing child overweight and obesity: a survey of primary care physicians at four clinics in southern Appalachia. South Med J 2011;104(1):14–9.
114. American Dietetic Association (ADA). Position of the American Dietetic Association: individual-, family-, school-, and community-based interventions for pediatric overweight. J Am Diet Assoc 2006;106(6):925–45.
115. Latzer Y, Edmunds L, Fenig S, et al. Managing childhood overweight: behavior, family, pharmacology, and bariatric surgery interventions. Obesity 2008;17: 411–23.
116. Wilfley DE, Tibbs TL, Van Buren DJ, et al. Lifestyle interventions in the treatment of childhood overweight: a meta-analytic review of randomized controlled trials. Health Psychol 2007;26(5):521–32.
117. Young KM, Northern JJ, Lister KM, et al. A meta-analysis of family-behavioral weight-loss treatments for children. Clin Psychol Rev 2007;27:240–9.
118. Gunnarsdottir T, Njardvik U, Olafsdottir AS, et al. The role of parental motivation in family-based treatment for childhood obesity. Obesity (Silver Spring) 2011; 19(8):1654–62.
119. Wilfley DE, Kass AE, Kolko RP. Counseling and behavior change in pediatric obesity. Pediatr Clin North Am 2011;58(6):1403–24, x.
120. Vander Wal JS. Night eating syndrome: a critical review of the literature. Clin Psychol Rev 2012;32(1):49–59.
121. Glass TA, McAtee MJ. Behavioral science at the crossroads in public health: extending horizons, envisioning the future. Soc Sci Med 2006;62(7):1650–71.
122. Huang TT, Drewnosksi A, Kumanyika S, et al. A systems-oriented multilevel framework for addressing obesity in the 21st century. Prev Chronic Dis 2009; 6(3):A82.
123. Kumanyika SK, Obarzanek E, Stettler N, et al. Population-based prevention of obesity: the need for comprehensive promotion of healthful eating, physical activity, and energy balance: a scientific statement from American Heart Association Council on Epidemiology and Prevention, Interdisciplinary Committee for Prevention (formerly the Expert Panel on Population and Prevention Science). Circulation 2008;118(4):428–64.
124. Wilfley DE, Stein RI, Saelens BE, et al. Efficacy of maintenance treatment approaches for childhood overweight: a randomized controlled trial. JAMA 2007; 298(14):1661–73.
125. Dorsey KB, Mauldon M, Magraw R, et al. Applying practice recommendations for the prevention and treatment of obesity in children and adolescents. Clin Pediatr (Phila) 2010;49(2):137–45.
126. Smith RE, Smoll FL, Curtis B. Coach effectiveness training: a cognitive-behavioral approach to enhancing relationship skills in youth sport coaches. J Sport Psychol 1979;1:59–75.
127. Smoll FL, Smith RE. Coaching behavior research and intervention in youth sports. In: Smoll FL, Smith RE, editors. Children and youth in sport: a biopsychosocial perspective. Dubuque (IA): Kendall-Hunt; 2002. p. 211–33.
128. Coatsworth JD, Conroy DE. Enhancing the self-esteem of youth swimmers through coach training: gender and age effects. Psychol Sport Exerc 2006;7: 173–92.
129. Barnett NP, Smoll FL, Smith RE. Effects of enhancing coach-athlete relationships on youth sport attrition. Sport Psychol 1992;6:111–27.

130. Allender S, Foster C, Scarborough P, et al. The burden of physical activity-related ill health in the UK. J Epidemiol Community Health 2007;61:344–8.
131. Hughes L, Leavey G. Setting the bar: athletes and vulnerability to mental illness. Br J Psychiatry 2012;200(2):95–6.
132. Telama R, Yang X. Decline of physical activity from youth to young adulthood in Finland. Med Sci Sports Exerc 2000;32:1617–22.

Effects of Obesity on Obstetric Ultrasound Imaging

Loralei L. Thornburg, MD

KEYWORDS

- Ultrasound scan • Obesity • Anatomic evaluation • First-trimester screening
- Genetic sonogram • Anomaly • Nuchal translucency

KEY POINTS

- Obesity, especially morbid obesity, limits the ability to complete screening in pregnancy.
- Obese patients are at higher risk for fetal anomalies and failure to detect anomalies before birth than their normal-weight counterparts.
- Birth weight prediction in obese patients by the gestation-adjusted prediction method seems to be accurate and allows evaluation of the fetus at a gestational age when visualization is improved.

INTRODUCTION

Obesity is increasing worldwide, with most of the industrialized world having obesity rates of 20%–30% in the adult population and some selected populations, such as the southern Pacific, reporting obesity rates of 44%–80%.[1,2] Obesity is defined as a body mass index (BMI) of greater than 30 and is generally divided into classes, with class I consisting of BMI of 30.0–34.9 kg/m^2, class II BMI of 35.0–39.9 kg/m^2, and class III BMI of $\geq$40 kg/m^2. Class III has also been called *extreme obesity* and represents body weights 50%–100% higher than ideal.[1,3] According to the World Health Organization, "(obesity) is now so common that it is replacing the more traditional concerns...as one of the most significant contributors to ill health."[1] Weight, age, and parity all tend to increase in concert, and obesity can lead to increase medical concerns; therefore, the obese woman often tends to have additional medical concerns and may be of advanced maternal age.[4,5]

The ability to penetrate an obese patient can be limited in ultrasound scan; therefore, understanding the limitations of visualization in this population is important for the clinician counseling patients regarding their pregnancy risks. Obesity is also a

This article originally appeared in Ultrasound Clinics, Volume 8, Issue 1, January 2013.

Disclosures: None.

Conflicts of interest: None.

Division of Maternal Fetal Medicine, Department of OB/GYN, University of Rochester Medical Center, University of Rochester, 601 Elmwood Avenue Box 668, Rochester, NY 14642, USA

E-mail address: Loralei_thornburg@urmc.rochester.edu

2352-7986/14/$ – see front matter © 2014 Elsevier Inc. All rights reserved.

major risk factor for numerous obstetric complications and may limit a clinician's ability to assess the health of the fetus by ultrasound scan.

GENERAL APPROACH TO ULTRASOUND IN THE OBESE PATIENT

There is no question that with increased depth of penetration, there is increased absorption and dispersion of the sound waves, such that the reflected signal is distorted and weakened, resulting in backscatter and an increased noise-to-signal ratio.[6] Therefore, when performing ultrasound scan on the obese patient, the sonographer must take into account the altered habitus and plan accordingly. In general, the sonographer should make an effort to find and use the best acoustic windows for a woman's habitus. Adjusting approaches to improve ultrasound visualization has been suggested, most with little prospective data (**Box 1**). In general, abdominal adiposity tends to cluster centrally below the umbilicus and above pubis, with little at the inferior abdomen, umbilicus, or laterally.[6] Therefore, for some morbidly obese women, visualization may be best underneath the pannus at the pubis, whereas for others, the skin apron may be relaxed and inferiorly displaced enough that the depth of penetration is actually better above the fold. If an under-the-pannus approach is taken, the sonographer may need to request help from the patient or family in holding or retracting her abdomen to allow hand movements once within the fold. Additionally, care should be taken to fully dry this area after completion, because it is prone to breakdown with increased wetness. Rolling a patient onto her side may improve visualization (**Fig. 1**), as can using the iliac fossa, which generally also has less adipose tissue (**Fig. 2**). Prior abdominal scarring from cesarean delivery or multiple gestation, both more frequent in obese patients, can also decrease visualization.[4,6]

For some women, the umbilicus may provide a window, and a narrow probe or even transvaginal probe within a deep umbilicus may improve visualization. However, the angles and mobility of the probe are limited. Using the maternal bladder as a window

---

Box 1
Tips for scanning obese patients to improve visualization

- Use of the lateral, inferior, or periumbilical regions, because abdominal adiposity tends to cluster centrally below the umbilicus and above pubis

- Retraction of skin apron to allow visualization within the superpubic fold

- Rolling patient onto her side

- Making use of the iliac fossa

- Use of a narrow probe or even the transvaginal probe within a deep umbilicus

- Use of the maternal bladder as a window and to raise the uterus out of the pelvis

- Combined transvaginal/transabdominal approach with the transvaginal probe used to elevate the uterus out of the pelvis, and the transabdominal approach to visualize the fetus

- Upright scanning with the patient sitting to displace adipose inferiorly

- Transvaginal assessment for those fetal parts near the cervix

- Use of harmonic imaging, spatial compounding, and speckle reduction filters

Data from Paladini D. Sonography in obese and overweight pregnant women: clinical, medicolegal and technical issues. Ultrasound Obstet Gynecol 2009;33:720–9; Bromley B, Shipp TD, Mitchell, et al. Tricks for obtaining a nuchal translucency measurement on the fetus in a difficult position. J Ultrasound Med 2010;29:1261–4; Thornburg LL. Antepartum obstetrical complications associated with obesity. Semin Perinatol 2011;35:317–23.

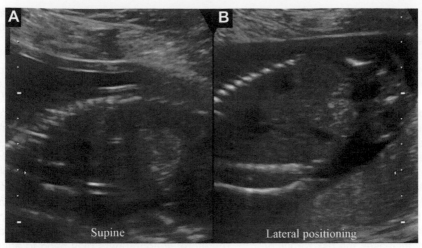

Fig. 1. Lateral positioning. The supine position (*A*) may have decreased visualization compared to lateral positioning (*B*), which can allow use of the thinner lateral abdomen and shift a pannus away from the fetal parts. In the image obtained in the lateral position (*B*), there is markedly better visualization of the fetal abdomen, chest contours, and bladder without changing any other settings.

is critical, especially in the first trimester, and in later pregnancy, a full bladder may serve to raise the uterus out of the pelvis and move the fetal target closer to the surface of the maternal abdomen.[6] Other suggested strategies include combining transvaginal/transabdominal approach, using the transvaginal probe to elevate the uterus out of the pelvis, and the transabdominal approach to visualize the fetus.[7] Upright

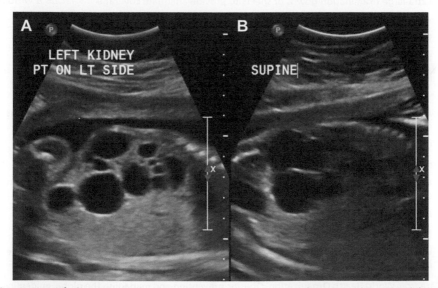

Fig. 2. Use of the iliac fossa. Because adiposity tends to cluster in the central lower abdomen, using the iliac fossa (*A*) where there is less thickness may improve visualization. In visualizing this multicystic abnormal fetal kidney, the views obtained through the central abdomen (*B*) lack the clarity of those images obtained through the lateral iliac fossa (*A*), where individual cysts become clearly visible.

scanning with the patient sitting may further displace the adipose inferiorly and provide acoustic windows, and for those fetal parts that are near the cervix, transvaginal assessment may also be valuable.[8]

Visualization may be limited even with the best equipment, and scanning of the obese patient can represent a physical challenge to the sonographer, with the literature suggesting that scanning obese patients contributes to injury.[9,10] Making sure that the physical environment is not contributing to sonographer burden is important (**Box 2**), and ideally alterations should include higher stools and high-rated, motorized patient beds so that patients can be easily positioned and repositioned as the scan proceeds. If patients lack mobility, ultrasound scans can be performed in motorized wheelchairs and scooters, especially if these can be reclined, to avoid staff having to transfer patients. If a transvaginal approach is used, the weight rating of the bed should be checked against the patient weight, because if a morbidly obese patient is placed in stirrups on an unbolted, underrated bed, weight readjustment can cause the bed to tip. The larger the patient, the pressure a sonographer will have to apply over likely a prolonged period of time is higher, and this prolonged orthopedic strain likely increases the risk for injury.[6,9,10] Therefore, sonographers may need to adjust their body position frequently or, in the case of particularly long ultrasound examinations, such as an anatomic survey in twins on a morbidly obese patient, change operators midway through the examination.

Box 2
Alterations to care for obese patients in the ultrasound environment

Create an accessible and comfortable office environment

- Sturdy, armless chairs and high, firm sofas in waiting and examination rooms, because obese patients often have obese family members

- Extra-large examination gowns or sheets to provide adequate coverage

Use medical equipment that can accurately assess patients

- Sturdy, wide examination tables bolted to the floor to prevent tipping

- Stool or step with handles to help patients get on the examination table

- Hydraulic beds that easily allow patients to easily get on and off the table

Reduce patient fears about weight

- Avoid the term *obesity*—many patients may be more comfortable with terms such as *difficulties with weight* or *being overweight*

- Only ask about weight or weigh patient when medically appropriate and do so in private

Protect the safety of the ultrasound staff

- Examination chairs for sonographers with adjustment to support arms and allow position changes

- Rotation of sonographers during ultrasound examination if particularly long or difficult

- Maximization of settings to minimize time and effort required to obtain images

- Use of assist devices and beds that easily allow patients to be repositioned to improve imaging

Data from World Health Organization. Obesity: preventing and managing the global epidemic. WHO technical report series 894. Geneva (Switzerland): World Health Organization, 2000; Paladini D. Sonography in obese and overweight pregnant women: clinical, medicolegal and technical issues. Ultrasound Obstet Gynecol 2009;33:720–9; Thornburg LL. Antepartum obstetrical complications associated with obesity. Semin Perinatol 2011;35:317–23.

Ultrasound equipment should have optimized obesity and penetration settings to aid in completing scans more comfortably and quickly, which may help reduce the risks of sonographer injury because of needing to use less pressure and time to adequately visualize. Harmonic imaging (**Figs. 3** and **4**) and spatial compounding and speckle reduction filters can markedly improve the visualization in these women and should be part of this "obesity" setting (**Fig. 5**).[6,11] Doppler imaging may also help with visualization of cardiac inflows and outflows.[6] Regardless, before any imaging, the patient should be counseled regarding the technical limitations, from obesity and other medical conditions, and the increased risk of undiagnosed fetal anomalies.[6,8,12]

Obesity and First-Trimester Screening

As obesity increases with maternal age, early and accurate screening ultrasound scan for aneuploidy screening is important. Although first-trimester screening is offered to all women, there is a failure rate associated with this test. The First and Second Trimester Screening (FaSTER) trial had a failure rate of only 7.1% for nuchal translucency (NT) measurement.[13] However, other studies have found higher failure rates outside of the study setting, with Wax and colleagues[14] showing a 20% NT failure rate on first attempt among all comers (taking into account that some patients will be referred at an inappropriate gestational age or have a nonviable pregnancy), which is more of real world failure number. Repeated attempts did seem to improve completion rates to at least 84% and as high as 97% when removing no-shows.[14]

For obese women, the completion rates for NT screening seem to be much lower. The largest series on NT failure rates among obese women suggest that obese women are less likely to be able to complete NT screening ultrasound scans, even with the addition of extra time and repeat assessments (**Table 1**), and this clearly trends with class of obesity.[15] Several other studies have also found that the time per patient is longer with obese patients for NT screening, adding to the burden of sonographer work.[15,16] Obesity also increases the need for transvaginal assessment for the NT

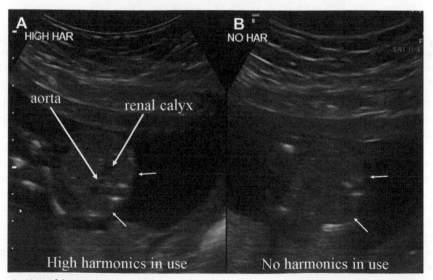

Fig. 3. Use of harmonics. Use of harmonics may improve visualization of fetal structures, such as the fetal kidneys in this image. When harmonics are in use (*A*), the kidneys (*arrows*) are much better visualized, and the renal calyxes and even aorta become visible, which are not visible without harmonics (*B*).

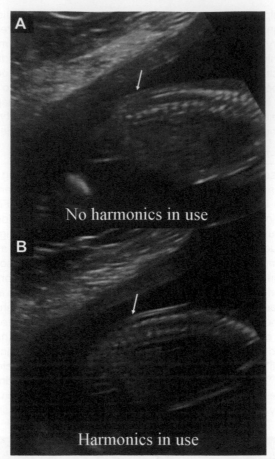

Fig. 4. Use of harmonics to visualize the spine. Compared to images without harmonics (*A*), use of harmonics (*B*) improves the visualization of skin line and sacral spine (*arrow*) over the images obtained without harmonics (*A*), which is important, as obese patients are at high risk for neural tube defects.

(23% vs 41% in obese patients), and also reduces the likelihood of visualizing the nasal bone (NB), with 97% of normal-weight patients having adequate visualization of the NB compared with 87.3% of obese patients.[16]

This is particularly important when patients are trying to decide on the use of invasive testing techniques. Although the data suggest that most obese women who desire NT screening will be able to obtain it, there is a stiller higher risk of NT screen failure. This is especially true with the morbidly class III obese patient, in whom, even after repeated attempts, greater than10% will fail to have an NT measurement obtained.[15] These patients should be counseled before the NT assessment and should be prepared for a longer examination, high likelihood of transvaginal assessment, and the possibility of repeat visit.[14–16] Even in the best of circumstances, they should be prepared for the possibility of having to await second-trimester screening.

Obesity and Second-Trimester Genetic Sonogram

For many ultrasound units, the initial aneuploidy risk assessment is determined by maternal age, serum analytes, and NT screening and then is further tailored at the

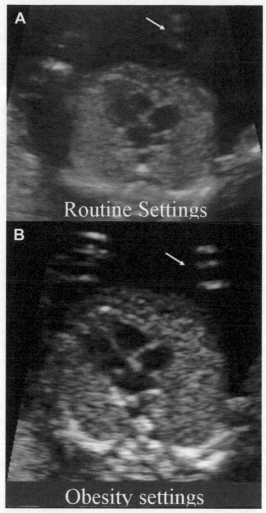

Fig. 5. Obesity-specific settings. Images without obesity-specific settings (A) lack clarity compared to those that, use obese specific settings (B) which include the use of harmonics and spatial compounding and speckle reduction filters can markedly improve visualization over standard settings (A). Note also the improved visualization of the umbilical cord (arrows).

Table 1					
Failure rates for NT ultrasound scan by BMI class					
				Obese	
	Normal Weight	**All Obese**	**Class I**	**Class II**	**Class III**
First attempt	2.2%	9.7%	5.4%	8.8%	22.7%
Repeated attempt	1.6%	6.6%	3.9%	6.7%	13.5%

Data from Thornburg LL, Mulconry M, Post A, et al. Fetal nuchal translucency thickness evaluation in the overweight and obese gravida. Ultrasound Obstet Gynecol 2009;33:665–9.

time of second-trimester screening ultrasound scan by the use of soft-marker assessment. These findings vary in their association with aneuploidy and can help guide the use of invasive fetal testing. Importantly, the absence of these markers is also used to reassure many patients with borderline positive screening. Several studies have looked at the genetic sonogram among obese patients and found poor completion rates. Tsai and colleagues[17] showed that on the first attempt at soft marker screening, 60% of normal-weight women completed the examination compared with only 49% of obese women, with the rates decreasing to as low as 38% in class III obese women. Even after repeated attempts, normal-weight women had significantly higher rates not completing the genetic screening sonogram, with 63% completing the assessment compared with 55% of obese women (47% of class III obese). Additionally, even in women completing the scan, the rates of finding some markers, including short humerus and femur, varied by class of obesity, suggesting that visualization was likely suboptimal.[17] The FaSTER data showed similar results, with obese women having a lower sensitivity (22% vs 32%) of the genetic sonogram, a higher false-negative rate (78% vs 68%), and higher missed diagnosis rate compared with normal-weight patients.[18] If an obese patient is using ultrasound soft marker screening as her only screening method to guide the need for invasive testing, she should be aware of the limitations. Conversely, if the lack of soft marker findings is being used to reassure an obese patient with abnormal screening, the ultrasound detection limits for these should also be discussed.

Obesity and Second-Trimester Assessment For Anomalies

Obesity is clearly associated with an increased risk of fetal anomalies. Defects of the neural tube are markedly increased with reported odds ratios (OR) of 1.7–3.5 for spina bifida and 7.3 for encephaloceles, with these risks rising even higher when obesity is complicated by diabetes.[19–25] Cardiac defects are also increased, with ORs of 1.4–2.0 over those of the normal-weight population.[20–22] However, for some specific cardiac anomalies, the risks may be even higher, such as abnormalities of the great arteries (OR, 4.4) and common arterial truck defects (OR, 6.3) over those of the normal-weight population.[25] These data suggest that adequate visualization of the fetal heart and spine in obese patients is of particular concern.

However, maternal BMI has been noted by multiple authors to limit the ability to visualize fetal structures in the second trimester, and therefore limit ultrasound-based risk screening in this population.[26–30] In 2 of the largest studies, Dashe and colleagues[27] (>10,000 women) and Thornburg and colleagues[29] (>6500 women) noted similar results, with completion rates of anatomic ultrasound decreasing as maternal BMI increased (**Table 2**). Both also noted a poor ability to complete the survey at the first attempt, with Dashe and colleagues noting a completion rate of 50% on the first attempt for obese patients, while Thornburg and colleagues noted a first attempt completion rate of 41% for class I, 23% for class II and 17% for class III obese patients.[27,29] During these ultrasound anatomic evaluations, the spine and heart were the structures most likely to be poorly visualized.[29,31] As discussed earlier, these are also the structures most likely to be anomalous in the obese patient, especially if there is associated diabetes.[21,22] Rates of completion of the cardiac anatomy, including outflows, seem to be particularly limited, with the data from Thornburg and colleagues[29] showing that only 72% of patients with class III obesity ever completed the 4-chamber view (64% right outflow, 70% left outflow) even after repeated attempts, compared with a 91% completion of the 4-chamber view (89% right outflow, 90% left outflow) in normal-weight patients. Hendler and colleagues[31] also showed a high suboptimal visualization rate for obese women for cardiac anatomy, with 18.7% of normal-weight women having suboptimally visualized fetal cardiac

Table 2					
Completion of anatomic ultrasound evaluation (multiple attempts)					
			Obese		
Type of Ultrasound Survey	Normal Weight[a]	Overweight	Class I	Class II	Class III
Basic (10 structures)	72%	68%	57%	41%	30%
Basic (12 structures)	79%	76%	72%	61%	49%
Comprehensive (18 structures)	43%	40%	38%	41%	31%

[a] Dashe et al. included underweight patients within the normal-weight category.
Adapted from Dashe JS, McIntire DD, Twickler DM. Maternal obesity limits the ultrasound evaluation of fetal anatomy. J Ultrasound Med 2009;28:1025–30; and Thornburg LL, Miles K, Ho M, et al. Fetal anatomic evaluation in the overweight and obese gravida. Ultrasound Obstet Gynecol 2009;33:670–5.

structures compared with 29.6% of class I, 39% of class II, and 49.3% of class III obese women, and other studies have had similar results.[31,32] Both studies also showed poor visualization of the craniospinal structures, with Hendler and colleagues[31] reporting suboptimal visualization in 29.5% of normal-weight women compared with 36.8% of class I, 43.3% of class II, and 53.4% of class III.

Multiple strategies have been suggested to improve visualization in the obese gravida, especially for the heart and spine. Improvement of ultrasound equipment did not seem to improve completion rates for these critical structures in an earlier study Hendler and colleagues,[33] but this study was completed before some of the more recent technologic advances. Because of this, other investigators have questioned this conclusion and suggested that harmonic imaging as well as spatial compounding and speckle reduction filters may markedly improve the visualization of cardiac views (see **Figs. 2–4**).[6] Senior sonographers are also more likely to obtain adequate visualization.[26] Repeat examination seems to decrease the rate of suboptimal visualization and improve completion rate.[28,29]

The timing of examination has also been evaluated to attempt to improve visualization. Transvaginal assessment for an early anatomic assessment between 12 and 14 weeks has been suggested as the optimal time to visualize extremities and hands, as there are reports that limb reduction defects are higher in obese patients, with then a follow-up assessment for the remainder of the anatomy later in pregnancy.[6,22] However, to minimize visits, other studies have suggested delaying the initial assessment to 18–20 weeks to improve completion rates.[29,34] One small study (245 obese women) suggested delaying until 22–24 weeks to further improve completion, as they noted a single examination completion rate of 92% at this gestational age compared with completion rate of 88%–89% at 18–22 weeks.[26] Both of the larger studies addressing this question have found 18–20 to be superior. Lantz and colleagues,[34] in a study of 1444 women (448 obese), concluded that the 18- to 19-week window was optimal with completion rates of 68% at 18–20 and 76% at 20–22 weeks compared with 46% at 15–18 and 65% at 22–24 weeks. Thornburg and colleagues,[29] in a study of 7140 women (1952 obese), found that completion rates improve for each class of obesity until 20 weeks then decline. Therefore, given the preferred gestational age for aneuploidy testing and the legal limits of pregnancy termination for anomalies, 18–20 weeks is likely a better window. Regardless, patients should be aware that they are likely to require additional imaging options, including repeat visits, position changes, and use of transvaginal assessment.

After completion of the anatomic survey, there remains a substantial residual risk of anomaly in the obese patient. The most recent data suggest that routine and targeted ultrasound scan has a detection rate at least 20% lower in obese compared with normal-weight women (**Table 3**), giving a residual risk of anomaly of 0.4% for normal-weight patients, and 1% for obese patients.[12] Even when referred for targeted ultrasound scan because of a prior abnormal ultrasound scan or high-risk indication, detection rates are markedly lower for obese women (see **Table 3**).[12] The detection rate was also lower in pregestational diabetic women (38%) compared with 88% in those without diabetes but with other high-risk indications.[12] In the FaSTER study, detection of cardiac anomalies was 21.6% in normal-weight women compared with 8.3% in obese women with a much higher false-positive rate in obese women (91.7% obese vs 78.4% normal weight women).[18] The OR for sonographic detection of anomalies in obese patients was 0.7.[18] Given these data, the obese patient should likely be made aware of the increased residual risk of anomaly despite normal ultrasound screening.[6,12,29]

Fetal Weight Estimation in the Obese Gravida

Obese patients are at risk for macrosomia, especially if they also have excessive weight gain or diabetes, with maternal obesity alone giving at least a 2-fold increased risk of macrosomia.[35] Prediction of macrosomia may be especially difficult in obese women given their habitus and the inability to accurately assess the fetal weight through Leopold's maneuvers, fundal heights, or other clinical assessments. There are data that indicate intrapartum and late pregnancy estimates of weight may be less accurate than those done earlier (34–36 weeks) in pregnancy and then projected forward, known as the *gestational adjusted prediction* (GAP) method.[36] The GAP method extrapolates estimated fetal weights forward using Brenner's median fetal weight curves and has the advantage in the obese gravida of measuring the fetal weight when the infant is higher in the pelvis, making head measurement easier, and when the amniotic fluid volume is greater, making acoustic windows better. There is evidence that fetal weight estimations using Hadlock's formulas may become less accurate when fetal weights are greater than 4500 g, a more common occurrence in the obese, especially obese diabetic woman at late term, giving additional value to estimating the fetal weight earlier in the pregnancy.[37] The GAP method has also been shown to be accurate in both diabetic and obese women.[38,39] However, there seems to be a tendency to overestimate weight in class I and II obese women and underestimate those with class III obesity. Regardless, the systematic and random error of the GAP method suggests that for obese patients, this method would predict birth weight within 20% over 90% of the time regardless of the obesity class.[38] Importantly, this method also had an excellent negative predictive value (>90%) for exclusion of macrosomia.[38] Regardless, all methods of fetal weight estimation have an associated error; therefore, clinical assessment of the entire patient picture is imperative.

Table 3 Detection of fetal anomalies in the obese gravida			Obese		
	Normal Weight	Overweight	Class I	Class II	Class III
Standard ultrasound	66%	49%	48%	42%	25%
Targeted Ultrasound	97%	91%	75%	88%	75%

Data from Dashe JS, McIntire DD, Twickler DM. Effect of maternal obesity on the ultrasound detection of anomalous fetuses. Obstet Gynecol 2009;113:1001–7.

SUMMARY

Obese women require additional considerations when planning the ultrasound approach. Typically, they require additional time, effort, and ultrasound examinations than their normal-weight counterparts. Screening options may be limited, and there is a higher risk for a missed diagnosis for all prenatal sonographic approaches. There is also a risk that anatomic evaluations cannot be completed, and even when completed, will have a higher residual risk for fetal anomalies. Birth weight prediction and following fetal growth will also be more difficult. Therefore, the clinician must partner with patients to assure that they understand the risks and benefits of different approaches and the technical limitations from obesity and other associated medical conditions on ultrasound evaluations.

REFERENCES

1. World Health Organization. Obesity: preventing and managing the global epidemic. WHO technical report series 894. Geneva (Switzerland): World Health Organization; 2000.
2. Popkin BM, Doak CM. The obesity epidemic is a worldwide phenomenon. Nutr Rev 1998;56:106–14.
3. NAoS IoM. Nutrition in pregnancy. Part I. Weight gain. Part II nutrient supplements. Washington, DC: National Academies Press; 1990.
4. Yu CK, Teoh TG, Robinson S. Obesity in pregnancy. Br J Obstet Gynecol 2006; 113:1117–25.
5. Heliovaara M, Aromaa A. Parity and obesity. J Epidemiol Community Health 1981; 35:197–9.
6. Paladini D. Sonography in obese and overweight pregnant women: clinical, medicolegal and technical issues. Ultrasound Obstet Gynecol 2009;33:720–9.
7. Bromley B, Shipp TD, Mitchell MA, et al. Tricks for obtaining a nuchal translucency measurement on the fetus in a difficult position. J Ultrasound Med 2010; 29:1261–4.
8. Thornburg LL. Antepartum obstetrical complications associated with obesity. Semin Perinatol 2011;35:317–23.
9. Magnavita N, Bevilacqua L, Mirk P, et al. Work-related musculoskeletal complaints in sonologists. J Occup Environ Med 1999;41:981–8.
10. Schoenfeld A, Goverman J, Weiss DM, et al. Transducer user syndrome: an occupational hazard of the ultrasonographer. Eur J Ultrasound 1999;10:41–5.
11. Paladini D, Vassallo M, Tartaglione A, et al. The role of tissue harmonic imaging in fetal echocardiography. Ultrasound Obstet Gynecol 2004;23:159–64.
12. Dashe JS, McIntire DD, Twickler DM. Effect of maternal obesity on the ultrasound detection of anomalous fetuses. Obstet Gynecol 2009;113:1001–7.
13. Malone FD, Canick JA, Ball RH, et al. First-trimester or second-trimester screening, or both, for Down's syndrome. N Engl J Med 2005;353:2001–11.
14. Wax JR, Pinette MG, Cartin A, et al. The value of repeated evaluation after initial failed nuchal translucency measurement. J Ultrasound Med 2007;26:825–8 [quiz: 29–30].
15. Thornburg LL, Mulconry M, Post A, et al. Fetal nuchal translucency thickness evaluation in the overweight and obese gravida. Ultrasound Obstet Gynecol 2009;33:665–9.
16. Gandhi M, Fox NS, Russo-Stieglitz K, et al. Effect of increased body mass index on first-trimester ultrasound examination for aneuploidy risk assessment. Obstet Gynecol 2009;114:856–9.

17. Tsai LJ, Ho M, Pressman EK, et al. Ultrasound screening for fetal aneuploidy using soft markers in the overweight and obese gravida. Prenat Diagn 2010;30: 821–6.

18. Aagaard-Tillery KM, Flint Porter T, Malone FD, et al. Influence of maternal BMI on genetic sonography in the FaSTER trial. Prenat Diagn 2010;30:14–22.

19. Hendricks KA, Nuno OM, Suarez L, et al. Effects of hyperinsulinemia and obesity on risk of neural tube defects among Mexican Americans. Epidemiology 2001;12: 630–5.

20. Waller DK, Mills JL, Simpson JL, et al. Are obese women at higher risk for producing malformed offspring? Am J Obstet Gynecol 1994;170:541–8.

21. Watkins ML, Rasmussen SA, Honein MA, et al. Maternal obesity and risk for birth defects. Pediatrics 2003;111:1152–8.

22. Waller DK, Shaw GM, Rasmussen SA, et al. Prepregnancy obesity as a risk factor for structural birth defects. Arch Pediatr Adolesc Med 2007;161:745–50.

23. Shaw GM, Velie EM, Schaffer D. Risk of neural tube defect-affected pregnancies among obese women. JAMA 1996;275:1093–6.

24. Watkins ML, Scanlon KS, Mulinare J, et al. Is maternal obesity a risk factor for anencephaly and spina bifida? Epidemiology 1996;7:507–12.

25. Queisser-Luft A, Kieninger-Baum D, Menger H, et al. Does maternal obesity increase the risk of fetal abnormalities? analysis of 20,248 newborn infants of the Mainz Birth Register for detecting congenital abnormalities. Ultraschall Med 1998;19:40–4 [in German].

26. Chung JH, Pelayo R, Hatfield TJ, et al. Limitations of the fetal anatomic survey via ultrasound in the obese obstetrical population. J Matern Fetal Neonatal Med 2012;25(10):1945–9.

27. Dashe JS, McIntire DD, Twickler DM. Maternal obesity limits the ultrasound evaluation of fetal anatomy. J Ultrasound Med 2009;28:1025–30.

28. Hendler I, Blackwell SC, Bujold E, et al. Suboptimal second-trimester ultrasonographic visualization of the fetal heart in obese women: should we repeat the examination? J Ultrasound Med 2005;24:1205–9 [quiz: 10–11].

29. Thornburg LL, Miles K, Ho M, et al. Fetal anatomic evaluation in the overweight and obese gravida. Ultrasound Obstet Gynecol 2009;33:670–5.

30. Maxwell C, Dunn E, Tomlinson G, et al. How does maternal obesity affect the routine fetal anatomic ultrasound? J Matern Fetal Neonatal Med 2010;23: 1187–92.

31. Hendler I, Blackwell SC, Bujold E, et al. The impact of maternal obesity on midtrimester sonographic visualization of fetal cardiac and craniospinal structures. Int J Obes Relat Metab Disord 2004;28:1607–11.

32. Khoury FR, Ehrenberg HM, Mercer BM. The impact of maternal obesity on satisfactory detailed anatomic ultrasound image acquisition. J Matern Fetal Neonatal Med 2009;22:337–41.

33. Hendler I, Blackwell SC, Treadwell MC, et al. Does advanced ultrasound equipment improve the adequacy of ultrasound visualization of fetal cardiac structures in the obese gravid woman? Am J Obstet Gynecol 2004;190:1616–9 [discussion: 19–20].

34. Lantz ME, Chisholm CA. The preferred timing of second-trimester obstetric sonography based on maternal body mass index. J Ultrasound Med 2004;23: 1019–22.

35. Jolly MC, Sebire NJ, Harris JP, et al. Risk factors for macrosomia and its clinical consequences: a study of 350,311 pregnancies. Eur J Obstet Gynecol Reprod Biol 2003;111:9–14.

36. Pressman EK, Bienstock JL, Blakemore KJ, et al. Prediction of birth weight by ultrasound in the third trimester. Obstet Gynecol 2000;95:502–6.
37. Alsulyman OM, Ouzounian JG, Kjos SL. The accuracy of intrapartum ultrasonographic fetal weight estimation in diabetic pregnancies. Am J Obstet Gynecol 1997;177:503–6.
38. Thornburg LL, Barnes C, Glantz JC, et al. Sonographic birth-weight prediction in obese patients using the gestation-adjusted prediction method. Ultrasound Obstet Gynecol 2008;32:66–70.
39. Best G, Pressman EK. Ultrasonographic prediction of birth weight in diabetic pregnancies. Obstet Gynecol 2002;99:740–4.